Dimensions of Psychotherapy, Dimensions of Experience

Dimensions of Psychotherapy, Dimensions of Experience explores the three basic elements of psychotherapy – time, space and number – summarising theory, setting it in context and bringing concepts to life with clinical illustrations.

Michael Stadter and David Scharff bring together contributions describing how each of these elements, as well as their simple and direct manifestations in the physical world, also combine to form the psychological dimensions of symbolic reality both in the inner world and in the transactional world. They also reveal how, in encounters between patient and therapist, the combination of inner worlds form a new, uniquely psychological, fourth dimension that saturates the activity and experience of the other three elements. This book aims to increase understanding of the action of the three dimensions of psychotherapy by looking at the elements that constitute the setting and process in which clinicians engage every day. The contributors, all of whom are experienced psychotherapists and psychoanalysts, connect their thinking on the dimensions to clinical practice by illustrating their ideas with case material and examining their impact on general treatment issues.

This clear and readable investigation into the impact of the dimensions of time, space, number and state of mind will be of interest to practising psychotherapists and psychoanalysts and students of psychoanalysis and philosophy.

Michael Stadter is a clinical psychologist and a member of the faculty and Board of Directors of the International Psychotherapy Institute. He is also Clinical Psychologist-in-Residence at the Department of Psychology at American University in Washington, DC.

David E. Scharff is Co-Director of the International Psychotherapy Institute and a psychoanalyst in private practice.

Contributors: Geoffrey Anderson, Charles Ashbach, Carl Bagnini, Susan E. Barbour, Christopher Bollas, Hope Cooper, Sheila Hill, Earl Hopper, Theodore J. Jacobs, Leslie A. Johnson, James L. Poulton, Kent Ravenscroft, Judith M. Rovner, Jill Savege Scharff, Lea Setton, Sharon Zalusky.

Dimensions of Psychotherapy, Dimensions of Experience

Time, space, number and state of mind

Edited by Michael Stadter and
David E. Scharff

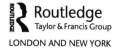

Routledge
Taylor & Francis Group

LONDON AND NEW YORK

First published 2005 by Routledge
2 Park Square, Milton Park, Abingdon, Oxfordshire OX14 4RN

Simultaneously published in the USA and Canada
by Routledge
711 Third Avenue, New York, NY 10017

Routledge is an imprint of the Taylor and Francis Group, an informa business

Typeset in Times by Garfield Morgan, Rhayader, Powys, UK
Cover design by Sandra Heath

British Library Cataloguing in Publication Data
A catalogue record for this book is available from the British Library

Library of Congress Cataloging in Publication Data
Dimensions of psychotherapy, dimensions of experience : time, space,
number, and state of mind / edited by Michael Stadter and David E.
Scharff.
        p.   cm.
    Includes bibliographical references and index.
    ISBN 1-58391-863-9 (hbk)
    1. Psychoanalysis. 2. Time. 3. Spatial ability. 4. Mathematical
ability. 5. Consciousness. I. Stadter, Michael. II. Scharff, David E.,
1941–
    RC506.D56 2005
    616.89'17–dc22
                                                            2004030448

ISBN 13: 978-1-58391-863-0 (hbk)
ISBN 13: 978-1-138-88148-8 (pbk)

Reflections on dimensions of psychotherapy

Jill Savege Scharff

Please to remember
That inner and outer
Aren't places, they're just points of view
There's me and there's not-me
And who I appear to be,
False self belying the true

Please to reflect
On your self, and accept
All your parts, don't disintegrate yet
For all states of mind
Be they nasty or kind
Enrich your relational set

Please to agree
One is you, one is me
And the you that's in me is in you
So do take the trouble
To see that you're double
And one's the expression of two

Please to remember
The fiction of number
Complex, simple, or prime
From one to seven
Start counting to heaven
While we are still here marking time

Contents

Notes on contributors

EDITORS

Michael Stadter, PhD is a clinical psychologist and a member of the faculty and Board of Directors of the International Psychotherapy Institute (formerly the International Institute of Object Relations Therapy) in Chevy Chase, MD. He is also Clinical Psychologist-in-Residence in the Department of Psychology at American University in Washington, DC, and on the faculty of the Washington School of Psychiatry.

He is the author of a number of publications including the book, *Object Relations Brief Therapy: The Relationship in Short-term Work* (1996). His most recent publication is 'The consultants as part of the drama in a family business', in *Self Hatred in Psychoanalysis: Detoxifying the Persecutory Object* (2003). Dr Stadter maintains a private practice in Bethesda, MD, that includes long-term and brief psychotherapy as well as clinical supervision and organizational consultation.

David E. Scharff, MD is Co-Director of the International Psychotherapy Institute (formerly the International Institute of Object Relations Therapy). He is Clinical Professor of Psychiatry at the Uniformed Services University of the Health Sciences and also at Georgetown University. Dr Scharff is a Teaching Analyst at the Washington Psychoanalytic Institute. He is a former president of The American Association of Sex Educators, Counselors and Therapists (1988–1989), and former Director of the Washington School of Psychiatry (1987–1994).

Dr Scharff's 15 books include *The Sexual Relationship* (1982), *Refinding the Object and Reclaiming the Self* (1992), *Object Relations Theory and Practice* (1995), and *Fairbairn: Then and Now* (1998). He has also written 50 articles and chapters and is widely sought as a lecturer on the topics of family and couple theory, object relations theory, and sexual development, disorders and their treatment. He maintains a private practice in psychoanalysis and psychotherapy in Chevy Chase, MD.

CHAPTER CONTRIBUTORS

Geoffrey Anderson, PhD is a Clinical Psychologist in private practice in Omaha, NE. A fellow of IPI he is also a Lecturer in Psychiatry at Creighton University and Director of the Center for Psychotherapy and Psychoanalysis.

Charles Ashbach, PhD is a psychologist in private practice in Philadelphia. He is a faculty member and the Director of the Philadelphia satellite of IPI. He is author of several articles on object relations and narcissism and co-author of the book, *Object Relations, the Self and the Group: a Conceptual Paradigm* (1987).

Carl Bagnini, MSW, BCD is chair of IPI's Program on Child, Couple and Family Therapy, and directs the Institute's Long Island Satellite Center. He is also visiting faculty at the Suffolk Institute for Psychotherapy and Psychoanalysis, and clinical faculty at the Postdoctoral Program in Family Therapy of St John's University. His latest publication is 'Object relations stepfamily therapy: expanding the frame' (2004) in *The Journal of Advanced Psychoanalytic Studies*. Mr Bagnini is in private practice in Port Washington, NY.

Susan E. Barbour, EdD is a psychologist in private practice in Appleton, WI, and is a graduate of IPI's Object Relations Theory and Therapy Training Program.

Christopher Bollas is a psychoanalyst in private practice in London, and a member of the Group of Independent Analysts of the British Psychoanalytical Society. He is author of *The Shadow of the Object* (1987), *Forces of Destiny* (1989), *Being a Character: Psychoanalysis and Self Experience* (1992), *Cracking Up: the Work of Unconscious Experience* (1995), *The Mystery of Things* (1999), several other books and numerous articles. He is widely held to be among the most creative and influential psychoanalytic writers of our day.

Hope Cooper, MSW is a child psychotherapist in private practice in Williamsburg, VA, and a fellow and member of the Board of IPI. Her article, 'The sibling link' was published in the *International Journal of Infant Observation* (2003).

Sheila Hill, MSW is a clinical social worker in private practice in Chevy Chase, MD. She is a faculty member of IPI and has taught at training institutes in St Louis and Boston.

Earl Hopper, PhD is a psychoanalyst, group analyst and organizational consultant in private practice in London. He is a supervisor and training analyst for The Institute of Group Analysis, The British Association of

Psychotherapists and The London Centre for Psychotherapy. Dr Hopper is also an honorary tutor at The Tavistock and Portman NHS Trust and a member of the faculty of the Post-Doctoral Program at Adelphi University, New York. His most recent books are *The Social Unconscious* (2003) and *Traumatic Experience in the Unconscious Life of Groups* (2003).

Theodore J. Jacobs, MD is Clinical Professor of Psychiatry at the Albert Einstein College of Medicine and a training and supervising analyst at the New York Psychoanalytic Institute and at the Psychoanalytic Institute at New York University. He is author of *The Use of Self: Countertransference and Communication in the Analytic Situation* (1991) and is on the Editorial Board of *Psychoanalytic Quarterly*.

Leslie A. Johnson, PhD, LPC is in private practice in Charlottesville, VA. She is a fellow of IPI and a contributor to the collection, *Self-Hatred in Psychoanalysis: Detoxifying the Persecutory Object* (2003). Formerly a teacher of Russian language and literature, she has written two studies on Dostoevsky.

James L. Poulton, PhD is a psychologist in private practice, a faculty member of IPI, and co-director of IPI's Salt Lake City Satellite Center. He is also an Adjunct Associate Professor in the Department of Psychology, as well as a Clinical Instructor in the Department of Psychiatry, at the University of Utah.

Kent Ravenscroft, MD is Associate Clinical Professor at George Washington and Georgetown University Medical Schools. Based on work at the Tavistock Institute, he has recently co-edited two volumes on eating disorders in children and adolescents. He currently lives in Washington, DC, where he supervises and teaches on the faculty of IPI and is in full-time private practice.

Judith M. Rovner, MSW is a Clinical Assistant Professor of Psychiatry at Georgetown University, an adjunct faculty member of the Georgetown University Counseling and Psychiatric Services, and a consultant faculty member of the Clinical Social Work Institute. She is on the faculty of IPI and is also Chair of Supervision and the Clinical Application Program. She is in private practice in Chevy Chase, MD.

Jill Savege Scharff, MD is Co-Director of IPI, Clinical Professor of Psychiatry, Georgetown University, Teaching Analyst at the Washington Psychoanalytic Institute, and Series Co-editor of the Library of Object Relations at Jason Aronson. Her latest book co-edited with S. Tsigounis is *Self Hatred in Psychoanalysis: Detoxifying the Persecutory Object* (2003).

Lea Setton, PhD is a faculty member of IPI, professor at the University Santa Maria La Antigua and at the State University of Panama. She practices individual, couple, and family therapy in Panama City.

Sharon Zalusky, PhD is a member of the California and Southern California Psychoanalytic Societies and has written extensively on the issues raised in the conduct of psychotherapy and psychoanalysis by telephone.

Acknowledgements

First and foremost, we want to thank the authors of the chapters for their wisdom, creativity and generosity. Without them, the book would only be an internal object. Next, we are indebted to all of the authors' patients and clients who have been co-creators in the therapy process. We also want to express our enduring gratitude to the students, fellows and faculty of the International Psychotherapy Institute (formerly the International Institute of Object Relations Therapy) who for over 10 years have nurtured and challenged our thinking and clinical work. We would particularly like to acknowledge three people at IPI: Stan Tsigounis who hosted and co-chaired the conference with us in Sarasota, FL, where most of the chapters were initially presented and Anna Innes and Ana Granados who helped us with the preparation of the manuscript.

We each have a few additional people that we want to thank. I (MS) want to express my gratitude to my wife, Jane Prelinger, to the Albemarle Psychoanalytic Study Group and to Dr Abigail Lipson and her staff at the Counseling Center at American University for their professional and creative help at various points in the project. I also want to give special thanks to my family – Jane, Greg, Chris, Joanna and Laura – for their support, good humor, and patience. I (DES) continue in my gratitude to Jill Scharff for her wise support in this as in so many other projects. Hope Cooper and I also thank Ross Skelton and Earl Hopper for critically commenting on an early version of our two number chapters.

Lastly, we are very grateful to the editorial staff at Routledge, especially Joanne Forshaw for her encouragement and promotion of the project, Claire Lipscomb for her help in bringing the book to its completion and Zoë Smith and Imogen Burch, our production editors.

Michael Stadter, PhD
Bethesda, MD

David E. Scharff, MD
Chevy Chase, MD
May 2004

Introduction: Exploring the dimensions

Michael Stadter and David E. Scharff

The therapist sits in a room with a patient for a period of time.

This simple sentence includes three basic elements of psychotherapy – time, space and number. Yet, we know that the interactions faced in the conduct of psychotherapy and psychoanalysis are intricate, unique, and often baffling human encounters. In our efforts to understand them, we have many ways of examining the complex interplay and synergy of the multiple elements that make up the whole experience. But, we rarely isolate the fundamental elements of the therapy process to reflect on each independently. This volume is an attempt to increase our understanding of the dimensions of psychotherapy by looking at fundamental but usually unexamined elements that constitute the setting and process in which clinicians engage every day.

When the therapist sits in a room with a patient for a period of time, the encounter is affected by their moment-to-moment conscious and unconscious internal states.

The three basic elements of time, space and number have simple and direct manifestations in the physical world, *and* combine to form the psychological dimensions of symbolic reality both in the inner world and in the transactional world. They characterize elements of these situations. When a therapist and patient interact, the encounter is affected by their conscious and unconscious internal states. The patient's and therapist's inner worlds – their states of mind – form a new, uniquely psychological, fourth dimension that saturates the activity and experience of the other three elements. Time, space and number are physical dimensions, but they become psychologically saturated as they take on the colors of the states of mind of the participants in the therapy encounter. State of mind itself possesses many different dimensions. It is complex, the heart of psychoanalytic inquiry, and, by definition, the dimensions of the mind and of minds in interaction have no literal equivalence in the physical world.

Nevertheless, we think there are corollaries and metaphors in physics and mathematics – and especially in the theories of self-organizing dynamic systems – that give us new ways to understand states of mind and their intrinsic quality of being in flux. For these reasons, we believe that state of mind can usefully be described as an overarching fourth dimension of psychotherapy that integrates the other dimensions.

What can we learn from basic questions posed by elemental and richly suggestive moments in therapy such as:

A therapist says with embarrassment, 'I thought the session was over, but we've actually got *10 more minutes.*'

A man says suddenly, 'I can't stand to be in my life. I just want time to stop.'

A woman says, 'Right now I am sitting in your bookshelf. Right in that little space down in the bottom shelf where it is dark and no one can see me.'

A patient acknowledges briefly that the therapist's new office is larger than the old one, then resumes her usual line of fire, ignoring the setting as if no move had occurred.

A patient describes his experience of self as moving between a singleton, a couple, and himself as a useless third wheel.

A therapist, hoping for new ways of seeing into the meaning of the therapy process, seeks supervision, and in this way the dyad of patient–therapist enlarges to become a triad of patient–therapist–supervisor.

A therapist who has never done family therapy before, sits for the first time with the chaos of a family group while the three children fill the physical and emotional space by fighting over the office toys.

A therapy expands to a new level of magnitude when a therapist presents a session at a conference and the privileged dyad is folded into the large conference group's excited examination.

This book came from our interest in elements that are primary to psychotherapy and, for that matter, to all human experience. As we have each done psychotherapeutic and psychoanalytic work for over 30 years, we have each found that the power of the fundamental, apparently simple, dimensions of these human encounters prominently emerged. We each had influences that stimulated our attention to these dimensions.

I (Michael Stadter) came to the theme for this book following several years of fascination with the concept of time. The clinical beginnings of this interest occurred while writing a book on the application of object relations concepts to brief therapy (Stadter 1996). I became intrigued with the variable uses and experience of time in brief therapy that contrasted dramatically with long-term psychotherapy. I was also struck by the unique impact that the termination phase of therapy has on patients' and therapists' sense of time. This initial curiosity extended to other temporal phenomena in therapy, health and psychopathology and then to an exploration of the philosophy (an old interest) and the physics of time and space. As I thought further, the dimensions of number and state of mind also emerged as elemental aspects of our clinical work and I thought a book on these four dimensions could make a fresh contribution.

I (David Scharff) was intrigued by Stadter's idea as it fit with my own theoretical and clinical interests. As I explored the dynamics of transference and countertransference I saw that they have their own geography of time and space that define their operating location (Scharff and Scharff 1998). Charting this helps to understand the interplay of two minds interacting. The dynamics of the pair in individual therapy is qualitatively and quantitatively different from the multiple dimensions of interaction in couple, family and group therapy. Some of the differences are relative and quantitative, but some involve the qualitatively different factors introduced by the size of the group in the therapeutic process – from the threesome of couple therapy to the five or ten people in family or group therapy. Later I became interested in how the principles of organization of groups of this size operate on a different order of magnitude than those of individual therapy.

Related to this problem – and so far not really considered by psychoanalysis or dynamic psychotherapy theory – is the question of the dynamic organization of complex systems in constant flux and characterized by constant feedback. In the process of writing a book on individual therapy (Scharff and Scharff 1998), Jill Scharff and I began to see how chaos theory, or the theories that study systems characterized by emergent self-organization, are new and useful models for the organization of complex psychological behavior, both internal and external. These theories describe previously unexplained aspects of the mathematical and physical world, but go beyond these to include problems in biological systems like population dynamics or the rhythms of the heart and nervous system. We began to see how they could also be useful to understand individual mental organization and psychological interaction of pairs and groups.

We believe this kind of theory is a bridge between the non-mathematical understanding of states of mind provided by developmental and psychoanalytic research, and the understanding of dynamic patterns of behavior and internal organization. It began to occur to me that chaos theory offers a physical model for the movement in postmodern philosophy to deconstructionism, a move paralleled in literary criticism that underscores how meaning is always subjective, dependent on individual experience and interpretation. In this view there is no place to stand in order to achieve certainty, and all meaning is relative. Chaos or complexity theory gives guidance in the physical sciences to a search for meaning in this new sea of uncertainty. Ultimately, I began to feel that we also need such theories to make number itself a useful concept in a complex way that does fuller justice to human psychology.

These dimensions of psychotherapy have all been written about, but we are not aware of any collection that has isolated and examined them as objects of study in their own right. We believe that such a focus offers a deeper appreciation of their action in psychotherapy although, of course, no book or collection can ever fully exhaust the richness of the inquiry. To pursue the study of these dimensions, we asked 18 psychotherapists and psychoanalysts to write essays focusing on one of the dimensions. We asked them to connect their thinking on that dimension to clinical practice through illustration with case material or by posing general treatment issues. The resulting chapters are both deconstructive and applied. Several of the chapters emphasize theoretical exploration and offer noteworthy conceptual contributions. The chapters are essays on the dimensions from the individual authors' unique points of view but no attempt is made to synthesize a general theory from them.

The book is divided into four parts: time, space, number, and state of mind. We have written a brief introduction to each part which sets the context for the dimension being studied, and provides a preview to and linkage among the chapters. All of the writers of the 19 chapters are experienced therapists or analysts and most have previously written about psychotherapy and/or psychoanalysis. We (MS and DES) have worked together for more than 15 years, and for the past 10 years at the International Psychotherapy Institute (formerly the International Institute for Object Relations Therapy). Early versions of 12 chapters were presented at an Institute conference 'Dimensions of Psychotherapy' in Sarasota, Florida, January 17–19, 2003. To these we have added the invited contributions of a number of notable writers.

The resulting collection offers an array of perspectives on the dimensions of psychotherapy. Some chapters focus on a single event (e.g., a therapist moving her office) while others investigate a general process (e.g., an unconscious developmental clock). As previously noted, complete study of these dimensions is well beyond the scope of any book. Our hope is that this volume will stimulate you, the reader, to view these fundamental elements in ways you previously had not, and to extend your reflection on them well beyond what we present here. We hope to stimulate you to think a little differently about your work and to ask more questions than we can hope to answer. Working on this collection has done that for us.

REFERENCES

Scharff, J. S. and Scharff, D. E. (1998) *Object Relations Individual Therapy*, Northvale, NJ: Jason Aronson.

Stadter, M. (1996) *Object Relations Brief Therapy: The Therapeutic Relationship in Short-term Work*, Northvale, NJ: Jason Aronson.

Part I

Time

Time, life and psychotherapy: an overview

Michael Stadter and David E. Scharff

Time is a basic ingredient of existence, studied for thousands of years by philosophy, for hundreds by physics, and for one hundred years by psychoanalysis. In this section, we hope to stimulate curiosity about its role and action in the clinical situation.

Time is one of the most common human dimensions through which we measure experience. Of course, time and experience are connected in complex and intimate ways. For instance, it is equally true that we measure time through experience just as we measure experience through time. Consider these mundane examples of time in our lives: most of us wear wrist watches, we see countless clocks in a given day, we look forward to having 'time off', we as therapists emphasize starting and ending our sessions 'on time', we detail in case presentations how long we've seen the patient and how frequently. Consider, too, how often people refer to time: time to kill, time on my hands, what time is it? how much more time do I have? time is on my side, time is working against me, the two-minute drill in football, the one-minute waltz.

Time is also one of the most profound of human experiences. The human awareness of time has been described as one of the most important capacities that differentiate us from other animals (Wright 2002). It gives us an ability to see a past, a future and, ultimately, our own mortality. The nature of time has been the subject of study and controversy by philosophers and physicists since the beginning of those disciplines. Aristotle asked whether time exists if no change occurs – a question still explored in philosophy (Le Poidevin 2003). Time has also been a central subject for the phenomenological philosophers such as Husserl, Heidegger, Sartre, and Merleau-Ponty. Indeed, Heidegger's (1927/1962) most influential work is titled *Being and Time*. As Dreyfus states:

> What Martin Heidegger is after in *Being and Time* is nothing less than deepening our understanding of what it means for something (things, people, abstractions, language, etc.) to be. He wants to distinguish

several different ways of being and then show how they are all related to human being and ultimately to *temporality* [italics added].

(Dreyfus 1991: 1)

We would just briefly note that historically there has been a complementarity and overlap between phenomenology and psychoanalysis. Moreover, Stern (2004) has noted that the phenomenological approach has been revitalized by current scientists and philosophers. In his fascinating book (Stern 2004) on the 'present moment' in life and psychotherapy (defined as a one- to ten-second duration) he describes the profound influence of the phenomenologists, especially Husserl and Merleau-Ponty, on his work. Similarly, Stolorow (2003) recently wrote a short paper that referred to concepts of Husserl and Heidegger and their impact on his thinking on time and trauma.

In the realm of physics, Newton famously declared that time was an absolute, that time flows steadily 'without reference to anything external' (Greene 2004: 45). This temporal perspective was dominant for the next 200 years. Then came Einstein and the physics of time took an enormous leap. His theories of relativity proposed that time is altered by the effects of motion and gravity. This shattered the idea that time could be an absolute, unchanging phenomenon (Galison 2003; Greene 2004). Moreover, quantum mechanics and string theory have presented new temporal notions to physicists. Currently, some time questions in physics and philosophy are (Callender 2002; Greene 2004; Le Poidevin 2003):

Does time actually exist?

Does time have a beginning or end?

Could time go backward?

Is every moment a time capsule and partial record of the past?

Our work as therapists and analysts is less concerned with the basic nature of time and more with the human experience of it. Consider, though, that these temporal questions of physicists and philosophers are very similar to the questions about clinical phenomena that we and our patients have – albeit at different and/or symbolic levels. The interested reader is referred to Callender (2002), Galison (2003), Greene (2004), and Le Poidevin (2003) for extended exploration of these other disciplines' perspectives on time. In our present brief overview we are simply noting that the questions that arise in analysis and psychotherapy are similar to ones explored in these other sciences as we all try to apprehend the world and being human in it. To illustrate, we have listed below just a few examples of these four questions in the clinical setting.

DOES TIME ACTUALLY EXIST?

Consider these phenomena from the clinical situation:

The 'stopping' of time by dissociative processes

An absence of a sense of time passing during an intense, engrossing experience

The obliteration of time by chemical intoxication

The 'transcendent' state in intense narcissistic gratification

The absence of time was noted by Freud (1933) in his well-known statement that the unconscious is timeless. While many contemporary writers (e.g., Hartocollis 1975; Stolorow 2003; see also, Ravenscroft, Chapter 1 in this volume) would argue that the unconscious is not truly timeless, and we would agree, the subjective experience of timelessness is pervasive.

DOES TIME HAVE A BEGINNING OR END?

Here are some experiences of temporal beginnings or endings:

The experience of having little or no time left

Following a trauma, the sense that time has ended

The experience that time began with a major event in a person's life

The sense that one has only *now* started to live

Such examples suggest the experience of the 'clock' stopping or starting in response to intense experience. They also demonstrate the strong connection between a sense of time and a sense of self, a connection Heidegger described in 1927.

COULD TIME GO BACKWARD?

The following are examples of the present moving back in time:

The frequent wish to return to the past

An adult living life as an adolescent

Traumatic flashbacks

Different varieties of regression

Of course, the phenomena of transference and countertransference are powerful instances of the past being lived in the present. Freud's concept of 'nachträglichkeit' (Kernberg 2001), now most often referred to by French analysts as 'après coup' (Birksted-Breen 2003), is an example of the present moving back in time, infusing the past with meaning it had not had at the time it occurred in the past.

IS EVERY MOMENT A TIME CAPSULE AND PARTIAL RECORD OF THE PAST?

Therapists often do not 'know' what factually happened in patients' pasts, but traces of the past are embodied in the present nevertheless.

> A patient noticing that he angrily answered a question like his father did
>
> A therapist being very directive and protective with a patient resembles the way the patient was treated as the parentified child in her family
>
> A patient telling the therapist how disappointing he is reenacts what the patient's mother said to her
>
> A therapist being unable to think just as she had with some previous patients and with her own parents

Transference, countertransference and emphasis on the here-and-now are built on the premise that the present moment contains remnants of the past. Much of our analytic work studies the contents of the past that have been brought into the present of the therapeutic relationship. Hopper, whose work is represented in Part II on space (Chapter 7), has established a four-cell square (Hopper 2003a, 2003b) to show the clinical relationship of space and time. The treatment space and time are the here-and-now of the present inside therapy. The past that existed outside the therapy and in another place, that is a patient's history, is the 'there-and-then.' The 'here-and-then' represents those moments the past enters the therapy, especially the past of the therapy itself. And the 'there-and-now' is the place outside therapy in which the patient's current life occurs.

Interestingly, physics questions whether the present actually exists (Greene 2004). Certainly, the sense of the present is a powerful subjective experience. In considering the clinical situation, though, we realize that we cannot actually make 'here-and-now' interpretations, important as this concept is. We actually are referring to a time that is very recent but is actually 'here-and-then', a few seconds or minutes past.

Jill Scharff and I (DES) (Scharff and Scharff 1998), have extended the concept of time that is not the 'now' of the present. Time both past and present are constructs of the mind. The past is carried as memory (the 'there-and-back then'), and in a similar way, the future is carried as fantasy, hope and fear (the 'if-and-when'). Just as our pasts guide us in the form of internal psychic structure and memory, the 'if-and-when' in a structure of fantasy serves to guide each of us forward from the current moment into our futures.

We have four chapters on time in this section. Kent Ravenscroft begins our exploration with the notion that there is an unconscious developmental clock that affects us not only in the familiar developmental sequences of individuals, but also in our group experience as families. His temporal focus sheds light on the nature of Freud's primary unconscious. Using child, family and couple cases, he illustrates time shifts in sessions, in variations in patients' narrative coherence, and during therapists' use of counter-transference.

In the next chapter, I (MS) consider the interrelationships among time, trauma and psychotherapy. I begin with a traumatized patient who wanted time to stop. For this patient, time was an intruder and a thief. I then describe the balance, oscillations and co-existence of time-centered versus timeless subjectivity: time-near and time-far. Finally, I explore how trauma profoundly affects temporality.

Leslie Johnson further examines attempts to stop or transcend time through the discussion of two narcissistic patients. Their relationships to time impaired their lives and their therapies. Emphasizing the connection between time and the experience of separation, she develops her ideas using the Greek concepts of chronos, kairos and pleroma.

Lea Setton and Jill Scharff also write of the link between time sense and separation. Additionally, they consider the concept of time sense developing from innate rhythms and from hunger. At the heart of their chapter, they present a detailed case history to illustrate the impact of time in a three-year treatment where sturdy consistency was required of the therapist *over time*. They describe how the patient played with time, and make the case for the necessity of a large quantity of time in the successful treatment of many patients.

As Bollas has written of psychoanalytic listening:

> This way of listening takes time, lots and lots of time. It takes time for the evocative movement of the patient's discourse to affect the analyst's unconscious life. This aspect of an analysis leads to a greater appreciation of unconscious time and unconscious thought: indeed, it gives its participants a new appreciation of time itself.
>
> (Bollas 1999: 186)

REFERENCES

Birksted-Breen, D. (2003) 'Time and the Apres-Coup', *International Journal of Psychoanalysis*, 84: 1501–1515.

Bollas, C. (1999) *The Mystery of Things*, Routledge: London.

Callender, Craig (ed.) (2002) *Time, Reality and Experience*, Cambridge, UK: Cambridge University Press.

Dreyfus, H. L. (1991) *Being-in-the-World: A Commentary on Heidegger's Being and Time*, Cambridge, MA: MIT Press.

Freud, S. (1933) 'Lecture XXXI: The Dissection of the Psychical Personality', *Standard Edition*, 22: 57–80, London: Hogarth Press, 1964.

Galison, P. (2003) *Einstein's Clocks, Poincaré's Maps*, New York: Norton.

Greene, B. (2004) *The Fabric of the Cosmos: Space, Time, and the Texture of Reality*, New York: Knopf.

Hartocollis, P. (1975) 'Time and Affect in Psychopathology', *Journal of the American Psychoanalytic Association*, 23, 383–395.

Heidegger, M. (1962) *Being and Time* (J. Macquarrie and E. Robinson, trans.), New York: Harper & Row. (Original published 1927.)

Hopper, E. (2003a) *The Social Unconscious: Selected Papers*, London: Jessica Kingsley.

Hopper, E. (2003b) *Traumatic Experience in the Unconscious Life of Groups*, London: Jessica Kingsley.

Kernberg, O. (2001) 'Freud Conserved and Revised: An Interview with David Scharff', in D. E. Scharff (ed.), *The Psychoanalytic Century: Freud's Legacy for the Future*, New York: Other Press, pp. 41–60.

Le Poidevin, R. (2003) *Travels in Four Dimensions: The Enigmas of Space and Time*, Oxford: Oxford University Press.

Scharff, J. S. and Scharff, D. E. (1998) *Object Relations Individual Therapy*, Northvale, NJ: Jason Aronson.

Stern, D. N. (2004) *The Present Moment in Psychotherapy and Everyday Life*, New York: Norton.

Stolorow, R. D. (2003) 'Trauma and Temporality', *Psychoanalytic Psychology* 20(1): 158–161.

Wright, K. (2002) 'Times of our Lives', *Scientific American*, 287(3): 58–67.

Chapter 1

Time and the unconscious life-cycle

Kent Ravenscroft

As human beings, we are capable of becoming deeply and finely attuned to each other for inborn and acquired reasons – attuned in ways far beyond our conscious awareness. I propose that we are also born attuned and prepared for our longer-range encounters with each other as human families and groups throughout the human life-cycle, as a result of human evolution. Through an interplay of our innate biological potential and good enough personal experience, we progressively develop the capacity for taking in personal and family life-cycle experiences, including a sense of time, calendar, narrative, and history from generation to generation.

Some of these structures and functions of our shared unconscious personal worlds are innate and part of our primary unconscious – our unconscious phantasy life which has never been conscious – and some are secondarily unconscious – taken in, and secondarily layered into these innate mental structures, and hidden from our awareness in one way or another. These phantasies make up hidden object worlds which are variably dynamic and evolving in structure and function – themselves undergoing unconscious life-cycle development, although by different psychological routes and rules than our conscious experience of the life-cycle.

TIME AND THE UNCONSCIOUS

First, I would like to outline the distinction between the primary and secondary unconscious, and between primary and secondary repression. The primary or inborn unconscious is composed of processes and inner representations that emerge into the mind from the body and brain and have never been conscious; primary repression is that mental mechanism that keeps them out of consciousness. The secondary or acquired unconscious is composed of two sets of processes and inner representations described in more detail later, one for metabolizing tolerable to good enough experiences, the other for managing intolerable traumatic experiences.

Freud (1933: 22: 74) originally described the unconscious as that part of the mind closest to the brain and body, with a set of special properties and processes, including 'timelessness'. Modern neurobiology informs us that all aspects of the body are a synchronized orchestra of biological clocks, with the brain being the master clock (Wright 2002). In most species, internal biological rhythms are deeply linked with their seasonal, procreative and family life-cycles. For the human animal, that aspect of the mind most closely linked to the body is the primary unconscious.

It is my contention that the primary unconscious has evolved adaptively as a partially open system in relation to the brain and body, on the one hand, and to the conscious mind and external world, on the other. The primary unconscious is, thus, linked both to the maturing psychobiological rhythms of the non-conscious body and brain, and to the developing psychosocial rhythms of the conscious mind and outer world. Through these unconscious linkages, our internal clock, our innate sense of time, becomes ready for, responds to, and shapes individual and family life-cycle evolution.

The Freudian 'timelessness' of the unconscious is only timeless relative to our conventional logical sense of time. The primary unconscious, much closer to the body and its growth, has its own relative sense of bodily time and rhythm. It is governed by its own variable primary process dream logic and its own maturation. The secondary unconscious is much closer to conscious time and experience, yet has its own dynamic structures, processes and development as a result of maturation, experience, and shifting states of repression and dissociation. This secondary or acquired unconscious sense of time can have healthy or pathological aspects, as can any internalized experience, function and set of object relations.

For example, on the healthy end of the spectrum, adults, families, subcultures, and entire nations are recognized as having differing 'senses of time', narrative, history and world view (Ezzell 2002: 74). And we all know that it is normal for young children to lack a sense of time, personal narrative, and history – capacities they develop over time as they mature.

On the pathological end of the clinical spectrum, all traumatically repressed or dissociated experiences are variably time-altered, time-dissociated, and time-linked based on the ambient altered states of consciousness and shifting projective and introjective identifications at the time of the traumatic experience (Scharff and Scharff 1994; see also Stadter, Chapter 2 in this volume).

As an example of the latter, one of my patients experiences shifting states of altered time-sense and bodily confusion as she achieves progressive recall of traumatic memories around being sexually abused by her father at age 6. She recalls her simultaneous sense of breathless excitement and frozen terror as her father comes slowly up the stairs during her 'nap', hoping 'this time he will be close and cozy, only kissing my lips' but fearing 'he will do that horrible thing again with his "peepee"'. For both of us time seems to race ahead and yet stand still at different points during these sessions as splitting and dissociation emerge. These shifting states are related to changes in projective and introjective identification, as she recollects and relives previously dissociated aspects of herself, at times in relation to me as the different sides of her father, at other times, aspects of her mother. At other moments I represent split-off aspects of her excited, loving, tense, hating, abused or abusing self. When she first came to me this patient had major disturbances in her sense of time, personal narrative and 'historicity' (Ogden 1989: 13), which resolved over time as a result of painful work in therapy.

EVOLUTION AND THE UNCONSCIOUS

Arising from our collective, often violent and dangerous experience during early primitive humanoid evolution, as individuals and as groups we have inherited through genetic selection two potentials which are both conscious and unconscious. The first deals with psychological impingements and trauma – from inside and outside ourselves – allowing us to cope cooperatively with inner and outer danger. The second potential involves the generative use of our internal and external objects, usually safeguarding the extended family group from patricide or murderous aggression. These dual capacities have provided us as individuals and family members with a powerful adaptive group advantage, leading to the selective evolution of our human family and its extended family life-cycle. Given both the routine expectable experiences of our life-cycle, as well as its unpredictable accidental aspects, these dual capacities prepare us to take advantage of both expectable continuities and traumatic discontinuities of experience, equipping us to cope adaptively with the good and bad in either situation.

In a Kleinian sense, the paranoid-schizoid as well as the depressive position (Klein 1946; Segal 1979) have their distinct adaptive advantages as well as significant risks. When being stalked by a carnivorous animal, an enemy, or a sexual predator, it helps to be vigilant and suspicious (paranoid-schizoid). But then afterwards, it is adaptive to regroup psychologically and socially by forgetting through flexible use of grief, repression and mild dissociation (depressive). We can also remember enough to be adaptively vigilant and prepared for future attacks, leaving room for generative personal and social healing, continuity, and growth – Winnicott's 'going-on-being' (Winnicott 1971: 80). At the same time, there are personal and group costs for repression and dissociation through the damage it does to narrative, history, and time sense. For instance, with the previous abuse case we would hope the predatory father's abuse of his daughter would stop through vigilant discovery or her own self-assertion, and that she would heal emotionally and socially, despite our also knowing there will be damage to her repressed or dissociated internalized father–daughter object pair which will affect her future relationships.

Another patient always came ten to fifteen minutes late, arriving with guilty apologies. She had a deep need to tell me every detail of her life, 'running her whole tape', as she put it, unedited and undigested. She left me no room for feedback. Moreover, giving her feedback threatened her with intrusive damage. Near the end of each session, she talked even faster, as if totally heedless that time was rapidly running out. She left me no way to end the session. I felt pent up, frustrated, guilty and trapped. She lived and related to me in a 'time-far' state of mind (Stadter, Chapter 2 in this volume).

One day, in exasperation, I found myself threatening not to see her the next session if she came late again. After blurting this out, I quickly back-pedaled, saying if she came on time, she might discover what she was avoiding. But the damage was already done. She came twenty minutes late to our next session, and I felt disarmed and speechless. Finally, I said I felt guilty and surprised by my abruptness last time, but also curious and concerned. I mentioned feeling trapped and frustrated, but also sad about never having time to give her much beyond a sympathetic ear. My acknowledgement of my countertransference enactment seemed to unlock something.

She became quiet, then began to tell me about her parents' chronic cold war, how tied she was to her mother, and her forbidden longing for her distant, secretive father. Despite his distance and financial troubles, he had a warm spot for his daughter, slipping her money on the side and telling her of his vintage cars, hidden from mother all around the neighborhood. She recalled wondering what else he might be up to. She also told me her mother was fearful, relatively house-bound and friendless, living vicariously through her. During her teenage years she and her mother would take sleeping pills, and then lie together on her bed in a delicious twilight state talking endlessly about her sensuous teen life before falling asleep together. The next day mother would dutifully punish her for her naughtiness.

She went on to tell me that in her later teenage years her mother developed multiple sclerosis, becoming more needful and controlling. My patient would run away to friends for hours, being chronically late and angrily neglecting her mother, only to come back with deeper guilt, apologies and confessions. When she began college her mother neared respiratory death. The patient interrupted college and grudgingly came home to be with her, intensifying her conflict. As mother's breathing became more labored one day, she and her father gave mother the prescribed injection of morphine to ease her terrible distress. Unfortunately, the injection turned out to be lethal. She died in front of them, leaving my patient feeling she had actually killed her, ending up alone now with her father, fueling terrible guilt.

All of this came into conscious view for us. As it did, her lateness, manic 'running of her tape', her avoidance of me – all began to change. She felt time to be less her enemy and endings less traumatically intrusive. As we uncovered and reworked her unconscious adolescent life-cycle issues, she arrived on time, began mourning, and allowed us to end sessions more comfortably.

Moreover, her personal narrative became increasingly coherent.

UNCONSCIOUS OBJECT RELATIONS

Extending Freud's view of the unconscious, Klein (1946), Segal (1964), and others have proposed that there are primary unconscious phantasies which shape and determine our external object relations through projective and introjective identification, although we only know them through their derivatives as they appear in our minds as conscious fantasies, and/or in our behavior.

Not all that enters our secondary or acquired unconscious represents the traumatically repressed. Much of our expanding internal world represents our healthy generative encounters with 'good enough' objects (Winnicott 1971: 11) through which we express our essential desires, our 'idiom' as Bollas (1992: 68) would say. According to Bollas, these generative experiences are 'received' into our secondary unconscious and held there through an atraumatic form of repression. They are transformed there through a dream-like primary process, called the work of reception. This builds up increasingly complex internal object representations and interrelationships in the secondary unconscious through the layering of self and object representations onto unconscious phantasy structures originally deriving from the primary unconscious.

These unconscious phantasies and their evolving inter-relationships provide the basis for receiving, processing and influencing not just the range of current object selections and interactions, but also, I would propose, the whole evolving human life-cycle, with all its stages. As our bodies and brains mature, we develop increasing capacities for more complex personal and interpersonal group object relationships. At each stage of our life-cycle, as new brain-based unconscious phantasy[1] capacities emerge we are able to consciously imagine more complex ways of being and relating in our conscious fantasy life. Of course we soon begin to add layers to these emerging/evolving unconscious phantasies from our secondarily repressed self-object experience from earlier stages. Let me give a clinical example from oedipal child development.

---

1 Kleinians use 'phantasy' for unconscious and 'fantasy' for conscious fantasies.

I was seeing a 4-year-old girl because of severe tantrums occurring in the context of regressive sado-masochistic marital struggles. Her 'terrible twos' were lasting too long. Suddenly, the mother and father began reporting that their previously defiant child had changed dramatically, becoming increasingly clingy, refusing to go upstairs unless accompanied by one of them. She 'feared being bitten by rats up there in the dark'. When we reviewed their fights, it was at night after they put her to bed. They were loud and she had big ears. After we worked on their marital and parental issues a bit, they became less 'biting' and 'ratty' with each other, especially in their daughter's presence or earshot.

As I helped them recognize her nascent oedipal yearnings, especially her budding romantic bids for father, he recognized that his daughter's romantic approaches actually aroused and made him anxious. Mother chimed in that she was jealous and irritable about losing her baby to father. And the daughter confused them both when, at one moment, she seemed to love them being together, only to wedge herself between them and hate them being together. Splitting them apart, she would snuggle up to dad, rubbing herself against him, only to switch and get clingy with mother. What confused them more was that her phobic concern about rats seemed to come and go somewhat independently of their marital fighting, reflecting her inner dynamics and not only reality circumstances.

Their daughter's dramatic switch from fearless to fearful, with all its fluctuations, reflects the appearance of a higher level phobic oedipal defense. Instead of disruptive raw murderous aggression towards her parents (or later, towards group authority figures), she inhibits, displaces, and projects her anger, experiencing it coming from outside her, from 'the rats'. By her unconscious sparing and protecting her parents, she is able to enlist their sympathy and help instead of irritating and antagonizing them. This normal, newly emerging phobic defense adaptively protects her and her parents from her anger whether they are fighting or not. The emergence of phobic defense represents brain-based maturation leading to a new primary unconscious phantasy, a template for a new type of oedipal dyadic and triangular relating. She sees the world through new eyes, through the phobic oedipal lens.

THE DEVELOPMENTAL ASPECTS OF UNCONSCIOUS TIME

With each age and stage of development, there is a sense of time, including a sense of one's self and one's relationships in time and through time – the longitudinal pace and rhythm of things – representing a maturing and developing time-sense. One's maturing biologically based time sense and one's encounter with the timing of the external human family life-cycle have both independent and dependent time-linked aspects to them. We are driven separately (1) from the inside by our maturing brains and minds providing a readiness for taking in and giving shape to outside experiences, and (2) from the outside by the readiness of our families and cultures for receiving and providing social experiences. At the same time there is an innate and necessary matching and meshing of interaction between child, family and cultural interaction through age-appropriate timing and scheduling of experience. How the child matures and behaves determines what the family and society provide at home and at school, at the same time that family and society impose time and timing of socializing experience on a child. The parental couple invents the family for the child, even as the child stimulates, calls out and reinvents the social experience for parents and family (Scharff and Scharff 1987).

Extending the Kleinian (Segal 1979) perspective, primary unconscious phantasies undergo maturation and development over the course of the emerging unconscious internal life-cycle, forming the evolving predisposition and readiness for both receiving and shaping our conscious encounter with others within the shifting social context of the external life-cycle.

Unconscious phantasies, involving dynamic interrelationships among internal objects, have inherent within them a potential sense of time and timing – a readiness for social rhythms, seasonal cycles, continuities, and discontinuities – a built-in emerging competence for human chronicity and calendar. All this forms the inborn basis for the internal extended family life-cycle. Many animals have remarkable herd instincts involving time-related intra-group, migratory, procreative, and generational cycles. Similarly, we have a built-in capacity – albeit with *much more plasticity* – for internalizing intergenerational rhythms and cycles, including the universal human need for legacy and myth.

Anniversary phenomena are related to our primary unconscious life-cycle and sense of time. As a personal example, each year between October and early November, if I do not consciously remember the death of my parents, I become grouchy, depressed, and develop minor somatic symptoms. I cast about for reasons why – until I, or my wife, happens to recall that it is *that* time of the year, the combined October–November anniversaries of my father's and mother's deaths. In other years when I consciously remember them, in advance, none of these unconscious, time- and calendar-linked bodily or emotional reactions occur – though I am sad and reminisce, and call my sister.

THE INTERPLAY OF LIFE-CYCLES

So, there is an ever-evolving interplay among three interrelated life-cycles: (1) our internal primary unconscious life-cycle; (2) our acquired or secondary internal unconscious life-cycle; and (3) our external conscious personal and family life-cycle; The secondary unconscious life-cycle, acquired through experience and reinternalization, develops from two categories of experience in family and social life, as I have mentioned: (1) traumatic impinging experiences which are repressed or dissociated; and (2) generative 'good-enough' experiences which are 'received' into the unconscious (Bollas 1992: 73).

Based on our genetic heritage, our given family, and our experience, each of us will have particular valences for success and failure at each stage of our life-cycle. Additionally, married couples will share a unique set of unconscious basic assumptions coming from their courtship which will influence their relative success or failure as parents at different stages of their subsequent family life-cycle. Here is an example.

I worked with a Jewish couple both of whom had lost hated fathers before meeting each other. During the first year of treatment, as the date for the Jewish service for atonement approached, they slipped into a familiar, tense, deadly struggle with increasingly regressive levels of primitive paranoid/schizoid projection. As I tried to work with them they could agree on only one thing: that I was not helping them much, and, as a matter of fact, actually making things worse, because I kept wanting them to talk about their life and experience together. I began to feel anxious, inarticulate and deadened – and finally noticed my stomach was painfully tied in knots.

On the day after the Service of Atonement, as I cautiously began to explore their weekend and the Service, they bristled. Finally, we eventually discovered their shared guilt about their angry fantasies toward their dead parents. Slowly, after anxious talk about hating fathers in general, each slipped into goading the other to talk about awful experiences with their own fathers. I pointed this out, sharing my sense of tension and anxiety, saying I felt this must all be so hard to stomach. Things shifted slightly toward sadness as they began owning up to their personal experiences, each begrudgingly recalling a few good things about their parents.

The next year at the same time, as the fighting began to happen again, I recalled their anniversary experience and wondered with them if they might be forgetting something. At first they were angry and brushed my curiosity aside. But then it came out that both his father, who had stomach cancer, and her father, who had committed suicide, had died during their adolescence near the actual date of the Day of Atonement. As they reminded each other about this, they became angry with each other, then with me. With my patient inquiry, countering their irritable lack of curiosity, they began to recall painful memories of how absent and unsupportive each of their overwhelmed mothers had been around their teenage anger and grief when their fathers died. Feeling abandoned and angry, they each had resorted to passive-aggressive ways of driving their mothers away, consolidating a hostile stance toward dependency figures. I said I and the knot in my stomach knew something about that characteristic stance of theirs. As I said this, they cracked sheepish smiles that helped them open further discussion.

Through my somatic countertransference, via linked projections and introjections, this couple's unexpressed paternal (and maternal) transference behavior had gotten into my mind and my body that first year, and, much less so, the second time round. Recall my own personal valence for receiving and dealing with anniversary phenomena because of my own parental mourning experience. As we found words to express our immediate human experience together, more intimate details about their parallel and coincident histories emerged, and we moved from soma to psyche, co-creating a shared verbal narrative of their own experience apart and together (Ogden 1994). They had disliked their paranoid-schizoid position with each other, with its alienation, blaming, and sado-masochistic struggle, but feared entering the depressive position with its painful concern about past and present aggression, guilt and mourning. It always amazes me how people so well matched and mismatched find each other, given the uncanny timing of traumatic events in their unexpressed external life cycles – that is, until I recall how driven they both were by their secondary unconscious life-cycles to find each other to reenact their familiar pathological drama, and perhaps to work it out together.

Thus, in a fundamental sense, we, as human beings, all share an inborn unconscious family life-cycle predisposition to seek out similarly inclined mates congruent with our internal phantasy worlds. What is true of individuals is also true, of course, in a primary unconscious sense, for marital couples and their family groups. Beginning with the dance of mate selection, driven by projective identification and their unconscious life-cycle timing, couples progressively develop a shared system of mutual projective identifications.

As they relate to their families of origin and move into child-rearing, they share intimate, evocative experience together. As each stage of their external life-cycle reawakens their own past internal memories and phantasies, these in turn shape their outside experience and behavior. As a result they take in and develop an increasingly powerful congruence of shared secondary unconscious life-cycle. Through similar processes, their children also come to share the same secondary unconscious life-cycle congruence, acquired over their lifetime of experience with their parents and evolving family.

The interplay of all these factors sets in motion a two-way process: the externalization of the internal life-cycle, and the internalization of the external life-cycle. For example, a new baby or an adolescent, with his or her particular powerful biological and behavioral presence, takes over the parents and family, while the departure of a college-bound teenager or the death of a grandparent impact each family member's internal experience, reverberating through deep interior levels. Since most families provide a 'good enough', developmentally facilitating environment for children (Winnicott 1971: 11), positive generative encounters usually prevail during the family life-cycle. Extending Bollas's (1992: 73) concept of the 'received' to this positive life-cycle, I would emphasize that there is a constant unconscious reworking or transformation of our internal object representations and their dynamic interrelationship.

This normal generative life-cycle process, based in biological maturation and actual experience, constantly remodels our internal world, even as our internal phantasies mold and remodel our experience of our external world. As the Scharffs so succinctly put it, the 'infant reinvents the family' even as the 'family reinvents the infant' (1987: 101).

Because of unconscious basic assumptions, parents usually share a mutual developmental level and frequently have stage-specific strengths and vulnerabilities throughout the life-cycle, even though they may seem to be at different levels because of taking on complementary roles.

If co-parents both happen to have their inner conflicts stirred up at the same time by current circumstances, there is a much higher co-determined likelihood of distorted projective identification, distorted delineation (Shapiro and Zinner 1971/1989: 83), and distorted holding and caring for developing children. Failure of holding by one parent is bad enough, but failure by the co-parental pair is particularly damaging.

As a brief example, the daughter of the sado-masochistic couple mentioned above did reasonably well until adolescence. However, at that point, she began to have trouble with friends and especially with boys. As a result she fell back on her parents, especially her mother, but in an off-putting argumentative way. Her parents found her hostile dependent behavior particularly obnoxious, and had little sympathy for her failed forays with boyfriends. They disliked her constant blaming and especially her talk about sadness and loneliness. It was too reminiscent of their own chronic problems. As the parents resolved similar issues, grieved their fathers, forgave their mothers, and became better partners and parents, their empathy and holding for their daughter began to facilitate her own growth in these stage-specific interlocked life-cycle conflicts.

Thus, with shared co-parental distress, there is an increased probability the parental pair will regress to the paranoid-schizoid mode of functioning. Increasing levels of primitive projection take place. Parents find themselves returning emotionally to intolerable child-self experiences – experiences originally encountered with their own parents but now projected into spouses and children. This reveals vulnerability for stage-specific regression to a more primitive, paranoid-schizoid mode around similar life-cycle-specific childhood developmental issues. It is precisely these grandparent–parent–child experiences that transmit these phase-specific life-cycle problems to the children of the next generation. This accounts for the co-evolution of shared, transgenerational life-cycle pathology, including phase-specific conflicts, secondary repression, arrests in developmental level, and pathological shared basic family assumptions.

During treatment, the therapist attends to transference and countertransference distortions of time, feeling, and body states, as well as to breaks in personal narrative, and can sense the presence of repressed or dissociated experience. Attunement to the mutual interplay between internal and external life-cycles, both conscious and unconscious, in oneself and in patients, will facilitate more effective therapeutic process, increasing its scope, intimacy and accuracy.

CONCLUSION

Far beyond our conscious awareness, we humans resonate and relate with each other through our unconscious mind, using the full register of our human instrument. A major part of this mental capacity is our shared sense of the human life-cycle, our mutual sense of time, personal narrative, family calendar and shared history. Our collective human evolution has equipped us with this life-cycle capacity consciously and unconsciously. From birth on, through interplay of our innate potential and good enough developmental experience, we take in personal and family life-cycle experiences.

Major aspects of our evolving life-cycle capacity are structures and functions of our shared unconscious personal worlds. Some are innate and primarily unconscious – part of our unconscious phantasy life which has never been conscious – and some are secondarily unconscious, taken in, and layered into primary phantasies, hidden from our awareness. All these hidden worlds are dynamic in structure and function, and themselves undergo unconscious life-cycle development, although each by different psychological rules and routes.

Through our conscious and unconscious hopes and desires, we seek another to complete our selves, and to repeat our inner dramas. Finally, we select our mates, for better or for worse, someone with sufficient complementarity of fit, sharing our basic needs and unconscious assumptions, whether they emerge from healthy or traumatic experience. To the degree that there is a congruence of unconscious co-parental life-cycle pathology, there will be serious co-determined distortions of children's evolving life-cycles, both conscious and unconscious, shaping their development, subsequent mate selection and families, including distortions of time sense, social calendar, narrative, and history. Though we can only know the surface behavior emerging from unconscious life-cycles, we, as clinicians can enhance treatment through the use of our own human instrument. This fuller attunement of our selves with our patients then opens new aspects of transference and countertransference and treatment possibilities.

REFERENCES

Bollas, C. (1992) *Being a Character*, London: Routledge.

Ezzell, C. (2002) 'Clocking Cultures', *Scientific American*, 287(3): 74–75.

Freud, S. (1933) 'Lecture XXXI: The Dissection of the Psychical Personality', *Standard Edition*, 22: 57–80, London: Hogarth Press, 1964.

Klein, M. (1946) 'Notes on Some Schizoid Mechanisms', *International Journal of Psycho-Analysis*, 27: 99–110.

Ogden, T. H. (1989) *The Primitive Edge of Experience*, Northvale, NJ: Jason Aronson.

Ogden, T. H. (1994) *Subjects of Analysis*, Northvale, NJ: Jason Aronson.

Scharff, J. S. and Scharff, D. E. (1987) *Object Relations Family Therapy*, Northvale, NJ: Jason Aronson.

Scharff, J. S. and Scharff, D. E. (1994) *Object Relations Therapy of Physical and Sexual Trauma*, Northvale, NJ: Jason Aronson.

Segal, H. (1964) *Introduction to the Work of Melanie Klein*, London: Heinemann (enlarged edition, 1973).

Segal, H. (1979) *Klein*, London: Karnac Books.

Shapiro, R. L. and Zinner, J. (1971) 'Family Organization and Adolescent Development', in J. Scharff (ed.) (1989) *Foundations of Object Relations Family Therapy*, Northvale, NJ: Jason Aronson, pp. 79–108.

Winnicott, D. W. (1971) *Playing and Reality*, London: Routledge.

Wright, K. (2002) 'Times of Our Lives', *Scientific American*, 287(3): 58–67.

Chapter 2

Time-near and time-far: the changing shape of time in trauma and psychotherapy

Michael Stadter

We have a very complex relationship with time. Through awareness of it, we can function in the world, choreograph the intricate dance of modern society and 'be on time'. However, awareness of time is one of the great sources of human suffering as well. Through the knowledge of time we anticipate losses, see the aging process, and, ultimately, recognize our own mortality. We experience mourning and the unidirectional flow of past to present to future. We see, how in this temporal sense, we can never go home again.

In this chapter, I reflect on the concept of time and its changing shape. First, I will present a clinical vignette of a patient stuck in time. Second, I will describe a typology of time applicable to experience in and out of psychotherapy. Third, I will examine the important and complex relationship between trauma and time. Finally, I will offer some clinical implications of this discussion of time.

'I WANT TIME TO STOP'

Martin was referred to me due to a major depressive episode triggered by his only son's leaving home to attend college. This 56-year-old physician has been painfully feeling the passage of time – in his son growing up and away from the family, in his wife's aging and chronic physical problems, and in the limitations on his career. He has repeatedly declared that he doesn't want to grow old and prides himself on looking young for his age (he does) and on being in excellent physical shape (he is). When I asked him whether he had a vision for the future, he said with a mixture of annoyance and guilt, 'Yeah, I want to fuck teenage girls.' He has no other vision for his future.

Within two months, with the help of Celexa, Martin's depression lifted revealing an angry, empty sense of self and much existential anxiety about the future. When he was depressed, he was dependent on me, asked frequently for direction and was grateful for the help and relief he got. Four months later, I still felt his dependence on me and on the therapy but there was an angry, demanding quality to him – 'Am I getting any better?', 'How long is this going to take?', 'Eleven years of psychoanalysis didn't do much for me.' I felt alternately touched by his suffering, angry at his frequent demands, and had some feelings of inadequacy.

In a recent session, he complained that he was still depressed. I actually didn't think that he seemed particularly depressed; he felt like a passive, demanding baby to me and I found myself again being irritated with him. I said that I thought the dominant feeling he was struggling with was more anger than depression. He said his wife frequently says he's angry but he doesn't get it. I said maybe he's angry with me for not helping him more and faster. I also suggested that he might be angry with himself for being in such a state at this time of his life. He paused and said maybe there's something to that and that he just wanted time to stop.

I asked him if he had ever wanted time to stop before. He said at least two times: when his sister fell to her death in front of him on a family hiking trip (he was 10, she was 17) and when his mother died (he was 18). He had done much processing of this in his previous analysis but he still had a considerable amount of work to do on it and on the angry empty self that was generated by these traumas. He has developed a good understanding of his vulnerability to depression and to anniversary reactions. But, he has split off awareness of his frequent states of hostile dependency and angry protest against the passage of time and death. He HAS tried to stop time since those deaths. His son going to college shattered his unconscious fantasy that time can be stopped. In a way, it has stopped for him, since he can't think about a future. His obsession with teenage girls symbolized his sense of self in frozen time.

PSYCHOANALYTIC PERSPECTIVES ON TIME

Several psychoanalytic writers have investigated the role of time in our lives. The development of a time sense has been most notably connected with separation (Sachs 1925) and hunger (Spitz 1965). Time has also been considered to be an intruder (e.g., Schiffer 1978). The infant is seen as initially experiencing a timeless, endless union with the mother. The awareness of time, with its passage and limits, is experienced as an intruder into this union. Because of this Schiffer (1978) described time as the earliest target for elimination. Time is frequently portrayed as a father figure with imagery that has a negative charge: Father Time (elderly, enfeebled man with a scythe). Consider how differently Mother Nature is often represented (powerful woman, abundant nurturance). Moreover, while time is one of the core dimensions within which we live, it is also the dimension that measures our aging and eventual death. For example, the only data inscribed on many Western tombstones is the deceased's name and dates of birth and death – these are the most basic facts, the time of our lives. It is not a coincidence that Father Time and the Grim Reaper both carry scythes. It is interesting to note that the other common information on Western tombstones has to do with relationship '. . . devoted son of . . .', 'loving mother of . . .'. Together, these inscriptions highlight the times of one's life, past relationships and present separations.

Many writers have described two states of time perception. Bonaparte (1940) wrote a particularly insightful, early psychoanalytic paper on time in which she describes these two temporal states. One state is a timeless, endless experience where the passage and duration of time are not even noted by the person; the other state is time-centered where passage and duration are felt and measured, as with clocks. She describes these states in child development:

> Children wake from their slumbers, get up, run about, eat, play, laugh and cry in a 'time' whose sweep is of a very different order from that of the brief, pathetic time enjoyed by adults . . . However, as the child's perception of objects in the outside world, at first vague and all-embracing, constantly gains in precision, he becomes better able to situate objects in time. He is obliged to reckon with this master and from this standpoint it marks an important date in his young life when he has learnt to understand the language spoken by watches and clocks and in former times, no doubt, by sun-dials and hour-glasses.
>
> (Bonaparte 1940: 427)

Timelessness is a function of primary process and clock time is a function of secondary process. The awareness of time as limited and forward-moving has been named objective time, adult time, clock time, categorical time, reality time, secondary process time, and sequential time. The timeless experience has been labeled subjective time, child time, existential time, unconscious time, non-linear time, and Freudian time. The different names for the two states do not describe exactly identical experience but each pair does divide temporality in a similar time-aware versus timeless manner.

While there are already various terms for this dichotomy, I suggest that the simple terms of time-near and time-far may be useful for two reasons. First, the near/far pairing highlights the individual's subjective relationship to time *in the moment*: is the person predominantly, in the moment, closely sensing time or is the predominant experience one of temporal awareness being either non-existent or distant? Second, I hope also to suggest a different, co-existent relationship between the two states. Many writers, including Bonaparte, conceive of either one of the temporal states as active at a time, not both states. Certainly human temporal experience does shift and even rapidly oscillate between the two. However, I also think of the two as often simultaneously co-existing although one may be more prominent at a given moment. Sabbadini (1989: 307) has also written about the 'paradoxical coexistence' of these two states.

TIME-NEAR, TIME-FAR AND EPOCHAL TIME

Time-near

When we are aware of time and its passage, when we are in the domain of clocks, calendars and schedules, we are in time-near states. Mention of being late, early, on time, and out of time occur in these states. The therapist and/or patient notice:

The session began five minutes late

It has been three weeks since a friend was seen

It is the anniversary of a father's death

There will be two more weeks until the vacation

The therapy will end in one month

The session is going slowly

Time-near states keep us grounded in the experience of the passage, speed and duration of events. This awareness can be comforting or can cause anxiety, sadness, etc. There is a unidirectional flow from past to present to future and time-near functioning helps to keep a sense of self-continuity and of temporal continuity as well as providing a way to manage the impact of change over time. In the section on trauma, I will examine how time-near experiencing can be powerfully employed to prevent psychological disintegration.

Time-far

Time-far states of mind have either or both of the following characteristics. First, time passage, duration and speed are not noticed. The experience is timeless, endless, without limits and there is no awareness of endings or mortality (see also Johnson, Chapter 3, and Scharff and Cooper, Chapter 14 in this volume). Second, time is not experienced linearly or unidirectionally. The past and/or future may be experienced in the present and the present altered and even intruded upon by it. Transference and countertransference are time-far examples of the past intruding into the present and future. The Hindu, Buddhist and other philosophies that look at time as cyclical emphasize a time-far perspective. The following are additional examples of time-far states of mind:

Being totally engrossed in a here and now experience

Sleep

Some dreams, daydreams and fantasies

Re-living the past as if it were actually happening now (common in transference and trauma)

Free association

Some states of intoxication

Being in love or hate: 'I will love you always.' 'I will hate you forever.'

Strong affective states: 'He'll never forgive me.'

Dissociation

The therapist 'forgetting' to end the session on time

When Martin (in the clinical vignette) was going through the major depressive episode, he was experiencing time painfully as both near and far. He was intensely feeling the slow passage of time both in and out of the sessions. While he felt each tick of the second-hand on his watch, he also had the conviction that he would be in this state forever.

For an effective and rich life, we need to live with a balance or an oscillation between these time states. Consider two points relevant here to psychotherapy. First, patients may have an imbalance between these time states. On the one hand, they may so often experience time-near that they are overwhelmed with the burden of schedules, deadlines and endings and have little or no access to the fullness and depth of their inner worlds (e.g., obsessive-compulsive defenses). On the other hand, time-far experiencing may be so dominant that they may become preoccupied by the here and now (e.g., impulsivity) or by the intrusion of the past (e.g., traumatic flashbacks) and are ineffective in managing life. Second, the process and structure of psychotherapy can facilitate or inhibit the evocation of time-near or time-far states. In conducting treatment, it is therefore important to be cognizant of the impact of our approach and actions on patients' and therapists' time sense.

Epochal time

An additional time experience is epochal time which powerfully combines time-near and time-far states of mind. These are 'Events or epochs that have a monumental impact on history' (Engelman *et al.* 1992: 123). Examples would include the birth of Christ (years becoming measured as BC or AD), the Declaration of Independence, and the Holocaust. However, Engelman *et al.* (1992) are also referring to personal history. Examples would be: the birth of a child, the death of a parent, or a traumatic event.

They occur within the matrix of sequential time, but radically influence all events that precede and are subsequent to the given epoch. Through such dramatic impact, the events that occur in the epoch have a timeless quality as they transcend the constraints imposed on them by sequential time.

(Engelman *et al.* 1992: 123)

This is especially salient and important in working with patients who have been traumatized. Mary, 24, suffered a severe trauma when her mother was murdered before her eyes at the age of 10. They had been walking home from a grocery store when her mother was robbed and shot to death. She described this as a 'tear in time.' Not only did she feel that her life was dramatically different after that but that the experience of her self was radically different after the murder.

Leonard, a man in his mid-40s, suffered the loss of his mother when he was 4. Since he was a man who put an extraordinarily high premium on self-control, he was shocked that he cried uncontrollably in an early session when he recounted it. Later in therapy, we explored his inability to feel love and strong emotion for any woman. He dated this to age 20 when he had been rejected by a girlfriend in college. The epochal event that first became conscious was this rejection in college. Of course, it helped us to understand the power of this rejection by seeing it as having elements of a more fundamental epochal event – his early loss of his mother.

TRAUMA

Overwhelming, inescapable experience injures the individual in a multitude of ways and its distortion of the person's time sense is particularly damaging. Several writers have detailed the neurobiological impact of trauma (Cozolino 2002; Siegel 1999). Stolorow noted that the disruption of 'the unifying thread of temporality' (Stolorow 2003: 158) is so central that it disrupts the sense of self. Herman (1992) stated that temporal distortions are very common among victims of confinement. We do see many time sense distortions in non-traumatized patients but they can be especially strong when trauma has been experienced. Using Ornstein's (1969) work on perceptual time functions, Terr (1984) has described how trauma can disrupt all four of the major elements of temporal functioning which are crucial for basic orientation and psychological regulation. Briefly, the four are:

1   Short time sense
2   Duration
3   Simultaneity and succession
4   Temporal perspective

Short time sense

This involves very brief, momentary durations and rhythms. Terr notes that most traumatized patients do not spontaneously report such phenomena and they may not register in memory. 'Yet awareness of the beat of the heart, of the in and out of breathing, of hunger, or of the need to eliminate are reminders of life, of living – and as such they serve as reassurances during traumatic events' (Terr 1984: 638). For instance, traumatized patients may rhythmically rock, sing songs to themselves, or count to endure a traumatic event and to keep from disintegrating. Such activities have a basic internal clock function that measures the passage of time. I suggest that this gives the victim a time-near focus that assists in managing the overwhelming experience. It is also useful to think of these behaviors as instances of regression to Ogden's (1989) autistic-contiguous functioning. In this primitive mode of experience, dissolution of self is the predominant anxiety. To ward that off, the person organizes self through a focus on sensory experience. That return to the basic awareness of rhythms, skin surface and bodily functions affirms the existence of self and helps the traumatized individual to not 'fall apart'. Similarly, at times in therapy we help disorganized patients 'pull themselves together' by time-near interventions (e.g., 'We have five more minutes;' 'What will you do with yourself for the next two hours?').

Duration

Trauma commonly distorts the perception of the speed of time and how long an event lasted. This can involve accelerated or decelerated time. People who have suffered a sudden, brief traumatic event (e.g., a car crash) frequently report that time seemed to go in slow motion and it was hard to believe that all that they experienced occurred in just a few seconds. On the other hand, Terr notes that some people who have been trapped for prolonged periods (e.g., miners, skiers in an avalanche) often report that the time passed much faster than normal. Patients who have been sexually abused over an extended time may remember it as having gone on for a much longer or shorter period of time than had actually occurred. These temporal accelerations and decelerations may function to help the individual bear the trauma. For example, the slow motion perception of a car accident permits the experience of taking in the traumatic event more slowly.

Simultaneity and succession

Two basic temporal perceptions are simultaneity and succession: whether events occurred at the same time or whether events occurred before or after other events. Traumatized patients may distort whether the trauma occurred before, during, or after another important event. These twists of memory can become important in the nature of the patient's personal narrative and may either aid containment of the damage from the trauma or intensify it.

These distortions can also be prominent in later non-traumatic experiences. Tom, who had been repeatedly physically abused by his older sister during childhood, described at age 40 frequently feeling that 'time was all mixed up in a bucket' – the idea of sequencing different parts of a task, setting priorities and developing time lines seemed impossible to him. This greatly contributed to procrastination and work paralysis. Additionally, the intrusion of past, present and future can break down sequencing. Individuals may be going about their daily business and a stimulus evokes an intrusive thought from the past that is experienced with the force of it happening in the present. Leslie, 55, who had been repeatedly sexually abused in childhood, was walking to my office when she absent-mindedly noticed a plastic chain draped so as to keep people from walking on a grass plot. This physical object reminded her of a particular time in her childhood which, in turn, suddenly threw her into a flashback of a childhood sexual trauma at that time. Much of the session was spent with her viscerally re-living that abusive event. On the other hand the future can intrude on the present as well. Anxious patients can become so paralyzed by their fear of future catastrophes that they cannot live in the present (Hartocollis 1975).

Temporal perspective

Temporal perspective refers to the change in the perception of the future in victims of trauma and is often, according to Terr (1984: 658), a 'time foreshortening'. Following trauma, the patient may expect a smaller future – a shorter life, no marriage or children, little joy, few job prospects, etc. Terr quotes a patient of hers two years after suffering a traumatic loss as saying, 'Now I simply exist – one day at a time' (1984: 659). As I write this, three traumatized patients immediately come to mind (including Martin) who are afraid to, or unable to, have fantasies about their futures. They are mired in the time-near experience of the present and the time-far intrusion of the past into the present. In their experience, they have no future. In the novel, *Einstein's Dreams*, Lightman (1993) described life without a future, 'In a world without future, each parting of friends is a death. In a world without future, each loneliness is final. In a world without future, each laugh is the last laugh. In a world without future, beyond the present lies nothingness, and people cling to the present [*or, to the past, in the case of our patients*] as if hanging from a cliff' (1993: 130). On the other hand, some trauma patients develop an expansive or transcendent time-far view of the future. This may involve a religious or philosophical belief – that now they are destined for greatness, God's will be done, that they will be reincarnated into a better life, that they can now just wait for heaven.

TRAUMA AND FROZEN TIME

Other effects of trauma on time sense include the state of frozen time and the desire to bring back the past. Many writers have described a freezing, a stopping, of time and parts of the personality as a response to trauma (see Scharff and Scharff (1994) for a survey of perspectives). As part of the complex effects of splitting and dissociation, the traumatic memory may be frozen and unchanging and a part of the self associated with it is frozen and unable to grow or develop. Davies and Frawley (1992: 21), in describing survivors of incest, have written of the child part of the patient being 'frozen in time' and isolated from the rest of the personality. Such patients continue to think, feel and act as they had in their lives at the time of the trauma. Van der Kolk (1996) has reported that despite the evidence of frequent distortions in the memory of trauma victims, they consistently claim that their memories and perceptions are exact representations of sensations at the time of the trauma. We might consider that this belief in the exact preservation of these sensations and memories serves as an obsessional defense giving the impression of certainty and control. Many other writers have described related phenomena – for example, Fairbairn's (1958) frozen tableau, Guntrip's (1969) regressed libidinal ego, and Hopper's (1991) encapsulation.

In his novel, Lightman (1993) also evocatively describes how the state of stopped time in itself destroys human connection and relationship: 'The tragedy of this world (of stopped time) is that no one is happy, whether stuck in a time of pain or of joy. The tragedy of this world is that everyone is alone. For a life in the past cannot be shared with the present. Each person who gets stuck in time gets stuck alone' (1993: 65). As Stolorow (2003: 158) notes, the breaking up of the 'unifying thread of temporality' disrupts the basic sense of self. It also disrupts and even destroys human relatedness.

TRAUMA AND BRINGING BACK THE PAST

Frequently traumatized patients are obsessed with the desire to return to a time prior to the trauma. For instance, they may be haunted with thoughts and longings for the time before the rape or the death of the spouse. The pre-trauma time may be idealized, making it larger than life. Such a passionate desire for the time-far of the past is a way to manage the overwhelming experience of post-traumatic life. Shakespeare dramatized such a state of mind with Richard II's lament, 'Oh call back yesterday, bid time return' (*Richard II* 3.2). We might think of this as investing temporal hope in the wrong direction – in the past rather than in the future. There is a saying, I don't know the attribution, that, 'You have to give up the hope of a better yesterday.'

The need to bring back the past can also cause trauma victims to persistently look for omens or turning points (Terr 1984). Omens are events that victims now believe could have forewarned them of the impending trauma. Turning points are events in which a choice was made and, had it been made otherwise, the trauma would not have happened: the present and future would be different. We can look at this as another example of obsessional defenses to manage the impact of overwhelming experience that the person could not control. It is an attempt at some mastery. The movie, *Sliding Doors*, with its double narrative after a seemingly insignificant event, and the many dramas about time travelers who change the past reflect this wish to control or undo the past – to kill time and/or to obliterate the epochal event.

APPLICATIONS AND IMPLICATIONS

The central premise of this chapter is that the therapeutic process can be enhanced by attention to the dimension of time – its quality and quantity, and its role in organizing psychological experience and a sense of self – as a specific ingredient in therapy. Particular attention to the temporal contours of the transference/countertransference matrix is valuable: the time-near and time-far states for both patient and therapist, temporal distortions and shifts (see also Ravenscroft, Chapter 1 in this volume), and epochal therapeutic events.

Here are some additional recommendations:

1 Simply listen for temporal references in the content and associations (therapist's and patient's) and consider their meaning. For example:

'I will *never* talk to him again.'

The patient repeatedly looks at the clock.

'She'll be in my heart *forever*.'

'It's been an *eternity* since our last session.'

'It seems like yesterday I was here.'

'So, that's that – *the beat goes on*.'

'It's been 50 minutes already?'

'The longest hour in my week is with this patient.'

In my work with Martin, our examination of his desire to have time stop has proven productive. Interestingly, he has an unconscious tendency to rub the face of his wristwatch and our curiosity about that has been helpful. Stolorow (2003: 158) noted that his simple statement to a traumatized patient 'Trauma destroys time!' helped her to feel less fragmented.

2   Note when the patient moves from predominant states of time-near to time-far or vice versa. Such transitions may indicate a defensive temporal shift to avoid an uncomfortable affect or state of mind. What is being warded off? What is being organized or disorganized? What is going on between us?

3   Ask: what is the impact of your approach, structure and process on time states? Is this a long-term therapy, at this point in time, or is it short-term or termination phase? These different contexts can profoundly affect the experience of time. For example, I believe that short-term therapy pulls patient and therapist into more time-near states (Stadter 1996). How does your style and approach affect the evocation of different temporal states? Does it more promote time-near or time-far experiencing? Would it be more effective to facilitate more of time-near or time-far functioning?

4   Consider the role of loss and blocked mourning in patients who have a great deal of difficulty in handling time. As I reflected on my practice and the patients who had issues with time, they so often were patients with traumatic losses who had had difficulty grieving the losses.

5   Be attuned to the profound impact that trauma can have on the experience of time. Be aware of and investigate the time-alterations of traumatized patients. Distortions in time sense can be particularly sensitive indicators of psychic trauma because time perception is relatively new on the phylogenetic tree and is especially vulnerable to overwhelming stress (Terr 1984). Does the degree of temporal distortion in your patient suggest a past traumatic experience? Remember it is estimated that over three-quarters of U.S. adults have had overwhelmingly stressful life events (van der Kolk *et al.* 1996). Yet, these events and their impact may be overlooked in treatment (McFarlane and de Girolamo 1996). Are there epochal events in your patient's life that were traumatic? Have there been epochal events in the therapy? In Part II of the present volume, on space, both Anderson and Hopper explore trauma as well.

6   Be sensitive to end-of-time phenomena. Consider the nature of the material that sometimes arises at the end of a session (so-called 'door-knob comments') or shortly before an anticipated interruption to the treatment (e.g., vacations, holidays) or during the termination phase of therapy. At times, these are moments during which little apparent work is done but they can initiate breakthroughs, as material comes in that has either not been mentioned before, or is presented in a less defended manner. Some writers have examined the effects when a whole culture

deals with an end-of-time event. For instance, Y2K at the end of the last millennium evoked this experience in many people (David *et al.* 1999).

7   Finally, at certain times, consider the creative use of time. Our object relations approach emphasizes the uniqueness of each individual patient and the particular relationship developed with each specific therapist at a distinct point in time. No matter how experienced the therapist is, each patient must be approached with an attitude of not knowing and of hopeful discovery (Stadter and Scharff 2000). This is the opposite of a 'one size fits all' approach, yet the firmness and stability of the therapeutic frame are also crucial. How might we use time creatively with a particular patient? Here are some creative uses of time in therapy:

A   Winnicott (1971), writing about therapy with few or infrequent sessions, argued for it being provided on demand, when the patient needs it and requests it. The therapy can then capitalize on the readiness and timely motivation of the patient.

B   Budman and Gurman (1988) recommend, on a case by case basis, that therapists consider changes in duration and frequency of sessions to enhance treatment. Of course, we routinely look at frequency (once, twice, three times per week therapy) in improving the effectiveness of therapy. Consider how changing the frequency or session length for a brief period would affect the treatment.

C   Lacan (Evans 1996) has developed the controversial technique of the therapist unilaterally ending the session early. This may occur when the therapist believes that either nothing will be accomplished if the session were to continue or that it will be more therapeutic for the patient to end the session with their inner state as it is at that particular moment. This is a very creative use of time although I do not recommend it myself.

D   I have, as a counterpoint to the Lacanian technique, a personal example from my own therapy of talking about an important but very uncomfortable issue. I noticed that the 50 minutes was up and I said, with relief, that we had to 'leave it here.' My therapist surprised me by saying, 'It is raining awfully hard outside; I don't mind continuing our session a bit.' She had never done that before. We did continue and quite deeply, and painfully, further explored my issue – the time was right to overcome my resistance.

IN CLOSING

To be fully alive, we must effectively live with the balance and co-existence of time-near and time-far states. We must face the nearness of time and also dive into the associative states of time-far. The same is true about psychotherapy. But, whatever our perception of time, our lives and our relationships with our patients are all, in fact, time-limited. As Bonaparte noted:

> We destroy time from the moment we begin to use it. To be master of one's time can only refer to time which lies before one, which has not yet done service, which one has not yet enjoyed. For in living our time we die from it.
>
> (Bonaparte 1940: 432)

REFERENCES

Bonaparte, M. (1940) 'Time and the Unconscious', *International Journal of Psycho-Analysis*, 21: 427–468.

Budman, S. H. and Gurman, A. S. (1988) *Theory and Practice of Brief Therapy*, New York: Guilford.

Cozolino, L. (2002) *The Neuroscience of Psychotherapy*, New York: Norton.

David, C., Lenoir, F. and de Tonnac, J. P. (1999), *Conversations about the End of Time*, New York: Fromm International.

Davies, J. M. and Frawley, M. G. (1992) 'Dissociative Processes and Transference–Countertransference Paradigms in the Psychoanalytically-Oriented Treatment of Adult Survivors of Childhood Sexual Abuse', *Psychoanalytic Dialogues*, 2(1): 5–36.

Engelman, T. C., Day, M. and Durant, S. (1992) 'The Nature of Time and Psychotherapeutic Experience when Treatment Duration Shifts from Time-Limited to Long-Term', in J. S. Rutan (ed.), *Psychotherapy for the 1990s*, New York: Guilford, pp. 119–137.

Evans, D. (1996) *An Introductory Dictionary of Lacanian Psychoanalysis*, London: Routledge.

Fairbairn, W. R. D. (1952) *An Object Relations Theory of the Personality*, New York: Basic Books.

Fairbairn, W. R. D. (1958) 'On the Nature and Aims of Psycho-analytical Treatment', *International Journal of Psychoanalysis*, 39: 374–385

Guntrip, H. (1969) *Schizoid Phenomena, Object Relations and the Self*, New York: International Universities Press.

Hartocollis, P. (1975) 'Time and Affect in Psychopathology', *Journal of the American Psychoanalytic Association*, 23: 383–395.

Herman, J. L. (1992) 'Complex PTSD: A Syndrome in Survivors of Prolonged and Repeated Trauma', *Journal of Traumatic Stress*, 3(1): 377–391.

Hopper, E. (1991) 'Encapsulation as a Defense against the Fear of Annihilation', *International Journal of Psycho-Analysis*, 72(4): 607–624.

Lightman, A. (1993) *Einstein's Dreams*, New York: Warner Books.

McFarlane, A. C. and de Girolamo, G. (1996) 'The Nature of Traumatic Stressors and the Epidemiology of Posttraumatic Reactions', in B. A. van der Kolk, A. C. McFarlane, and L. Weisaeth (eds.), *Traumatic Stress: The Effects of Overwhelming Experience on Mind, Body, and Society*, New York: Guilford, pp. 129–154.

Ogden, T. H. (1989) *The Primitive Edge of Experience*, Northvale, NJ: Jason Aronson.

Ornstein, R. (1969) *On the Experience of Time*, New York: Pelican Books.

Sabbadini, A. (1989) 'Boundaries of Timelessness: Some Thoughts about the Temporal Dimension of the Psychoanalytic Space', *International Journal of Psycho-Analysis*, 70: 305–313.

Sachs, H. (1925) Quoted by S. Harnik in 'Die Triebhaftaffektiven Momente in Zeitgefühl', *Imago* 78: 453–468.

Scharff, J. S. and Scharff, D. E. (1994) *Object Relations Therapy of Physical and Sexual Trauma*, Northvale, NJ: Jason Aronson.

Schiffer, I. (1978) *The Trauma of Time*, New York: International Universities Press.

Siegel, D. J. (1999) *The Developing Mind*, New York: Guilford.

Spitz, R. (1965) *The First Year of Life*, New York: International Universities Press.

Stadter, M. (1996) *Object Relations Brief Therapy: The Therapeutic Relationship in Short-term Work*, Northvale, NJ: Jason Aronson.

Stadter, M. and Scharff, D. E. (2000) 'Object Relations Brief Therapy', in J. Carlson and L. Sperry (eds.), *Brief Therapy with Individuals and Couples*, Phoenix, AZ: Zeig, Tucker and Theisen, pp. 191–219.

Stolorow, R. D. (2003) 'Trauma and Temporality', *Psychoanalytic Psychology*, 20(1): 158–161.

Terr, L. C. (1984) 'Time and Trauma', *Psychoanalytic Studies of the Child*, 39: 633–665.

van der Kolk, B. A. (1996) 'Trauma and Memory', in B. A. van der Kolk, A. C. McFarlane, and L. Weisaeth (eds.), *Traumatic Stress: The Effects of Overwhelming Experience on Mind, Body, and Society*, New York: Guilford, pp. 279–303.

Winnicott, D. W. (1971) *Therapeutic Consultations in Child Psychiatry*, New York: Basic Books.

Chapter 3

Bad infinity: narcissism and the problem of time

Leslie A. Johnson

The experience of time is a function of separation. We care about time, we suffer from it, because birth separates us from the inorganic substrate from which we arise and to which we know we will return. Time is the awareness of this relation between being and nonbeing, a relation that defines us existentially, even as it insults and challenges our narcissism.

The existential awareness of time depends, however, on another prior separation: the achievement of psychic birth or subjecthood, whereby a stable self-representation is differentiated from the internal world of objects, in particular from the maternal object. This process of separation and differentiation may be thought of metaphorically as the opening up of space – real space but also internal mental space structured by the gaps that begin to emerge in the earliest discriminations of 'me' from 'not me'. Only when psychic birth has opened up this interior does experience become saturated with temporal significance. Feelings such as desire, dread, grief or frustration heighten the awareness of time – they are, in a sense, awarenesses of time – because their cathected objects are acknowledged as separate from, rather than coextensive or identical with the self. From a psychoanalytic point of view the experience of time is thus above all a function of intrapsychic space or separation. Time opens up and comes to matter in so far as we can bear to sustain the gap between the self and its internal objects. There is always a countervailing tendency exerted by omnipotent mental processes to implode this space, to shrink or close these gaps. Ultimately, it is the capacity to undergo the depressive position which keeps space open, respects the integrity of the object, and, in a matter of speaking, lets time temporalize, i.e., be experienced as subjectively real and moving.

Two Greek philosophical terms help to clarify how human beings typically adapt to the temporal exigencies of existence. Time understood as *chronos* emphasizes the ubiquity of change and transience. Personified in the ancient god Kronos, ruler of the cosmos who propels genealogical process (and eats his children), *chronos* designates time as an ever-flowing stream whose regular motion we objectify and measure (Peters 1967). The concept of *kairos*, on the other hand, refers to a span of time that is shaped or made significant by decisive actions which bring it to fulfillment. In Ecclesiastes, the seasons of life are called *kairoi*, while the Crucifixion is taken to be the *kairos* par excellence, the accomplishment of God's plan whereby Old Testament prophecy is fulfilled and human history redeemed (Kittel and Friedrich 1985). The concepts of *chronos* and *kairos* inform many aspects of experience. They describe, for example, the phenomenon of music, where the *chronos* of beat is shaped into deeply satisfying kairotic structures and resolutions. Likewise, psychotherapy begins by doling out 50-minute portions of *chronos*. But if it can release the idiom of the self and better structure intrapsychic space, the patient lives more creatively in and with time, turning *chronos* into *kairoi* of work and love.

TIME AND NARCISSISM

This chapter originated in my work with two narcissistic patients who could not make this creative accommodation to time. For them, time tended to expose the gaps and thus the vulnerabilities of the differentiated self. They defended themselves by foreclosing temporal awareness. As I considered the vicissitudes of their temporal experience, it seemed to me that the narcissistic patient (and the primitive narcissistic core of all individuals regardless of pathology) strives to escape the relentless horizontal flow of *chronos*, to break out in a vertical thrust, a seemingly 'transcending' movement that opens onto another kind of duration (see also Ashbach, Chapter 18 in this volume).

To conceptualize this narcissistic move I borrow another Greek term, *pleroma*, from the Christian and Gnostic traditions. Signifying fullness, *pleroma* designates the plenitude of God that comprises the aeons, the infinite sphere of deity, 'home of all that is perfect, godlike, eternal, imperishable' (Hastings 1919: 64). References to the *pleroma* occur in Jung (1969) in his ruminations on the mythologies of the Self. I use the term to connote the illusion of God-like self-sufficiency at the heart of narcissism. The *pleroma* connotes a state of mind in which the self savors eternity understood as an infinitely expanding duration of fullness where time seems neither to pass nor to pass away.

The *pleroma* is reminiscent of the 'oceanic feeling' of Freud, with its 'restoration of limitless narcissism' (1930: 72). In *pleroma*, however, the accent is on grandiosity and power, rather than on passivity and mystical oneness. In so far as the *pleroma* is not a delusion, but rather an illusory heaven where the self feels full and without gaps, it also resembles Steiner's 'psychic retreat', a hideaway governed by a state of mind in which painful realities can be 'simultaneously accepted and disavowed' (Steiner 1993: 89). Most of all, the *pleroma* pertains to the zonal geography of narcissism theorized by Meltzer (1992).

In this work, Meltzer transforms the classical notion of zonal fixation into a type of narcissistic part-object relation supported by the persistence of omnipotent phantasies of projective and introjective identification. In the classical conception, the ego organizes the discharge of energy around oral, anal or genital zones of its own body. In Meltzer's conception, the self is intimately involved with the body and the corresponding zones (or part-objects) of the phantasied maternal imago, in such a way as to resist the integration of that imago into a whole object and also, which amounts to the same thing, to resist the anxieties of the depressive position in relation to it. The three erogenous zones thus become in Meltzer's conception three phantasied spaces inside the internal object – Meltzer calls them life-worlds or claustra – inhabited by parts of the self: the so-called head/breast, the genital and the rectal compartments of the maternal body (see also Hill, Chapter 17 in this volume).

Despite the indifference narcissists often exhibit toward external objects, Meltzer indicates how incessantly they are engaged with their internal objects through omnipotent mental acts of projective identification. The phantasied inside of the maternal body exerts a fascination on the self. To be inside of it, to be in control of it, is to inhabit the idealized source of plenitude and power where vulnerabilities disappear and all gaps are sutured. In order for the self to exploit this power, however, the exterior of that internal imago – the boundary which secures its integrity in the imagination – must be breached. Meltzer shows that omnipotent phantasies of intrusion, rape, robbery, and appropriation are rampant in the claustral zones of narcissistic object relations. These phantasies, however, are not merely mental figments of omnipotent thinking. Projective identification into the internal object is energized and made psychically convincing because it is linked to masturbatory excitation and the fullness of orgastic sensation (Meltzer 1992). 'The act of masturbation,' Meltzer stipulates, 'of whatever orifice or body part, derives its urgency and often compulsive force from its capacity to generate omnipotence' (1992: 30). Penetration into 'the imaginary world of the inside of an internal object,' he specifies elsewhere, 'is based on nothing but the omnipotence of masturbatory processes' (1992: 102).

The idea of *pleroma* overlaps with the head/breast compartment in Meltzer's taxonomy – that life-world inside the internal object associated with self-idealization, sensual delight and omniscience. The *pleroma*, however, with its connotation of transcendence of time, highlights the specifically temporal vicissitudes of narcissistic adaptation. The clinical material below, which illustrates the attainment of *pleroma* through masturbatory processes, indicates how narcissistic object relations are a defense against time and time-saturated awareness. The *pleroma* functions to scotomize time, i.e., to make the perception of time disappear. In so far as the self exploits omnipotent masturbatory processes to breach the integrity of the internal object, it closes the gap which separates it from the object –

the very separation out of which the experience of time arises. Thus the narcissistic self avoids loss and mourning by effacing the tension between 'now' and 'no longer'; it avoids dependency and frustration by effacing the tension between 'now' and 'not yet'; it avoids dread by effacing the tension between being and nonbeing. Fueled by the omnipotence of masturbatory processes, the narcissistic self exploits the internal object in order to dwell in a *pleroma*, a nontemporalizing duration that fosters the illusion of plenitude and self-sufficiency.

CASE MATERIAL: MARSHA AND ALAN

Two patients fostered my thinking about time and narcissism. Both came to therapy depressed and unable to work productively. Marsha, a graduate student in French, began when she was 31 and left almost two and a half years later to take a one-year teaching job. Alan, who taught high-school Spanish, began when he was 24 and stopped four years later to get married. Both took extensive time away from treatment for study or research abroad. Alan came once a week, sometimes less. Marsha came twice a week during the last ten months. The brief notes that follow are meant to provide a feeling for the grandiosity and omnipotence of these patients, a glimpse into their sexual proclivities, and a sense of their difficulties coping with time. The next section illustrates the problems that ensued when their narcissistic adaptations collided with the time limits of the clinical hour.

Marsha had a secret ambition 'to be the greatest French professor in the world.' For years, however, she had been spinning her wheels on her dissertation. She could not tolerate deadlines, often throwing a tantrum or fit the day before. Orgastic events, these fits would break the tension of relating to *chronos* and to an impending future. I never knew Marsha to mail an application in on time – yet rejection letters didn't seem to faze her. 'Somehow,' she said, 'I don't really worry about the future.' I remember thinking, 'Why bother, if you're already one of the elect?' We began to notice how little time seemed to matter.

Alan, on the other hand, became a Spanish teacher mainly because Latin Americans had celebrated him as a 'special' tourist, 'the best of all'. Convinced of his 'charm' (it was an explicit part of his self-description), he often complained when I didn't gratify him: 'No adult has ever not praised and flattered me!' Whatever his abilities, Alan scarcely coped with the time pressures of teaching, because every time he sat down to work he initiated a masturbatory ritual which continued until bedtime, producing nothing but ejaculate. It was high anxiety in class the next day, but while he was masturbating, he explained, 'I seem to have all the time in the world.' Alan's conscious fantasies seldom involved intercourse. Typically he'd be masturbating in the face of a woman, whose 'WOW!' would fill him with a sense of POWer. Then he would drink the actual ejaculate, thereby becoming his own breast and sealing the pleromatic illusion of gapless self-sufficiency.

Marsha never reported masturbating at her desk, but she did subvert her writing in a masturbatory way. She never got anywhere because she couldn't stop fussing, i.e., playing with her sentences. Nor could she resist playing with her dog. Projecting her idealized object onto the poor beast, she dwelled on his 'greatness' and 'perfection', seeming to identify with the timelessness of canine consciousness. Two weeks before her dissertation was due, she even bought another – as if puppy training were a way out of the temporal stream. Occasionally, Marsha had sex with her husband, but only subject to certain rules. '*Never*,' she informed me, 'on Sunday,' and '*never, never* before bedtime.' Intercourse was 'boring', and she didn't much care for foreplay. She did, however, enjoy 'orgasming and afterwards' – so long as the 'afterwards' did not involve sleep. Virtually non-relational and anti-sensual, Marsha's sexuality seemed atemporal as well, as if in defiance of instinctual processes whereby excitation builds to release over time. Far from describing the temporal structure of desire, sex for Marsha was a masturbatory process. She exploited it to attain the illusion of *pleroma*, which is why she had to not sleep but remain conscious 'afterwards'.

TEMPORAL VICISSITUDES IN THE CLINICAL SITUATION

Because the therapeutic encounter is time-limited, it frustrates the very needs and desires that it awakens. This is especially so for the narcissistic patient who cannot tolerate dependency. By creating a pleromatic state of mind in the sessions, Marsha and Alan persistently sought to make time disappear. There were several signs that this was happening.

Masturbatory motor activity

What first linked these patients in my mind was the fact that neither could sit still. I now view this activity as a masturbatory process going on before my eyes. Alan's habit, though subtle, was less displaced. Using his fingers, he would lightly tap or rub the arm of the chair; then, unobtrusively dropping his hand down to his thigh, he'd ever so lightly trace the folds in his pants. A compulsive masturbator from eight-years-old, as a teen he began to stage this activity inside the walk-in closet in his bedroom. By projective identification, my consulting room, and my mind within it, became such an interior space into which Alan deeply embedded himself to control my mind, my gaze, and my attention. Whatever the precipitant for therapy, Alan stayed because he had found another walk-in closet. I became his refuge from a frantic life, the place where he could levitate to *pleroma*. Toward the end, I took a more interpretive stance, thereby enacting our separateness. He wouldn't think with me about this, but chose instead to quit the masturbatory chamber, terminating treatment.

Marsha, on the other hand, did what I thought of as Rumpelstiltskin's dance. I'd watch in amazement as the feet beneath her chair would jab, stomp or twirl. For instance, the day she confided her vaunting ambition her ankles were twirling like pinwheels. Transferentially, Marsha exploited this masturbatory movement, I believe, to assert omnipotent control over me. Aware of my degree in literature, she coveted my mind and sought to kick her way into it in order to identify with my supposed power and omniscience. By thus closing the gap between self and object, she could cancel out time-saturated feelings of longing and envy, the awareness of immaturity and lack. When she was charged up and kicking, my room – the interior of her object – became hers, suffused with her *pleroma*.

Behavior at the boundaries

The time boundaries of a session are those points where the narcissistic self comes up most jarringly against the reality of *chronos* and separateness. For Alan and Marsha these boundaries required special negotiation. In Alan's case, the intriguing thing was that he never lingered before leaving. Was he indifferent to time? He certainly seemed indifferent to space: he alone, of all my patients, never commented when I moved to another (much nicer) office. I think that when Alan rubbed his 'magic lantern', he transcended space, time and desire. The exterior disappeared because in phantasy he was already in the interior, controlling my gaze, my WOW, to restore his grandiosity and power. Masturbatory phantasy was ubiquitous, propelling him into a *pleroma* that, from my point of view, seemed to float him out the door at session's end. And so it went, year in, year out, as Alan insulated himself against the winds of change.

Marsha did sometimes stumble at the boundary. When need would rustle in the transference, she'd scotomize the hour, coming late and explaining, 'I was playing with the dog and lost track of time!' Once I observed that dogs aren't conscious of time: they don't know that life, like a counseling session, comes to an end. 'I don't particularly want to think about my death!' she shot back, scorched by the very mention of the future as the harbinger of separation, loss, and mortality. When she came late, I encouraged her to describe her state of mind. A moment would come when she knew she had to leave, 'But somehow I get engrossed in something (usually dog-play) and time expands.' It sounded like a mystical technique: 'I feel sunken in, focused, like a point of illumination, with everything else blurred or dark.' A latter-day Gnostic, Marsha engrossed herself in a time-transcending *pleroma* when separateness and limitation threatened.

Time in the countertransference

The countertransferences evoked by Alan and Marsha were difficult and challenging, sometimes involving feelings of contempt and anger. For the purposes of this chapter, however, I limit myself to the experience of mind-numbing torpor described by Kernberg (1975) and other commentators, which often came over me when working with these patients. If they were 'transcending' time, I'd be clinging to the clock for a toehold in reality, trusting *chronos* to do its work and release me from this molasses of mindlessness. Because I had become for them, not so much the object as the internal location of their omnipotent control, I disappeared for them as a separate and exterior other. Profoundly unrecognized, I would lose the integrity of my own thoughts and become vulnerable to over-identification with them – not just empathizing, but somehow becoming them.

This happened on two occasions, when I 'woke up' to find that I too had made time disappear! Once with Alan I caught myself quietly rubbing my *own* thigh – then realized we were five minutes over. With Marsha, I fell into a similar trance the day she threw a fit. She had bent over, breathing convulsively, then hurled herself onto the couch (I thought of Pete Rose sliding into home), where she lay until I literally bethought myself and saw that we were ten minutes over. Lying there, Marsha recalled her recent fit at the vet's on seeing an X-ray of her dog. Gazing into this image of the interior of her object, she had beheld not the immortal Godhead, but a premonition of mortality. The glimpse of skeleton broke her illusion and demystified her identification with the object as a pleromatic refuge. So, nearing the chronometric limit of our session, she scotomized it by propelling herself deeper into my room, deeper into the inside of the internal object, deeper into my couch and my mind. Meanwhile, spellbound and, in a sense, reeling from this psychic attack, I was sucked into the *pleroma* as well, a state of bewitched fascination in which time had stopped.

The *pleroma* in dreams

Two dreams from late in treatment illuminate the narcissistic part-object relations on which the assumption to *pleroma* depends. Alan's dream illustrates the violence of the omnipotent phantasy. *He is observing an interior space similar to my office: two facing armchairs, a couch to the side. One chair is vacant. A man in his late 20s sits in the other. On the couch a bag of sugar is slashed open, sugar spilling out. A boy writhes in it, belly down, but the man won't let him leave.* Here, insinuation into me (my office) is doubled by the intrusive rape of my idealized head/breast (the sugarbag), source of everlasting admiration and approval.

Marsha also brought a dream of plunder in her quest for intellectual power and omniscience. *She enters an elegant atelier owned by a 'big queen'.*

Inside, she spots a gorgeous Kelly green hat in ribbons and tulle, but she doesn't buy it. The atelier refers to my sunny loft-like office; the hat to my green beret, fetish of mental potency, that sometimes hung on the chair by my desk. But rather than pay for the hat, i.e., work toward the *kairos* of separation and individuation so that she might have her own thinking cap, Marsha aimed to steal it – as her associations indicated. She complained about the fancy shops where she loves to browse but is frightened to enter because 'they always act as if I've st . . . st . . . st . . . something!' Three times Marsha stammered the give-away word, unable to speak the past participle of the verb 'to steal'.

Endings that weren't: bad infinity

Some months later, Marsha and Alan left treatment, but neither underwent the experience of termination. Neither was ready to mourn the loss of the object. Chronometric time ended, but there was no *kairos*. There was no 'sense of an ending' (Kermode 1967: title).

Sometimes, albeit rarely and painfully, these patients acknowledged the time that was passing. Marsha, who idealized the student movement of the 1960s, wished that she could have demonstrated and kicked over a few trashcans. 'But that's how two-year-olds behave,' I replied. Eyes widening, she blurted out, 'That time is *gone!*' She had caught the chilly draft of time passing – but she couldn't mourn the lost time of therapy. At the third-to-last session the masturbatory process resumed, only this time the toes wriggling away in her sandals were painted – like mine. 'Is she really ripping me off from head to toe?' I silently wondered, thinking of dream hat and the nail polish. Unconscious guilt about stealing probably drove her to 'forget' the next session in my atelier/boutique. 'What are patients supposed to *do* at the end?' she asked provocatively on the final day. I said it was customary to pay the bill and say goodbye, adding that her husband always signed the checks. She smiled knowingly, but a few days later it wasn't *her* check that came in the mail, it was her husband's, as usual. Staging another manic defense, she had kicked me in the can, hoping to get away with the goods.

What brought Alan back to earth was impending marriage and cohabitation: where would he masturbate? Suddenly he complained that I hadn't cured him after all these years. Refusing to face the end of our time together, he quit one weekend by phone. But his choice for a bride – a woman who like myself is also in the counseling profession – effaced the sense of an ending. A late dream, however, indicates the profound dilemma posed by the narcissistic solution to the problem of time. *He is seated at his desk in his apartment masturbating before the computer. He wakes up, still seated at his desk in his apartment masturbating before the computer.* The illusory *pleroma* maintained by omnipotent masturbatory processes may seal the gap of separateness and scotomize time. But without disillusionment, i.e., without acknowledging the separateness, the exteriority and the integrity of the Other, the self cannot experience the new. As Alan's nightmare uncannily premonitors, the *pleroma* is the claustrophobic realm of sameness – of more and more of the same: the selfsame Self. Seeming to vanquish time, it opens instead onto the ennui of 'bad infinity' (Mautner 1996: 209), an endlessly expanding duration unrelieved by the discontinuities of time, of difference, of otherness which signal meaningful change.

I sometimes think of these patients as closet revolutionaries. Marsha once dreamed *she was taking over the Dean's office, impacting the hall with filth.* Alan, for his part, was fascinated by Raskolnikov, Dostoevsky's nihilist hero in *Crime and Punishment* (1865). Like Raskolnikov, Alan believed he was special and aspired to *pleroma* by killing and robbing an old lady (*slashing my sugarbag*). Rosenfeld (1987), and Steiner (1993) after him, suggest that the citadel of narcissistic self-sufficiency is in fact guarded by an internal, powerful object gang. Meltzer (1992) argues that there is no projective identification into the head/breast of the object without an anal claustrum as well, a compartment for the split-off violence underlying narcissistic self-idealization. Alan's more ominous double in *Crime and Punishment* is not Raskolnikov, but the bored pervert Svidrigailov, who taunts Raskolnikov with a disturbing anal vision of the *pleroma*: 'Eternity is always presented [as] something enormous, enormous! But why should it necessarily be enormous? Imagine, instead, that it will be one little room . . . a bath-house . . . black with soot, with spiders in every corner' (Dostoevsky 1865: 277). The potentially unending, claustrophobic regression of Alan's nightmare in the masturbatory chamber echoes Svidrigailov's pornographic dream-within-a-dream-within-a-dream from which it is difficult to determine if he ever wakes up.

APPLICATIONS: OUT OF *PLEROMA* INTO *CHRONOS* TOWARDS *KAIROS*

Narcissistic defenses are profoundly resistant to change and all too often, as Steiner (1993) observes, intervention provokes deeper psychic retreat. By conceptualizing the narcissistic retreat or claustrum as a pleromatic duration, however, i.e., as a temporal vicissitude, it becomes possible to fashion interventions in the less-threatening register of reality-testing. Narcissistic patients are in and out of temporal awareness, maintaining a capacity simultaneously to accept and to disavow reality. By tactfully addressing their attempts to scotomize time, by describing or simply naming these evasions, we offer a standpoint outside of the omnipotent state of mind. From this standpoint we may point to the suturing of their gap without making it bleed. It is a matter of bringing *chronos* into the *pleroma*, in order to make the *pleroma* itself an object of consciousness and the experience of time something to think about. As always, one works with the counter-transference and the imagery at hand. For instance, I once caught myself giving a Japanese patient a little more time, a little too often. At first, I rationalized that she needed it because of the language barrier. Eventually, I realized that I was deeply identifying with her assumption that she had 'all the time in the world'. I discussed this with her, mentioning Peter Pan and Rip van Winkle. Into this transitional space she then brought the parallel Japanese story of Taro and the kingdom under the sea. She began to sense that part of her was hiding in my office, for years on end, in an effort to make time go away.

Of course, it is one thing to point out the clock; quite another to nudge a patient to the threshold of the depressive position from which the path to psychic change is a painful *kairos* of work and love, hate, guilt and reparation. Attention to these temporal vicissitudes, however, may also help the therapist, who otherwise runs the risk of being sucked into a timeless *pleroma*. The refusal of Alan and Marsha to mourn the termination of our relationship also deprived me of a satisfactory sense of an ending. In fact, this chapter arose out of a need to overcome the inertia I experienced after those endings that weren't. I had to write my way out of bad infinity by transforming my clinical work with these patients into a *kairos* of psychoanalytic meaning and learning. Such intellectual effort activates the true meaning of transcendence as a climbing across, rather than a soaring up. As Yeats reminds us at the end of his lyric, 'Ephemera': 'our souls / Are love, and a continual farewell' (1956: 15). There is no real escape from *chronos*. But there is deed, metaphor and narrative through which experience can be transformed into significant *kairoi* that bind the time.

REFERENCES

Dostoevsky, F. M. (1865) (ed. G. Gibian, 1964), *Crime and Punishment*, trans. J. Coulson, New York: Norton.

Freud, S. (1930) 'Civilization and Its Discontents', in *Standard Edition*, 21: 57–146, London: Hogarth Press, 1964.

Hastings, J. (ed.) (1919) *Encyclopedia of Religion and Ethics*, vol. 10, New York: Scribner's.

Jung, C. G. (1969) *Collected Works*, Bollingen Series XX, 2nd edn, vols. 9 and 11(ii), trans. R. F. C. Hull, Princeton, NJ: Princeton University Press.

Kermode, F. (1967) *The Sense of an Ending*, Oxford: Oxford University Press.

Kernberg, O. (1975) *Borderline Conditions and Pathological Narcissism*, Northvale, NJ: Jason Aronson.

Kittel, G. and Friedrich, G. (1985) *Theological Dictionary of the New Testament*, G. W. Bromiley (trans.), Grand Rapids, MI: Eerdmans.

Mautner, T. (1996) *A Dictionary of Philosophy*, Oxford: Blackwell.

Meltzer, D. (1992) *The Claustrum: An Investigation of Claustrophobic Phenomena*, Perthshire: Clunie Press.

Peters, F. E. (1967) *Greek Philosophical Terms: A Historical Lexicon*, New York: New York University Press.

Rosenfeld, H. (1987) *Impasse and Interpretation*, London: Tavistock.

Steiner, J. (1993) *Psychic Retreats: Pathological Organizations in Psychotic, Neurotic and Borderline Patients*, London: Routledge.

Yeats, W. B. (1956) *The Collected Poems of W. B. Yeats*, New York: Macmillan.

Chapter 4

Time and endurance in psychotherapy

Lea Setton and Jill Savege Scharff

INTRODUCTION

In this chapter, we explore the therapeutic effect of the passage of time and the therapist's relationship to time. We review the literature on the role of time in the development of psychic structure in childhood and in psycho-therapy, and then present the case history of Gertrude, a woman patient in psychodynamic once weekly psychotherapy with one of us (LS). Holding and containment over time, the main ingredients of Gertrude's treatment in the first two years, fostered a remarkable, unlikely degree of improvement in Gertrude. We will conclude with a vignette of a session from the second year of treatment to show how Gertrude's play with time delivered the problem directly into the transference and so provided material that will be the basis for interpretation to come – when the time is right.

THE ROLE OF TIME IN THE DEVELOPMENT OF THE PSYCHIC STRUCTURE

From the beginning of life, the passage of time provides a context and a marker for the development of the psyche. In the neonatal period, the experience of time is marked by physiological processes, which occur over time according to an innate rhythm of their own (Gifford 1960), from experiencing the time between hunger and feeding (Sachs 1925) and the length of separation from the mother (Spitz 1965). As the infant grows, feeling now this way and now that way, being held and lying alone, the passage of time marks the periods of hunger and satiation, separation and reunion in relation to the mothering person. Enduring delays imposed by the mother or enjoying gratification of needs, the infant participates in cycles of frustration and satisfaction in arriving at unity with the good object (Erikson 1956). When infants' active protests bring relief, they learn that the good object will come soon. This gradually establishes the sense of time (Hartocollis 1974) through waiting, anticipating pain and separation, and expecting satisfaction and connection. Primitive affective states connected to bad object experience differentiate over time into specific affects such as anxiety, depression, and boredom, in extreme cases leading to borderline personality disorder (Hartocollis 1972, 1975).

A sense of reality and a sense of time appear simultaneously in the system of perceptual consciousness once the infant is capable of conscious perceptions (Bonaparte 1940). In the unconscious, Freud thought, there is no awareness of time: mental processes revealed in dreams are not organized along timelines, and they are not altered by the passage of time (Freud 1915). Perhaps it is more accurate to say that the sense of time in unconscious processes is governed by primary process and so follows different rules than chronological time. An unconscious fantasy of timelessness is based in a wish that mother and child remain united (Bergler and Roheim 1946). When mother and child are not endlessly united, the infant's need is frustrated, and the ego is filled with its energy. The self may then feel threatened and helpless, as if flooded rather than filled with experience to process.

As time passes, the infant learns that distress leads to various outcomes. The infant self connected to a bad object by feelings of frustration which flood the self and lead to feelings of helplessness may disintegrate into a bad self. To maintain a good feeling inside the self, infants learn to hold on for future gratification by hallucinating a good object based on a memory of satisfaction. Then they learn that the same object can be experienced as good and bad at different moments. This attainment of object constancy is correlated with the achievement of a sense of time (Colarusso 1979). At the age of 15–18 months infants develop capacities for being aware of time and understanding concepts of object, space, and causality, which together enable them to understand objective time (Piaget 1937).

In Freudian theory, the sense of time is described as an autonomous ego function, deriving from repeated experience over the course of the psychosexual stages of development. During the anal phase, exploratory toddlers become increasingly aware of their mothers' 'No!' and 'Now!' The innate rhythm of physiological processes is shaped by the psychological task of producing on time to please the parent. Mastery over the body and the demands of time brings autonomy and self-esteem and has an organizing effect on the formation of the self. During the oedipal phase of psychosexual development, as the child identifies with the parental preferences, the superego develops and emphasizes the awareness of time and the need to follow its dictates (Hartocollis 1974). The internal representation of parental authority governs the realistic sense of time in the healthy person (Loewald 1962). The superego influences the ability to endure stressful experiences and think through decisions, and helps the organism adapt to and conceptualize time (Hartocollis 1974). In adolescence, there must be adequate resolution of superego guilt and ego problems of autonomy if there is to be a well-established sense of time; otherwise the teenager will be unconsciously late to court parental involvement and possibly punishment (Seton 1974). If time remains a diffuse concept, the young person's ego will not be able to maintain perspective on the functioning of self and other (Erikson 1956). Distortions in the sense of time and concomitant variables in affect, caused by unconscious fantasies and defenses, reflect the integrity of the person's object relations and ego organization (Hartocollis 1975).

THE IMPORTANCE OF TIME IN THE PSYCHOANALYTIC SESSION

The psychoanalytic therapeutic framework is closely involved with time (Abraham 1976). Attention to time sets the frame within which analysis or therapy can reliably occur. The time interval between sessions calls forth the psychic structure required for imposing delay between impulse and action (Freud 1933). The beginning and end of the session (and of the treatment as a whole) form a boundary that provides a hard edge against which to measure the patient's reactions to the requirements of the other. For instance, some patients come early; some are late; others do not accept the end of the session. Their attitudes toward the time boundary are products of their object relationships and conflicts. Time represents reality and otherness.

The therapeutic alliance assures the patient of continuity. For some patients, continuity gives the illusion of immortality and a timeless state of fusion, a fantasy that is interrupted by termination of treatment, or indeed by the end of each session. Acceptance of the reality of time undoes this illusion and leads to development and maturity. For other patients, commitment to continuity of care has to be proved over time before trust develops. For instance, a patient with insecure attachment requires a therapist who provides long-term availability, flexibility, and tolerance of chaos and fragmentation (Slade 1999). Feeling accepted and understood by the therapist as the years go by, the patient symbolically recovers the lost object (Anzieu 1970). The patient's resistance to the emergence of repressed issues slowly decreases in response to trust building over time as well as resulting from accurate interpretation.

THE TIMELINE OF INTERPRETATION

Interpretation occurs along a continuum from clarification, elaboration, and reconstruction, facilitating the patient's expressiveness, communication, and further associations. Exact interpretation of conflict in the transference makes conscious the patient's behavior and feelings and helps the patient gain insight into the origins of their difficulties (Gabbard 1994). But the therapist has to take time to get to know the patient before being in a position to make an interpretation. The therapist listens continuously for multiple levels of significance stemming from various stages in the patient's development, and then facilitates the working through of the effects of the interpretation (Schlesinger 1996).

TIME TO GATHER THE TRANSFERENCE

It takes time for the patient to focus the conflict on the person of the therapist, and for the therapist to take hold of the projective identifications in the here-and-now of the transference so that experiences from an earlier time can be reworked in the present. Some patients, like the one to be presented, fend off interpretations until they are ready, and need to hear them approached from different vertices, many different times, phrased in many different ways, before they can accept them and integrate them as insights that reorganize the mind.

TIMING OF INTERPRETATIONS

Becoming aware of the passage of time and of differences in the experience with the therapist and with the interpretive process from one time to another, the patient confronts a new reality within which to rebuild the self. Interpretation at the right moment provides the patient with a model of operating with awareness of the significance of time, understanding of the links between past and present experience and their influence on future hopes and fears, and sensitivity to the other's needs over time. The patient's internalization of the therapeutic attitude to time and timing moves the self toward reorganization in recognition of the self's relationship to others and to the demands of reality. The right moment for therapists to interpret is the moment at which they know what they think and can articulate it and the patient is at the point of comprehending the interpretation: the material has to be almost conscious and relatively accessible to patient awareness – and that takes time.

CLINICAL EXAMPLE OF GERTRUDE IN WEEKLY PSYCHOTHERAPY WITH LEA SETTON

Over the course of two years of weekly treatment with Gertrude, pathological organizations and psychic retreats were evident, but Gertrude would not engage in interpretive work on them. The main component of therapeutic action was the passage of time during which she experienced my (LS) consistent presence and containment of her stormy transference.

Gertrude is a 35-year-old lesbian with borderline functioning and frequent suicidal thoughts. She is obese and walks in a lumbering way. She came into treatment because of suicidal feelings connected to a repetitive post-traumatic memory, following a car accident in which her car was hit by a driver who then ploughed his car into her mother's beach house. This memory reappeared in Gertrude's recurring dream of a car accident in which she saw blood everywhere, which left her feeling suicidal. Gertrude said that she hadn't killed herself, only because she didn't want to make her father suffer. She said, 'It isn't the right time, my father would be left alone. I am waiting for the right time and the right place.' She was paradoxically timing her suicide to protect her from her self-destructiveness.

This dream is a replay of aggressive feelings toward her mother, and a longing to protect her father. She is pulled to suicide to kill off the angry internal mother. Her feeling that it was not the right time protected the internal father, and preserved the hope of a loving internal couple, and so there would never be a right time to kill herself. But it was not possible to say such things to Gertrude. I simply had to accept her desire to die, and the lack of a right time.

Gertrude comes from a highly dysfunctional family with a mother who criticizes her looks and her performance. Her mother is always angry and her father is bitter, silent, and preoccupied with work problems. Gertrude feels unloved. For instance, when I recommended a psychiatric consultation, her mother and her brother both refused to take Gertrude to the appointment even though they knew she was suicidal. They did not offer to pay for the therapy, they did not ask how it was going, and they did not ask her how she felt. This made her feel that they did not care about her. She had been in a relationship with a woman who has two children, and this was her only sexual relationship with a woman. It made her feel guilty to be replacing her mother's love with this woman's love. She said that she couldn't talk about it because she didn't understand how it happened. Gertrude did not accept that it was a homosexual relationship, and she pretended that the sexual aspect of their friendship was not continuing. On the other hand she drew attention to her genital experience by complaining how much she hurt after she awoke to find that she had scratched the top of her thigh so hard that she broke the skin. Because her self-inflicted wound was so close to the genital area, I had the impression that she wanted to remove her genitals from her body to get rid of what she was feeling there.

Process of the first year of therapy

Gertrude usually conversed about the happenings of the week in terms of her life at home with her mother, father, and brother, visits to her aunt, and occasionally her schoolwork, her lesbian friend/former partner, and any heterosexual dates she had. She worked on her difficulty becoming independent and succeeding at school, but she did open up on the issue of her homosexuality and its meaning for her.

Gertrude complained about her family being like a madhouse, always in chaos, with a mother who shouts, a father who stays silent, and a brother who stays out until midnight and returns like a ghost. She complained of the house not being clean, there being no food in the refrigerator, not even cold water. On the other hand she liked her room and felt comfortable there, but she did not sleep well, and she always felt hungry. The lack of provisions in the home reflected Gertrude's feeling rejected by her mother. Gertrude felt that her mother attacked her looks, devalued her work, and thought that everything she did was wrong. Gertrude felt sad, and yet she could not cry. She talked about being close to a supportive, motherly aunt on her father's side. She wished that her aunt could have been her mother, but she often refused invitations to her house or went there reluctantly, I think, because she was afraid of loving her, and then being rejected as happens with her mother. She used to hate her mother, but after a year of therapy she felt more separate from her and more able to love her.

Gertrude was generally rude and aggressive toward me, as her mother was to her. She was suicidal but she refused medication. She brought all her miserable behavior to me. I felt so put off by her that it was difficult to stay in touch with her suffering. She complained that she didn't feel well, that I didn't care, and that I didn't understand anything. In every session, she wanted to leave. She used to say, 'Can I go now?' and I would say, 'It's your decision, but if you want to stay, we have another 15 minutes to work.' And she always stayed. She was always fed up with treatment and sick of me. She tried to get rid of me by leaving the session, and yet so as not to miss me she sent me hundreds of e-mails. I did not want to encourage the e-mails, but I did read them. The only way I could tolerate her was to connect with her suffering as expressed in the e-mails because my countertransference to her in person was so burdensome. It was not that she said anything different in the e-mails; it was just easier because I could skim the electronic format and I did not have to be with her and look at her.

Like her mother, Gertrude gets angry easily and attacks herself as her mother did her. When Gertrude lost many documents and missed many classes in her first semester, I pointed out that this was an attack on herself and a way of undermining her ability to succeed. She dismissed my comments angrily, but in the second semester, she improved her attendance to meet the minimum so that she could receive her grades, and by the end of the first year she graduated with a Master's degree.

Process of the second year of therapy

Gertrude got a good job, but she continued to think of dying in a car accident and could not enjoy her accomplishment. I felt anxious, because her need to die so as to escape her desperate feelings seemed highly possible. Conversing and eating in company were difficult for her, because she ate slowly and got angry about the food. Gertrude was angry for months when one of her bosses kept teasing her about her weight, and she was tempted to quit the job. I addressed her dislike of herself, her inability to tolerate frustration, her embarrassment being with other people, and her fear of being out of control in public. Gertrude was still at risk for destroying the excellent opportunities at this company instead of learning to deal with the conflicts of the workplace. Nevertheless, she was doing well at work and getting lots of good feedback.

Gertrude cancelled her sessions if she did not like my comments about her self-destructive behaviors such as obesity, smoking, and missing staff meetings after she had been successful at work. She would not take the recommended medication, she would not move out to live independently, and she hid information from me. When I asked about her intimate life, she told me nothing, and said angrily, 'Why does the cat have to have a fifth leg?' This common Spanish idiom suggested a phallic intrusiveness that she experienced if I attempted to penetrate her defenses. She blocked my transference interpretations, sabotaged the therapy, and then complained that she did not feel any better. Her anger with her boss and her hatred of her mother were transferred to me in sessions where she continuously attacked our work. It wasn't easy to tolerate this, but I hung on believing that she needed continuing proof of my commitment to her, however awful she was to me, for however long it took, before this would yield to interpretation.

In the last four months of the second year, without apparent benefit of interpretive work, Gertrude became less aggressive and her positive qualities came forth. I took these improvements as a response to the benign quality of the time we spent together. Within the space of our time together, I had made a few interpretations, like the one about losing things as a way of undermining her success, but they were never well received and she did not work with them directly. I think it was my non-toxic presence, my relational stance, operating as an 'interpretation-in-action' that made the difference in her sense of self and in her behavior (Ogden 1994: 108). She became able to care for the welfare of the workers under her authority and considered living independently. Only now are we in a position to begin dealing with Gertrude's direct object transference to me. In the vignette that follows, we can see Gertrude's behavior within the constraints of time imposed by the session.

Vignette from the end of the second year: emergence of the focused transference

Before the session began, Gertrude, as usual, was hiding by the elevator rather than coming in to the waiting area, which she does ostensibly to avoid seeing someone she might know. This means that I always have to go out there to invite her into my office. She wants to know that I want her there, because of her fear of rejection. I noticed, as I often did, how obese she is, and it crossed my mind that she walks like a gorilla. I thought of how voracious and bullying she is. She wants to think that she is my only patient. I sensed her feelings of sexual attraction to me, but I didn't comment on them because she has found such comments ridiculous. She does not open up on her homosexual feelings in general, much less about me.

Once in the office, she dove into the cushions of the couch as if she wanted to be inside my womb, and at the same time not let me see her, as if to avoid any recognition of attraction. I felt that she wanted a lot from me. Continuing to look down into the couch, she began to complain about an employee whose exploitative need for too many hours of overtime cost him his job and her friendship. She associated to her parents excluding her from their bedroom. She then described with disgust their dirty house and meager provisions and she complained about their wishing she would leave. She didn't know what else to say. I said that she might be worried that if she told me what was on her mind, I, like her parents, would ask her to leave. The time was up. I didn't add that she might fear that I would want her to leave because I, like her mother, might not accept her homosexual feelings.

I ended the session on time. Gertrude got up slowly, looked at the disarray on the couch, and said provocatively, 'You will have to put this in order!' I asked her to help. Smiling, she walked past me to the door, the pillows still awry. She turned around and told me that she had seen her friend and that their homosexual relationship was still going on. The session being over, there was no possibility of working on this. I thought that Gertrude was telling me of her intimate involvement with her friend between sessions as a substitute for working intimately with me in the session. As she told me this and I bent over the couch to straighten the pillows, I felt as if we were together on the couch.

Gertrude played with the time boundary of the session. She brought her transference into therapy before the session began, during it, and at the end of it. She experienced reality as an intrusion (see also Chapter 2 by Stadter and Chapter 3 by Johnson in this volume). She did not want to recognize the need to separate and differentiate. She had trouble admitting her desire for engagement within the time boundary because of the intensity of her hunger and its sexualization and the accompanying fear of its rejection. Her manipulation of time reflects both a major resistance to the realities of the treatment process and an enactment that delivers her problems into the therapeutic relationship. In my countertransference image of us together on the couch, I respond to her longings to have all my time and to possess me sexually. This is the transference/countertransference dimension to which the passage of time has now brought Gertrude.

In the first two years of therapy, Gertrude, responding to the therapist's sense of time, became aware of the need to complete her studies in a timely way. She learned to accept the rhythm of the weekly sessions, no longer filling the interval with e-mails. She had learned to anticipate that her need for connection with the good object would be met in her next session. The therapist's concern was reflected in Gertrude's new-found concern for her employees. Gertrude got her life back on track, moved into a position of readiness to live independently, and made considerable gains at work, but she still needed more time to internalize a new way of being and of relating intimately. The therapist's provision of a steady presence and an extended opening phase set the context for further work on the intrapsychic dimension, and was helpful in effecting external change. Only then could she begin to open her focused transference issues to sustained interpretation.

Patient and therapist are now ready for the 'fifth leg' of the therapeutic journey as the patient begins to demonstrate her sexuality and claim her right to the relationship she wants. It would not have been possible to get to this point without the preceding time of continuity and containment. Analytic therapy simply takes a long time, and there is no shortcut. The combination of the quality of the time spent and the extended quantity of time produced a unique quality of relationship. Holding, continuity and containment in the treatment over time allowed the patient to create balance between the irreversible, indestructible past and the problems of the present, and gave her mental space to invest in the therapeutic process and think about a new facet of time: the future.

REFERENCES

Abraham, G. (1976) 'The Sense and Concept of Time in Psychoanalysis', *International Review of Psycho-Analysis*, 3: 461–472.

Anzieu D. (1970) 'Elements d'une Theórie de l'Interpretation', *Revue Française Psychoanalyse*, 34: 755–819.

Bergler, E. and Roheim, G. (1946) 'Psychology of Time Perception', *Psychoanalytic Quarterly*, 15: 190–206.

Bonaparte, M. (1940) 'Time and the Unconscious', *International Journal of Psycho-Analysis*, 21: 427–468.

Colarusso, C. (1979) 'The Development of Time Sense – from Birth to Object Constancy', *International Journal of Psycho-Analysis*, 60: 243–251.

Erikson, E. H. (1956) 'The Problem of Ego Identity', *Journal of the American Psychoanalytic Association*, 4: 56–121.

Freud, S. (1915) 'The Unconscious', *Standard Edition*, 14: 159–215, London: Hogarth Press, 1964.

Freud, S. (1933) 'New Introductory Lectures on Psycho-analysis', *Standard Edition*, 22: 5–182, London: Hogarth Press, 1964.

Gabbard, G. (1994) *Psychodynamic Psychiatry in Clinical Practice*, Washington, DC: American Psychiatric Press.

Gifford, S. (1960) 'Sleep, Time and the Early Ego. Comments on the Development of the 24-hour Sleep–Wakefulness Pattern as a Precursor of Ego Functioning', *Journal of the American Psychoanalytic Association*, 8: 5–42.

Hartocollis, P. (1972) 'Time as a Dimension of Affects', *Journal of the American Psychoanalytic Association*, 20: 92–108.

Hartocollis, P. (1974) 'Origins of Time: A Reconstruction of the Ontogenetic Development of the Sense of Time Based on Object Relations Theory', *Psychoanalytic Quarterly,* 43: 243–261.

Hartocollis, P. (1975) 'Time and Affect in Psychopathology', *Journal of the American Psychoanalytic Association*, 23: 383–395.

Hartocollis, P. (1988) 'The Psychoanalysis of Time', *Journal of the American Psychoanalytic Association*, 36: 985–1004.

Loewald, H. (1962) 'The Superego and the Ego Ideal: the Superego and Time', *International Journal of Psycho-Analysis*, 43: 264–268.

Ogden, T. (1994) *Subjects of Analysis*, Northvale NJ: Jason Aronson.

Piaget, J. (1937) *The Construction of Reality in the Child*, New York: Basic Books, 1954.

Rose, J. (1997) 'Distortions of Time in the Transference', *International Journal of Psycho-Analysis*, 78: 453–468.

Sachs, H. (1925) Quoted by S. Harnik in 'Die Triebhaftaffektiven Momente in Zeitgefühl', *Imago*, 2: 32–58.

Schlesinger, H. J. (1996) 'The Process of Interpretation and the Moment of Change', *Journal of the American Psychoanalytic Association*, 43: 663–688.

Seton, P. (1974) 'The Psycho-Temporal Adaptation of Late Adolescence', *Journal of the American Psychoanalytic Association*, 22: 795–819.

Slade, A. (1999) 'Attachment Theory and Research: Implications for the Theory and Practice of Individual Psychotherapy with Adults', in J. Cassidy and P. Shaver (eds.), *Handbook of Attachment*, New York: Guilford, pp. 575–594.

Spitz, R. (1965) *The First Year of Life*, New York: International Universities Press.

Part II

Space

Spatial metaphor and spatial reality: an overview

Michael Stadter and David E. Scharff

Marie Bonaparte described space as 'the atmosphere we breathe' (1940: 430). Like oxygen, space is essential for life and usually outside our conscious perception, yet, it is difficult to imagine how we could make sense of experience without spatial coordinates. While philosophers may debate the relationist versus absolutist argument of whether space exists independent of objects (does a spatial vacuum really exist?), there is agreement that space has at least three functions (Le Poidevin 2003):

1   Space as a point of reference: 'He was across the room.'
2   Space as a possibility: 'Put the book over there (in an unoccupied space).'
3   Space as a geometrical reality: 'My chair is 12 inches from the wall and 10 feet from the window.'

Similarly, psychotherapists study external and internal space as psychological experience:

1   Space as a point of reference: 'I feel so close to her even though she's 3,000 miles away.' 'Your anger pushed me away.'
2   Space as a possibility (or a lack of possibility): 'I can imagine you coming over to my side.' 'I can't be interested in anyone now – there's no room in my heart since she left.' 'Give me room to think!'
3   Space as a geometrical/psychological reality: 'I feel safe in your office.' 'I'm connected to her but you seem so distant to me.' 'I'm falling apart.'

Clinically, claustrophobia and agoraphobia are, at one level, directly about space – too little or too much. Psychoanalytic therapists are more concerned with the subjective, symbolic, relational and existential realities of space. The following are some psychoanalytic spatial perspectives: the projection of self into the world creating space (Freud 1941), potential space and transitional phenomena (Winnicott 1953), the container and the contained (Bion 1962), and the claustrum (Meltzer 1992). Space is also a key element in Ogden's (1989) three modes of experience. In the sensory dominated, autistic-contiguous mode (the most primitive), anxiety is about being unbounded and it can take the form of primitive terror of falling endlessly through space. In the paranoid–schizoid mode, there is no space between the symbol and the symbolized and anxiety is about falling apart, the self having spaces between its parts. In the depressive mode, there is space between the symbol and the symbolized and there is space to think and make linkages.

Perhaps no writer has discussed the internal/external spatial interplay more evocatively than Winnicott (1953). He saw the initial relationship between baby and mother as being a totally physical one, a psychosomatic partnership (Winnicott 1971), that began in utero where there is little physical space between mother and fetus, and the fetus occupies part of maternal space. After birth the increased physical distance between mother and baby creates potential space for the development of psychological experience and eventually for the development of transitional space and objects. Transitional space is a third area of experience, neither fully inside nor outside but between. It is in this space that the arts, culture and creativity itself develop. It begins as:

> . . . a developmental way station between hallucinatory omnipotence and the recognition of objective reality . . . Transitional experience is rooted in the capacity of the child *to play*; in adult form it is expressed as a capacity *to play* with one's fantasies, ideas, and the world's possibilities in a way that continually allows for *the surprising, the original, and the new* [italics added].
>
> (Greenberg and Mitchell 1983: 195)

We have six chapters in Part II on space. The first two examine the interplay between the external office space and the internal space of the patient and therapist. Geoffrey Anderson begins his chapter with a survey of the analytic writing on space, emphasizing the object relations theorists. He then presents how two patients made use of his office and the items in them. He details how this 'office usage' affected their development, their relationships with him and the treatment in general. Anderson shows how a patient with an unintegrated (never integrated) sense of self used him and his office differently and more primitively than a patient who was experiencing a disintegration of self. Judith Rovner explores the multiple levels of a simple situation: the therapist moving her office. She presents material from the psychotherapy of three patients to illustrate a range of developmental responses to this change in setting. Through discussion of her own countertransference reactions, Rovner also shows how some of the changes in the external space, the setting, involve changes in the therapist's own internal space.

Earl Hopper considers the dimension of space both theoretically and clinically, illustrated with a detailed case of a challenging patient seen in intensive individual and group psychotherapy. Expanding on Bion's (1961) work on group basic assumptions, he adds 'Incohesion: Massification/ Aggregation' as a basic assumption. He also illustrates how therapy group can give both patients and therapists the space to be able to think and therapists the space to reflect upon their countertransferences.

The next two chapters examine how the physical space of psychotherapy and teaching psychotherapy can be dramatically expanded through technology. Sharon Zalusky brings an intensely practical element for our study as she considers the impact on therapy when the patient and therapist are not even in the same room together and may be hundreds or even thousands of miles apart: when therapy is conducted by telephone. Her case vignettes demonstrate the usefulness, the technical issues, and the themes that are relevant to this increasingly accepted and important practice. I (DES) illustrate the unique aspects of teaching infant observation and psychotherapy by video-conferencing where the various students and teachers are working together from various geographically distant locations. Without this technology, it would ordinarily require a great deal of time, expense and travel to provide such training.

Finally, Susan Barbour expands on some of the themes about potential space by looking at them in an organizational setting. Beginning with Bion's (1961) group work and especially emphasizing the group-as-a-whole paradigm (Wells 1985), she presents the narrative of a professional workgroup whose previously successful functioning became seriously impaired when it experienced several staff changes and a change in leadership. Barbour shows how the workgroup's internal potential space collapsed and she gives suggestions for how leaders can create and maintain productive internal space for themselves and for their workgroups.

A NOTE ON SPACE AND TIME

For the purposes of study, we are isolating and focusing individually on the four dimensions in this book. However, as noted in the introduction, we know that there is a complex interplay and synergy among the various elements of psychotherapy and human experience. Perhaps, this is especially true about time and space. Indeed, there are ways in which these dimensions interact to create a single entity. For example, physics has the concept of a four-dimensional construct, space-time (Greene 2004; Galison 2003).

Consider how we experience the merger of space and time psychologically. Freud (1933) noted that in dreams, time was represented by space. Things that were far apart in the dreamspace could be understood to be separated in time, or an object that was very small and far away was being represented as being distant in time. In my chapter (Stadter, Chapter 2) on time, trauma and psychotherapy I found myself unconsciously using a spatial metaphor for different experiences of time: time-near and time-far. In Stern's (2004) exploration of the present moment, he frequently uses spatial metaphors. Grudin (1982) writes:

> . . . the use of metaphor – temporal metaphor for space and spatial metaphor for time – gives us a special sort of access to the space-time continuum. This is not because metaphor has anything particular to do with the physics of space-time, but rather because metaphor evokes both conscious and subconscious responses and produces . . . an awareness of the implicit connectedness of things.
>
> (Grudin 1982: 2)

Sabbadini (1989: 306) notes that a basic component of therapy practice, the waiting room, embodies time and space in the two words of its name: 'For instance, when we speak of the waiting room, we are referring to the space of the room but also to the time of waiting.' Grudin (1982: 5) writes that 'Rooms can be vessels of psychological temporality, silently encouraging specific attitudes toward time.'

REFERENCES

Bion, W. R. (1961) *Experiences in Groups and Other Papers*, London: Tavistock.
Bion, W. R. (1962) *Learning from Experience*, London: Heinemann.
Bonaparte, M. (1940) 'Time and the Unconscious', *International Journal of Psycho-Analysis*, 21: 427–468.
Freud, S. (1933) 'Revision of the Theory of Dreams. Lecture XXIX', *Standard Edition*, 22: 7–30, London, Hogarth Press, 1964.
Freud, S. (1941) 'Findings, Ideas, Problems', in *Standard Edition*, 23: 299–300, London, Hogarth Press, 1964.
Galison, P. (2003) *Einstein's Clocks, Poincaré's Maps*, New York: Norton.
Greenberg, J. R. and Mitchell, S. A. (1983) *Object Relations in Psychoanalytic Theory*, Cambridge, MA: Harvard University Press.
Greene, B. (2004) *The Fabric of the Cosmos: Space, Time, and the Texture of Reality*, New York: Knopf.
Grudin, R. (1982) *Time and the Art of Living*, New York: Houghton Mifflin.
Le Poidevin, R. (2003) *Travels in Four Dimensions: The Enigmas of Space and Time*, Oxford: Oxford University Press.
Meltzer, D. (1992) *The Claustrum: An Investigation of Claustrophobic Phenomena*, Worcester: Clunie Press.
Ogden, T. (1989) *The Primitive Edge of Experience*, Northvale, NJ: Jason Aronson.
Sabbidini, A. (1989) 'Boundaries of Timelessness. Some Thoughts about the

Temporal Dimension of Psychoanalytic Space', *International Journal of Psycho-Analysis*, 70: 305–313.

Stern, D. N. (2004) *The Present Moment in Psychotherapy and Everyday Life*, New York: Norton.

Wells, L. (1985) 'The Group-as-a-Whole Perspective and its Theoretical Roots', in A. D. Colman and M. H. Geller (eds.), *Group Relations: Reader 2*, Washington, DC: A. K. Rice Institute, pp. 109–126.

Winnicott, D. W. (1953) 'Transitional Objects and Transitional Phenomena', in *Through Paediatrics to Psycho-Analysis* (1958), New York: Basic Books, pp. 229–242.

Winnicott, D. W. (1971) *Playing and Reality*, London: Routledge.

Chapter 5

Right now I'm sitting in the bookshelf: patients' use of the physical space in psychotherapy

Geoffrey Anderson

Considering space from a psychoanalytic perspective, we are called to wonder about the nature of our experience of the physical world. What does the clinical evidence suggest to us about the nature of space as a human experience? In this chapter I explore how psychoanalysis and particularly object relations theory has viewed this question. I examine the notion of space as a relational construct governed by the earliest object acquisition. Then, clinical material is presented to demonstrate how the internal object world affects the perception and use of space in the transference. Finally, I explore what these uses of space in the transference mean for us as clinicians.

PSYCHOANALYTIC THEORIES REGARDING SPACE

Beginning with Freud, psychoanalysis has taken the approach that space is a developed characteristic of the human mind. Freud postulated that as the mind reached out to grasp the world around it, the mind projected its own sense of self into the unknown, creating the sense of space (Freud 1941). With this notion Freud brought to psychoanalysis the concept of space as the mind's relationship with the unknown. While physical space is not a frequent topic of psychoanalytic writers, there are many works which explore the phenomena associated with our subjective experience of space.

In an early paper by Schilder, it was postulated that humans perceived space dualistically (Schilder 1935). Specifically he stated that we not only experience an external space but also a space filled by the body. Schilder described the individual's subjective bodily experience as consisting of two types of space as well. The first of these he labeled perceptual space, which he linked to the ego. This is the conscious space of ordinary reality that we share with others. The second type of space he labeled the id space. Here reality breaks down under the influences of identifications, projections, and primal urges. Schilder's work goes on to explore how this id space was affected by different forms of psychological disturbance. The change within the id space brought on associated distortions of the use of the perceptual space by patients (Schilder 1935). Schilder saw these distortions in the use of space as attempts to control the distance between the ego and the object of desire. As I will show below, these types of distortions can be useful to the clinician in determining the course of the treatment.

In another paper on space, Berne (1956) looks at the regressive and creative uses of space depending on the psychic structure and development of the individual analysand. Berne described three psychological uses of space. These are: the exploration of space, the measurement of space and the utilization of space. Berne's incorporation of regression in the service of the ego into his concept of space indicates that internal representations of space are not static. In psychological health internal space has the flexibility to 'come apart' and return to an organized state in a different configuration. When internal space does become static, either through the impact of trauma or as a defense against anxiety, the individual may develop idiosyncratic perceptions of and reactions to both internal and external space.

These papers provide us with the beginnings of understanding space as an internal psychological construct. So far we see two types of internal space. One structured by the ego and the demands of reality and one structured by the id and the demands of internal needs and urges. Schilder in particular locates these needs and urges in relation to desired objects. So we have an internal space that is organized around our relationships to our objects. Space then is not only developed as a projection of the psychical apparatus as Freud suggested but is further developed by the introjection of objects into an internal relational space. With the development of the relational theories of the object relations theorists, space becomes an explicitly relational construct affected by the processes of projection and introjection.

Melanie Klein's work took psychoanalysis in an entirely new direction when she became one of the first clinicians to analyze children. Her theories led to understanding the earliest forms of psychological defenses (Klein 1946). One of the most basic of the psychological defenses illuminated by Klein was splitting. When splitting occurs the internal space is divided. The reason to divide the internal space is to protect a loved object from hateful feelings. In this way a good object (the caregiver or part of the caregiver's body) can be maintained even when it performs not-good acts. Once this division takes place, intolerable internal experiences such as rage against a loved caregiver can be projected into the external world. Another form of early defense is dissociation. In dissociation the intolerable internal state is left in the body and the subject or self leaves the body behind until the internal or external threat is over. While Klein did not specifically address this defense, it has become a much-discussed topic in recent years, especially in instances of trauma (Scharff and Scharff 1994). The difference in dissociation is that there is much less of an ego experience within the internal space than there is with splitting and the space usually held by the ego is also invaded by the bad object experience. The split-off ego is then experienced as being expelled from the body into a 'safe' place until the painful experience ends. These two examples of primitive defenses play an important role in the development of the experience of an internal space. Later object relations writers such as Winnicott and Bion added to our understanding of the relationship between space and object with new theories based in part on Klein's work.

Winnicott developed the concepts of the holding environment (Winnicott 1960) and the transitional space (Winnicott 1953). The holding environment includes the infant's experience of both the physical and emotional bond with the mother as a space in which the infant exists. In the holding environment, Winnicott has presented a notion of a relational space created by the caregivers that can then be taken in (introjected) by the infant. Transitional space on the other hand is an imaginary zone the infant creates between complete dependence on the mother and the independence of thought and experience of a separate self. Winnicott was clear in his belief that this was not inner reality, nor was it external life. It was a third space of between, one in which the boundary between subject and object is experienced. We can see here a relational concept that is very similar to Berne's notion of the use of space in which to build or create. If the holding environment is working well enough this space is one in which the child can begin to have its own thoughts and creations.

Bion (1962) added the concept of the container and the contained to the psychoanalytic theory of space. His idea is basically this: the infant will at times have overwhelming physical and emotional experiences. When such an event occurs the infant needs to have a container in the form of another human being who can take in the experience and make it tolerable by soothing the infant and giving back the affect as normal and survivable. We see in this theory a notion of the expelling (projecting) of unwanted affect out into an unknown nothing. The container (caregiver) who takes in the affect becomes an external object capable of incorporating the unwanted affect. The incorporated affect is then introjected or taken back into the psychic structure of the infant and creates an internal space capable of withstanding the affect from within. This 'new' internal space exists within an internal relationship between ego and object. It replaces the feeling of dread that is experienced when space can only be the experience of the unknown. The new experience is one of knowing and security in relationship with the internalized experience of care.

Expanding on Klein, Winnicott, and Bion, Bick (1968) postulated a theory regarding the formation of the internal psychological space in the developing infant. She concluded that in its most primitive form the personality has no sense of a binding force that holds it together and only a passive sense of a 'skin' boundary. The capacity to feel an active force holding the self together was dependent on taking in (introjection) an external object. The infant self's incorporation of (identification with) the binding function of the object (most likely the experience of being held together by the mother) gives rise to the experience of internal and external space.

Bick considered this introjection of a containing object to be of great diagnostic importance in terms of the level of functioning in patients and a predictor of their capacity to participate in treatment. Those persons who had not incorporated the containing object were subject to catastrophic anxieties and experiences of unintegration (no existence of a cohesive whole) of the self. In contrast, those persons who had incorporated the containing object were subject to active defensive operations such as projection and experiences of disintegration (the loss of a previously existing cohesive whole) of the self. Among patients who did not experience the containing object, Bick noticed a frantic search for a sensual object that could hold the attention and stave off the feelings of nonexistence. These patients often required some sort of tactile self-stimulation in order to soothe the tremendous anxieties associated with nonexistence.

The psychoanalytic theories reviewed above provide a picture of how human beings develop an internal space. It is a complex process of interaction with the external space of the perceived world and the internal space of conscious and unconscious experience. The successful development of a capacity to integrate and make use of space is dependent upon the negotiation of the early child/caregiver relationship. Disruptions in the early development of this internal/external space lead to impairment of the person's capacity for relationship as an adult. Depending on the timing, nature and severity of these disruptions serious impairment in cognitive and emotional processes may also result. Patients presenting for psychotherapy who display such disruptions are often unable to make direct use of the relationship in the therapy process. As a result they may shift their reactions to the experience of the physical space of the office of the therapist as the focus of the transference. In the next section I explore clinical material that illustrates these transference phenomena.

THE PATIENT'S USE OF THE PHYSICAL SPACE OF THE OFFICE

Patients who use a part of the office as a projective container often pick a feature or item in the office to represent some internal psychological conflict. They may be afraid to project the conflict into the person of the therapist, as then they would have to be in too close a relation to the therapist or perhaps feel guilty about the way they are using the therapist. It seems safer to project the conflict into a part of the physical space. The following example illustrates this use of the office space.

Use of the space as projective container

Mr D was a 47-year-old man with a long history of psychological treatment. He had seen a number of therapists prior to beginning treatment with me. As a child Mr D would come home from school to find his mother depressed and lying on the couch. All the drapes would be drawn and the lights off. He was terrified of the day he might come home and discover her dead body. He had repeated this arrangement in his current marriage where his wife had made numerous suicide attempts and was emotionally unavailable to him. Mr D's father was a silent angry man who would go out to the backyard when he was upset and chop wood for the fireplace. Mr D felt him to be entirely unavailable, 'almost like he lived on a different planet.' Mr D had recurrent periods of depression and severe anxiety, which at times bordered on agoraphobia. He could vividly describe the physical experience of depression and anxiety. The image of his persistent anxiety was 'There is a table that has a hump in the center. It is covered with marbles and I have to constantly run around the table pushing the marbles back into the center so they won't fall off.'

Mr D hated the process of psychotherapy. He truly felt miserable when relating his past experiences and felt that this was getting him nowhere. He was suspicious and mistrustful of me. He would say, 'Here I am all shitty and messy and there you are all clean and smug.' He would then retreat into silence. He could not make use of any interpretations about him feeling me as being unavailable like his father. The idea of being directly angry with me and seeing if I would survive this and remain available was outside his comprehension. He often complained about the décor of my office as being so gloomy and depressing.

One day I invited Mr D to tell me what was depressing about the office. Mr D looked around at the pictures in my office. One by one he described the persons depicted in the pictures. 'That one looks far away and not all there, like he would look right through you and not even see you. That one looks really mean and scary, almost evil. That one looks like my mother. I can't tell if she is angry or sad but just looking at it makes me feel really scared.' I suggested to him that his experience of feeling trapped with a depressed mother had been very sad and frightening for him. He started to weep briefly. Following this experience Mr D. began to slowly see more and more connections between his experiences with his depressed mother and how he related to people in his everyday life. He began to slowly understand how he viewed a relationship as being primarily the need to take care of an unavailable other whom he hated for giving him so little. Mr D's use of the paintings as a container into which he could project his fear and anger allowed him more room in his internal space to explore his feelings about his mother. Prior to this event he had been too afraid to use me in this manner. As a result of the experience of communicating how he used the office space he began to make use of me as a direct projective container. He started to directly express feelings about our relationship that contained the transference elements of his fear of abandonment and his fear that anger was irresolvable in relationships. With this shift in his use of me, Mr D experienced fewer episodes of disintegration during the therapy hour.

Use of the space as dissociative container

In contrast to the example above, patients who have experienced significant trauma in their early life frequently use dissociation as a defense. As noted previously, this is a defense in which they split off the traumatic experience as the self occupies an external space outside of the body. These patients often get a look in their eyes like nobody's home and the therapist may experience a boredom or deadening of sensation. When patients can later verbalize what occurred during these experiences they describe placing all or part of themselves into a space or external object in an attempt to escape from the terror and pain of the trauma. These patients frequently lack the ability to discriminate between 'there and then' and 'here and now'. As a result they may react to remembering trauma as if it is occurring in the present. They may quickly lapse into a dissociative state when trying to express what happened to them (see also Stadter, Chapter 2 in this volume).

Ms C was a 35-year-old woman who was violently abused by her biological father during a single episode as an infant. He threw her across the room because she wouldn't stop crying. He died shortly after that in an accident at work. Several years later her mother remarried and her experiences with her stepfather caused me to think of a concentration camp. He would watch her secretly at all hours when he was home. She was afraid of insects and rodents and he would torture her with them. Her stepfather would devise extreme punishments such as making her sit in one spot on her folded legs for hours without moving. If she moved or complained he would beat her. She had to sleep naked and he would enter her room at night and look at her body while she feigned sleep. He bathed her and penetrated her anally and vaginally with a soapy finger to 'wash them'. He beat her regularly for real and imagined infractions of his rules. He further humiliated her by not subjecting her brother to the same rules. She was singled out for punishment and abuse simply because she was a girl.

While describing the incidents of abuse Ms C would trail off and get a dreamy far away look in her eyes. She would take one of the pillows on the couch and crush it to her chest. She would then trace the embroidery on the pillow over and over with her finger. Some of the early sessions were excruciating for both of us, as they would lapse into long periods of silence filled with feelings of dread and horror. Later as Ms C began to verbalize her experience during these periods she would tell me 'Right now I am sitting in the bookshelf. Right in that little space down in the bottom shelf where it is dark and no one can see me.' 'Maybe if he can't see me he won't be able to hurt me anymore.' 'Maybe it will all go away and have never happened if I just sit out there long enough.'

As time went on in our work together, Ms C began to speak of her fear of our relationship. She longed for a connection with me but she was filled with dread that she would damage me if she became close to me. She had perverse fantasies of our being taken hostage by terrorists and her being forced to perform sexual acts on me at gunpoint. She was caught between her fears that I would hurt her and her fears that she would hurt me. Equally powerful were her fears of stimulating me or being stimulated by me. Her belief was that all human contact was an exchange of pain. Unfortunately she was also stimulated by pain and felt horror and shame about this. Her use of the physical space of the office as a container allowed her to keep coming back three times a week. Without the space in the bookshelf where she could keep her most vulnerable aspects of herself, she didn't feel safe with me. She could not have progressed in her work without having that spot in the bookshelf.

THE CLINICAL IMPORTANCE OF THE USE OF SPACE

These examples of the patient's use of the physical space provide a look at two different ways of organizing transference reactions. The example of Mr D illustrates the use of splitting and projection in an attempt to manage feelings of disintegration under stress. Objects in the physical space were used to contain the internal experiences of fear and rage that might either damage the needed object of the therapist or trigger a retaliatory attack. Mr D was able to experience an internal space that was threatened by his negative feelings. His desire to protect the good object (his hope that I might be able to help him) from the bad object (his own hatred and envy of me being able to help him) necessitated the split inside his internal space. He was able to hold himself together outside of therapy and did quite well at work and in caretaking for his depressed wife. Ms C, in contrast, seemed unable to hold herself together inside or outside of the therapy. Her experience under stress was one of unintegration (see also Hopper, Chapter 7 in this volume). She was unable to work or function in her marriage. She could not separate good and bad experiences as all stimuli and reactions seemed to flood together into a terrifying 'soup' inside of her. Her use of the pillow is clearly in the manner of the need for a sensual object to hold the attention as described by Bick above. In addition her use of the space in the bookshelf was in the manner of finding an external skin space, which would provide a safe haven for her disembodied self. Here, the function of the projection is the protection of good objects from bad feelings inside the internal space. The function of the dissociation is to frantically search for containment for an overwhelmed self with no internal space.

How do these findings affect the manner in which we work with such patients? With patients like Ms C who present an unintegrated self the psychotherapy must progress slowly and often entails long hours of sitting with the patient's massed confusion of affective experience (see also Setton and Scharff, Chapter 4 in this volume). Two primary tasks emerge in such cases. The first is to provide a safe space for the self by sitting without judgment and providing some measure of reality testing when asked. It is often my experience that such patients will present distorted notions of how life works and how other people think and then seek reassurance that everyone thinks this way. In those moments it is often possible to gently say: no, many people do not have the same thoughts or experiences as the patient does in that situation. Depending on the patient's response this may be the end of the exchange. Sometimes they will ask how others may respond in such situations and a normalizing response could be given. An example of this from Ms C's case was when she described how a 'friend' would come to her house and verbally attack her for behaving in a manner different from how the 'friend' would behave. In this case the friend attacked Ms C for not feeding her dog correctly (when she actually was). Ms C then made a statement that the friend must be correct in her criticism and that Ms C should not feel angry because 'everyone would act this way, right?' I responded, 'No, not everyone would treat others like this.' I also said that sometimes it is appropriate to feel anger at others when they treat us badly. Ms C seemed genuinely surprised by this.

The second primary task with unintegrated patients is to help them sort out their confused affective responses. These patients have little developed internal space which they often experience as filled with chaos. They may feel angry and sad at the same time. Or they may feel happy and unhappy about the same event. They are usually quite confused about having multiple or conflicting feelings. Having the feelings named and set next to each other by the therapist slowly helps them define their emotional reactions. At other times, patients may have a clearly defined emotional reaction that seems appropriate to the situation but they say they feel nothing. Sometimes just describing for them the behavioral antecedents of the emotion helps them to recognize that they are experiencing a feeling. The role of treatment here is to help the patient slowly incorporate an internal experience of cohesion and containment. Until this occurs, interpreting actions in light of resistance or defenses is often useless, or worse, and provokes a withdrawal, dissociation, or burst of unintegrated rage.

Mr D presents a different clinical picture and different needs in the psychotherapy. Mr D's anxiety provoked strong defensive reactions to the therapy and to his own aggressive and depressed feelings. By his own admission he was struggling to hold everything together and not disintegrate. His internal space was threatened by dangers from without. Mr D, however, could tolerate interpretations which highlighted internal conflicts. When the timing was right Mr D could be invited to move into his projections and verbalize them using the objects in the office. This in turn could be interpreted regarding his disavowed feelings of depression and pain. Mr D could cry and feel contained by the revelation of his pain rather than feeling overwhelmed by it. By building on such experiences, Mr D expanded his internal space in a way that allowed him to begin to see his projective process and the way it was affecting his current interpersonal relationships. A dialogue between the therapist and the patient about their interactions could begin at that point. As this occurred, the focus of the transference was moved from the physical space of the office to the relational focus of the interaction between the therapist and the patient.

By discriminating between those patients who have integrated a containing experience and those who have not, the therapist can make important decisions regarding the approach to treatment. With the examples given above, a picture of the ways in which patients make use of the office space has emerged. The manner in which patients with disturbed relational abilities do so can inform the therapist about the basic underlying structure of their inner world. Mr D and Ms C also demonstrate how seemingly non-relational behaviors often carry relational meaning. By accurately assessing such behaviors the therapist can choose whether or not it is appropriate to make an interpretation versus making an intervention designed to support and contain. Such distinctions in intervention are often subtle but are important to the patient who is struggling just to remain in the room with us.

REFERENCES

Berne, E. (1956) 'The Psychological Structure of Space with Some Remarks on Robinson Crusoe', *Psychoanalytic Quarterly*, 25: 549–567.

Bick, E. (1968) 'The Experience of the Skin in Early Object-Relations', *International Journal of Psycho-Analysis*, 49: 484–486.

Bion, W. (1962/1998) *Learning from Experience*, Northvale, NJ: Jason Aronson.

Freud, S. (1941) 'Findings, Ideas, Problems', in *Standard Edition*, 23: 299–300, London, Hogarth Press and the Institute of Psycho-Analysis, 1964.

Klein, M. (1946) 'Notes on Some Schizoid Mechanisms', *International Journal of Psycho-Analysis*, 27: 99–110.

Scharff, J. S. and Scharff, D. E. (1994) *Object Relations Therapy of Physical and Sexual Trauma*, Northvale, NJ: Jason Aronson.

Schilder, P. (1935) 'Psycho-Analysis of Space', *International Journal of Psycho-Analysis*, 16: 274–295.

Winnicott, D. (1953) 'Transitional Objects and Transitional Phenomena: A Study of the First Not-Me Possession', *International Journal of Psycho-Analysis*, 34: 89–97.

Winnicott, D. (1960) 'The Theory of the Parent–Infant Relationship', *International Journal of Psycho-Analysis*, 41: 585–595.

Chapter 6

Changing spaces: the impact of a change in the psychotherapeutic setting

Judith M. Rovner

A psychotherapist's move to a new office might seem like a simple, uncomplicated act. However, the act of changing the physical space, that is, the external setting, is really multi-layered and quite complex.

In this chapter, I define the psychoanalytic notion of setting and explore the implications of a change in setting. I use three clinical vignettes to illustrate how a change in the physical setting of my office generated a multitude of responses and unconscious phantasies in my patients. The patients' reactions reflected their levels of psychic functioning as well as the therapeutic issues with which they were dealing at the time of the change. My own fantasies, hopes, anxieties and reactions to the move formed the context in which I experienced the patients' reactions.

COMPONENTS OF THE SETTING

The terms setting and frame are defined and used in a variety of ways and even at times used interchangeably. From my perspective, frame is one of the components of the setting. The frame consists of those non-process, external constants which are needed for the process of psychotherapy to develop and within which it can. These constants, which define the therapeutic space, are made up of elements of place and time such as the location of the office, the furnishings in the office (see also Anderson, Chapter 5 in this volume), the stable schedule of appointments, as well as the treatment modality, and the fee arrangements.

In addition to the frame, the other dimension of setting is the therapist's attitude, state of mind and way of working. It involves the therapist's openness and emotional availability for unconscious communications, the therapist's conscious attitudes and unconscious phantasies and the therapist's theoretical orientation, which is the lens through which the patient–therapist interaction is understood. These two dimensions, the frame and the therapist's state of mind, make up the setting, are inseparable and reflect each other.

PSYCHOANALYTIC PERSPECTIVES ON SETTING

There are a number of different psychoanalytic perspectives on setting and frame. Winnicott described setting as 'the summation of all of the details of management' (Winnicott 1956: 297). It includes all of the ground rules for interacting, such as limiting communication to the consulting room, confidentiality, interventions geared toward interpretation, and anonymity.

Psychoanalytic theory stresses the importance of establishing and holding to a consistent setting. When the setting is stable and secure, it is the silent backdrop for the therapeutic work and although serving an essential function it goes unnoticed. In Bleger's terms the setting is 'dumb but not non-existent' (Bleger 1967: 511). He points out that while the muteness of the setting functions as a backdrop against which the process can develop, it still has unconscious meaning and serves as a container of psychotic anxieties.

Langs describes the frame as 'the psychological boundaries and agreed upon conditions under which therapy will take place' (Scharff and Scharff 1992: 92). The establishment and maintenance of a secure frame 'generate a trust of the therapist and a sense of safety that fosters the communication of the patient's unconscious fantasies . . .' (Langs 1978: 110).

A recurrent notion in the literature is that the setting contains and defines multiple realities. Modell asserts that 'the psychoanalytic setting frames a level of reality separate from that of ordinary life – an area of illusion; within this area of the psychoanalytic setting, there are further transformations of levels of reality' (Modell 1989: 71). For Bleger, the frame provides constraints and constants, which help distinguish the unique and illusory realities of the therapy from the reality of ordinary life (Modell 1989). McDougall uses the analogy of the theater as a metaphor for psychic reality and compares the illusion of theater with the illusion of transference (McDougall 1989). Milner uses the analogy of the frame of a painting to demarcate the separate realities:

> The frame marks off the different kind of reality that is within it from that which is outside it: but a temporal spatial frame also marks off the special kind of reality of a psycho-analytic session. And in psychoanalysis it is the existence of this frame that makes possible the full development of that creative illusion that analysts call transference.
>
> (Milner 1955: 86)

That demarcation is essential in safeguarding the transference and in allowing both therapist and patient to move from an ordinary relationship to the transferential relationship and back again.

The function and elements of the setting can also be understood in terms of Winnicott's (1965) concept of the holding environment and Bion's (1962) concept of containment. An analogy can be drawn between the holding environment provided by the mother for the infant and the physical space provided for the patient by the therapist. The infant comes to rely on the consistency and predictability of the holding environment to provide protection and a sense of safety. Winnicott described holding as the externally observable aspects of the caretaking provided by the mother to facilitate the infant's growth. It is through these external objects and interactions that the baby experiences the relationship with the mother. Similarly, the therapist's provision of a special holding environment provides the patient with the necessary support and safety to do the work of psychotherapy. The patient uses these external objects and interactions with the therapist to experience their relationship. The patient, like the infant, comes to rely on the consistency and predictability of the holding environment to provide protection and a sense of safety.

The concept of containment refers more to internal unconscious processes. Bion developed the notion to describe the unconscious process whereby the projected anxieties of the infant are taken in by the mother, digested and eventually returned in modified and less overwhelming form. The mother becomes the container and the anxieties are the contained. Containment in psychotherapy is the aspect of setting internal to the therapist. It is the process of taking in and metabolizing the patient's inner world and then giving meaning to unconscious experience.

PSYCHOANALYTIC PERSPECTIVES ON A CHANGE IN THE SETTING

When the setting is altered in any way, even when it is planned and when it would not be considered acting out, the silent background becomes a foreground that requires attention. In other words, when setting is disrupted it becomes process (Etchegoyen 1991; Bleger 1967). The disruption of the frame may bring into focus the more primitive, psychotic aspects of the personality. It may disrupt the phantasy of narcissistic fusion, and elicit unconscious and conscious feelings in the patient. The patient's sense of safety may be disturbed, not only because of the actual change in the arrangements but also because the change brings about the painful reality of the separateness between the patient and therapist as well as a shift in the therapist's state of mind. A change in the frame may alter the patient's experience and image of the therapist, both externally and internally. The patient feels he is no longer in the room with the same therapist.

Langs writes about the complexity of feelings that are generated by any change in the frame. The patient might feel that the therapist is intruding into his autonomy, is being controlling, seductive, hostile or disrespectful. Feeling less safe and more mistrustful, the patient might, at one extreme, deny the impact of the change. Conversely, the patient might need to exaggerate the impact of the change (Langs 1979).

Understanding the disruptive effect of a change in the setting becomes the pressing therapeutic task. The therapist must understand communication subsequent to a change in the setting as a reaction to that change. The patient's responses will include both accurate conscious and unconscious perceptions of the meaning of the change as well as distorted phantasies (Langs 1978).

The re-establishment of a safe therapeutic space and a feeling of containment cannot occur until the conscious meanings and unconscious phantasies of the patient are understood and addressed in language that is geared to the patient's level of psychic functioning at the time of, and in response to, the change. Patients functioning in the Kleinian paranoid/schizoid position would be impacted differently than those functioning in the depressive position. Those in the paranoid/schizoid position would be more prone to feel that something was being done to them and react with splitting, denial and feelings of persecution. Those in the depressive position would more likely have a more measured reaction and use introjection and repression and experience feelings of guilt and concern.

Setting changes give the therapist a unique opportunity to access issues unnoticed until then. In addition, the technique of interpretation is essential for reinforcing the frame and for providing safety to patients as they experience shifting levels of reality, including those of both time and space. Interpretation of the experience helps to reconstitute the patient and to re-secure the frame. The act of interpretation carries the implicit message that the therapist is still functioning and has a mind to think (Modell 1988). By taking in, and working with, the interpretation, the patient uses the space that has been created for thinking.

A CHANGE IN THE SETTING

For me, the move to my own office represented a significant and very positive change. A year earlier, I entered full-time private practice, leaving a faculty position in the Department of Psychiatry at Georgetown University, a position I had held for ten years. At that time, I decided to sublease space part-time in the city near the University in addition to the part-time space in the suburbs I had been using while at the University.

At the time of the move to my own office, I was consolidating my practice into one location. For the first time I selected, furnished and decorated a space to reflect my personality and my notion of a therapeutic environment conducive to clinical work.

THE IMPACT ON PATIENTS: THREE CLINICAL VIGNETTES

As I waited for the first patient I was to see in my new office space, I was feeling a great sense of satisfaction and exhilaration. In addition to being pleased with the location of my office, I thought I had created a comfortable and tasteful atmosphere. I was relieved that preparations had gone smoothly before I began seeing my patients. However, my office was considerably smaller than any of the spaces I had subleased.

George, a man in his early forties, who was being seen in twice-weekly individual therapy, had denied any feelings in anticipation of the move. He could not allow himself to be at all curious and insisted that the space where we met made no difference to him. While one might think that this could mean that only the relationship mattered, for this schizoid man who attacked links, even the relationship mattering was persistently denied.

On entering the office, George's first comments were 'I'm observing the room. It looks, I guess it's more convenient for me so it's nice. It smells freshly painted. It looks like you are sharing the office with other people. I guess I think that makes sense to do. Like before I got married I shared a house with four other guys. That made it affordable to be able to live there.' A moment later he likened my sharing a suite to his father's situation as he neared retirement from his medical practice. 'When he was nearing retirement he could barely pay the rent and the insurance. So, unless you are seeing ten patients a day, which would be hard, this makes sense.'

I understood this to mean that as a result of the change in space, George had a phantasy that he now had a therapist who could barely get by on limited resources and could only afford to do what people did at either end of their personal and professional development. I experienced George as putting me in a diminished position, making an envious attack on my capacities, and attempting to spoil the pleasure I could get from this move. His contempt reflected his envy of my growth, his pervasive difficulty experiencing good objects and his pattern of spoiling relationships and experiences. It was not that his reactions were unexpected, as I had many experiences of being devalued by George. This time I was hit in a different way. The difference had to do with my own narcissistic vulnerability. I was aware that his attack shook my own connection with this good experience. This example highlights the shared vulnerability of patient and therapist in the face of a change in setting. My psychological interior had also changed.

A second patient, Allison, a 40-year-old woman, had been in twice weekly individual treatment for a number of years, and therefore had seen me in my subleased offices as well as in my office at the university. Prior to the move she expressed excitement and anticipation at being able to finally see me in a space of my own which reflected my personality. I understood this as a reflection of her curiosity, her wish to know me in a more intimate way, and her phantasy of getting into my mind and my personal space.

Since a postcard of Freud's couch had been visible in my university office, Allison had wondered if my office would look like his, full of tapestries and interesting artifacts. She also looked forward to the office being closer to both of our homes, a feeling which reflected her phantasy that there would be less distance between us. There was some anxiety expressed as she noted that after so many years of stability I was making a second change just a year after the first one. She countered her anxiety that I was becoming unstable with the notion that I was making moves for the better. The therapy had enabled her to resolve her significant depression and to reduce her anxiety enough to add part-time employment to her roles of mother and wife. She hoped that she would feel strong enough to move to full-time employment and spoke of my being a positive role model for growth.

When Allison, who stands just five feet tall, entered the office, she noted with pleasure the return of the Freud postcard which she had not seen during the prior year in the subleased spaces. She was reconnecting with a lost good object. As she sat down on one of the two love-seats she uttered: 'Well. You obviously did not choose this furniture with me in mind,' reflecting her thought that the furniture was meant for taller people. Allison was expressing hurt and the phantasy that she no longer had a therapist who held her in mind. An additional statement that the desk was not the right proportion for the space reflected the feeling that things did not fit together and also reflected her feelings of hostility toward me.

I was surprised by this hostility and Allison, too, was perplexed by the intensity and aggression in her reactions. I recalled how differently I had experienced her negative comments about the furniture in the subleased office we had most recently been meeting in. I realized that it had been easy for me to not experience those comments as hostile since I shared her assessment of the office décor and since, after all, I could deny she was talking about me. Now, however, it was a different matter. I was being maligned and my space was being attacked. I experienced countertransference feelings I had not experienced when it was my colleague's office being attacked. I had missed the split.

When I addressed the hostility in her words, I knew and Allison appeared to feel that I was speaking from a different internal space. Allison then became anxious as she experienced me as a more threatening figure, which was partially a projection of her own anger and aggressiveness. She was able to own her aggressiveness and spoke of her capacity to spoil the accomplishments of others out of her strong envy as well as her feelings of inadequacy. I also understood that the feeling of things not fitting together not only referred to our relationship but also referred to her internal world and the way the more grateful, depressive part and the more primitive envious part did not fit together.

In discussing her deep hurt that my furniture selection meant she did not hold first place in my mind, she connected to feeling displaced by the birth of her younger siblings. She felt that I, like her mother, had rejected her and her needs in favor of the needs of her larger, that is, more important siblings. Allison elaborated on the feeling that she no longer fit into her mother's lap in the same way as she had before the birth of her siblings. For this patient, there was an alteration in her basic sense of security which had to do with the loss of closeness to the mother's body. The change in setting disrupted the illusion of being the most important, and brought up old painful memories which left her once again feeling betrayed and displaced.

Allison also expressed disappointment that the office décor was not more like Freud's, specifically that I had only one tapestry rug. Allison denied that there might be longing to lie on a couch and disappointment that there were two love-seats instead of a couch. I had to wonder silently about my own wishes and my own disappointment at not creating an analytic space with a couch like Freud's.

This patient is an example of the myriad of emotions which the change in setting can evoke: envy, anger, admiration, guilt, and identification with an object capable of growth and change. It shows how the change in location and in my internal ownership of the space influenced how both of us experienced the change.

I was seeing the third patient, Rebecca, a woman in her late forties, in four-times-a-week analytic psychotherapy. Rebecca, who had a PhD held a high-level position in organizational development. She was married to a mathematician, many years her senior, and they had an adolescent son. The marriage was characterized by conflict centering on space and time. Regarding time, the patient had the experience of a husband who couldn't keep time commitments and left her disoriented and unable to operate within a reliable time frame. In terms of space, the patient had the experience of an emotionally controlling, tyrannical husband who took over the physical space with objects that he could neither part with nor put away. It left her uncertain as to how to find an internal space for herself in the midst of the chaotic and unpredictable external space.

Rebecca was a bright, anxious woman, who worked hard in the sessions to try to figure things out. She spoke in a rapid, anxious manner, producing an abundance of rich material. The outpouring conveyed to me the patient's lack of internal space and her experience of being overwhelmed by her internal world. As the therapy progressed, my feeling of being continuously flooded subsided. The shift was related to an increase in the frequency of sessions as well as to my developing a greater capacity to introject the projected anxiety and, eventually, to interpret the experience to her.

At the time of my move, Rebecca was in the process of trying to extricate herself from her marriage and was in the throes of internal and external struggles to make that happen. She understood that she was terrified to be alone and that leaving the marriage meant facing both her claustrophobic and agoraphobic anxieties. Those anxieties were reflected in the way she navigated the world and the therapy.

Over the course of years of psychotherapy, Rebecca had threatened several times to terminate treatment. The threats occurred when she experienced overwhelming primitive anxiety, was overwhelmed by life circumstances and fearful that she was not up to the challenge of the therapy work. There were times when I was taken over by Rebecca's intense, disorganizing anxieties, experiences which at times were difficult to bear, in part because they threatened my own confidence in being able to do the work.

When I decided on the location of my office, I had some concern since it meant a longer commute for her from both home and work. In the transference, she was more openly acknowledging dependency and vulnerability, as well as her fears of rejection and retaliation. During the period when I knew but had not yet informed Rebecca of the move, she said, 'It's embarrassing to me for you to know I feel that way (dependent). You could use it against me. What if you go away? What if you moved? You're not going to move away, are you?' Rebecca was speaking to her fear that I would take advantage of her vulnerability and retaliate for her unconscious aggressive phantasies towards me. Rebecca was relieved to hear that the move she feared did not mean literally losing me.

Her intense anxiety and confusion were immediately apparent in the first session in the new space. As she took water from a water-cooler located outside my office, her confusion was reflected in not knowing which color spigot distinguished hot from cold. In the office Rebecca asked whether it mattered where she sat, reflecting her uncertainty as to the ground rules in the new setting and her searching to feel contained by having an element of the frame re-established.

As Rebecca sat down in the love-seat she said, 'Well, my first impression is I have to climb up to sit on here as though I'm a little girl. Isn't that interesting? I'm short but I imagine a little person climbing up on here.' I thought this was an expression of her experiencing a shift in status relative to me. That statement as well as concern she had expressed about being late and getting lost in time gave an Alice in Wonderland quality to Rebecca's thinking.

She felt appreciative that we had discussed the move over several months and that she could now acknowledge and express the anxiety, which she could not have done some time ago. Rebecca was speaking to the importance of being prepared for a change in the setting.

The following segments of the session give a flavor of the claustrophobic and agoraphobic aspects of the experience of getting to the new space. They reflect the primitive and disorganizing anxiety of getting lost in external and internal space and of not having any familiar signposts to deal with the disorientation. Rebecca's overwhelming anxiety is reflected in the verbal barrage and in the grammatical breakdown of her speech:

'Anyway, so I came down here to Georgetown Pike. My instinct was that I don't like this place at all. I really don't like this place at all. I don't like high buildings. I don't really like this city. This is really the city. And there is too many people. There is too many cars. Buildings are very high. I think I could hear myself say, hear you say, but we were in Georgetown. Look at all the people there. And I would say, yeh, but I didn't notice. I'm very aware. I actually think it is busier here, but I am aware of the busyness because I am not coming in on the tube I formed for myself in Georgetown. And I always liked Georgetown. I always disliked Bethesda. Just driving through it. I think that's because of the traffic and the congestion and the sense of it. And when you were in Georgetown you were in a building, although it was big it was all by itself and there was something and I loved the street because there was hardly anyone on it, just a few people. I got up here. I had to wait to make a right turn where there was all this traffic and all these lights. First thought, I don't really like this place. This is a bad place. Everything I saw made me feel anxious and worse. I saw these houses and I felt bad I didn't have a house like that. I saw the Bethesda Women's Country Club or whatever it was and I thought a women's club. Even a few months ago I would have gone yuck but now I went that is something I would long to be a part of instead of being rejecting of it. I was recognizing that the Women's Club evokes something in me and each thing I saw evokes, it was all very negative but it all made me feel funny. This is a new path. And it forces me to see new things. It forces me to see things I could close my eyes to. Sometimes when I see a Staples I go, oh good, there's a Staples in this neighborhood and it's like an orientation. And, I saw the Staples and I didn't even want to see it. I'm seeing too many things . . . I can't block enough of it out so I am threatened by it.'

Later in the session, I linked Rebecca's image of being a little girl climbing up on the furniture to her experience of being overwhelmed. I thought she was telling me that, like a little girl, she was being faced with more than she could manage and that I was the one who put her in that position. I spoke to her fear of telling me about her anger as an expression of needing to protect both her and me. Rebecca tentatively acknowledged the anger which we came to understand as due to her having no choice about the move. She felt that my choice of location simultaneously put more of a distance between us and brought us too close together. On the one hand she had to cover a greater distance to get to me and on the other hand she was in my home territory which put her very close and made her very anxious.

As the impact of the change in setting was explored, Rebecca became less anxious. 'It's as though I expected you to be threatened by what I am saying . . . my mother wouldn't allow me to be unhappy and deal with the things I was anxious about like where is the bathroom going to be. So maybe when I was little and was going to make any changes, going to school on the first day, going to the doctor's, maybe I could never talk about how anxious that made me. I can just hear her. Don't bother me. Not in so many words but in so many feelings.'

This vignette reflects the importance of helping the patient understand the impact of the change in setting and demonstrates the containment that putting words to the experience produces.

CONCLUSION

This chapter illustrates the importance of understanding the meaning of setting and the impact of any change to it. The situation of a change in office space was used to illustrate the impact on three different patients. It described a range of responses within the patients, within me and in the transference–countertransference relationships. It demonstrated the importance of keeping the internal space open for thinking. Setting changes, though disruptive, also provide an exceptional opportunity for new and deeper insight into aspects of the patients' inner worlds. Attention to the impact on both patient and therapist is crucial.

REFERENCES

Bion, W. (1962/1994) *Learning from Experience*, Northvale, NJ: Jason Aronson.

Bleger, J. (1967) 'Psycho-Analysis of the Psycho-Analytic Frame', *International Journal of Psycho-Analysis*, 48: 511–519.

Etchegoyen, R. H. (1991) *The Fundamentals of Psychoanalytic Technique,* London: Karnac.

Langs, R. J. (1978) 'Validation and the Framework of the Therapeutic Situation: Thoughts Prompted by Hans H. Strupp's Suffering and Psychotherapy', *Contemporary Psychoanalysis*, 14: 98–124.

Langs, R. J. (1979) *The Therapeutic Environment*, New York: Jason Aronson.

McDougall, J. (1989) *The Theaters of The Body*, New York: Norton.

Milner, M. (1955) 'The Role of Illusion in Symbol Formation', in M. Klein, P. Heiman, and R. Money-Kyrle (eds.), *New Directions in Psychoanalysis*, New York: Basic Books, pp. 82–108.

Modell, A. H. (1988) 'The Centrality of the Psychoanalytic Setting and the Changing Aims of Treatment: A Perspective from a Theory of Object Relations', *The Psychoanalytic Quarterly*, 57: 577–596.

Modell, A. H. (1989) 'The Psychoanalytic Setting as a Container of Multiple Levels of Reality: A Perspective on the Theory of Psychoanalytic Treatment', *Psychoanalytic Inquiry*, 9: 67–87.

Scharff, J. S. and Scharff, D. E. (1992) *Scharff Notes: A Primer of Object Relations Therapy*, Northvale, NJ: Jason Aronson.

Winnicott, D. W. (1956) 'Clinical Varieties of Transference', in *Collected Papers: Through Paediatrics to Psychoanalysis* (1958), New York: Basic Books, pp. 295–299.

Winnicott, D. W. (1965) *The Maturational Processes and the Facilitating Environment*, London: Hogarth Press.

Chapter 7

Pandora in time and space

Earl Hopper

INTRODUCTION

In this chapter I will argue that, just as helplessness is at the heart of the human condition, the fear of annihilation in the context of the traumato-genic process is the distinguishing characteristic of 'difficult' patients. In my practice as a psychoanalyst and group analyst I tend to see all my patients individually and then to bring them into one of my twice-weekly groups. I see them individually for varying periods of time, but eventually, after a lengthy transition, during which they are in both individual and group treatment, they will be in group treatment only. Groups help the group analyst with troublesome countertransference responses, which are typical of work with our most difficult patients, precisely because countertrans-ference responses make understanding them difficult (Gans and Alonso 1998; Alonson and Rutan 1990; Caligor *et al.* 1993; Kauff 1991). Provided that the group analyst is prepared to listen to and learn from the group, he can usually find support and insight from them. However, it is uniquely important that through their enactment of the constraints of group basic assumptions, difficult patients are likely to repeat their traumatic life experiences and to 'tell' the group about their key problems and symptoms. Containing and compassionate understanding of these processes can be used in the service of psychotherapy. It is especially important to work with 'Incohesion', which I regard as the fourth basic assumption in the uncon-scious life of groups. In making this argument I will draw on work that is both old and novel in its implications for the study of personality, for the study of groups, and for clinical work in groups and dyads: my own studies of the social unconscious, and of traumatic experience in the unconscious life of groups (Hopper 2003a, 2003b).

SOME OF THE CORE FEATURES OF OUR MOST DIFFICULT PATIENTS: NARCISSISTIC AND BORDERLINE STATES OF MIND

Difficult patients are usually diagnosed in terms of pathological narcissism and borderline personality organization. First and foremost they are characterized by the fear of annihilation. The phenomenology of the fear of annihilation involves psychic paralysis and the death of psychic vitality, characterized by fission and fragmentation, and then fusion and confusion of what is left of the self with what can be found in the object. Fusion and confusion are a defense against fission and fragmentation, and vice versa. There is oscillation between these two psychic poles, because each is associated with its own characteristic psychotic anxieties. For example, the fears of falling apart and of petrification are associated with fission and fragmentation; of fear of suffocation and of being swallowed up are associated with fusion and confusion. Both disassociation and encapsulation occur as a defense or protection against psychic paralysis.

These bipolar intrapsychic constellations are associated with two types of narcissistic and borderline character disorder: one, the 'contact shunning' or 'crustacean'; and two, the 'merger-hungry' or 'amoeboid'. These two types of character disorder have often been delineated in similar terms, for example, schizoid reactions against the fear of engulfment and/or clinging reactions against the fear of abandonment.

The fear of annihilation and its vicissitudes are caused by traumatic experience of failed dependency, leading to damage, abandonment and loss. Moreover, traumatized and difficult patients have not been able to mourn and symbolize their traumatic experience. Many have been able to engage only in various forms of inauthentic and perverse mourning characterized by schizoid ritualization and sado-masochism.

Traumatized patients tend to use projective and introjective identification of malignant kinds, involving the repetition compulsion and traumatophilia, in the service of expulsion of horrific states of mind, and attempts to attack and control their most hated objects, because the symbolic process has failed. However, these processes are also used in the service of communication of experience that is not available through conscious narrative. Thus, traumatized patients are exceedingly vulnerable to role suction, because specific roles offer them skins of identity.

These features of narcissistic and borderline states of mind are illustrated by my patient Pandora, who can be described as having a merger-hungry, amoeboid character:

> Shortly after Pandora was born, her mother was hospitalized for a depressive illness. When she was approximately three months of age, Pandora was looked after by family friends for six months. When she

was two years of age, Pandora was again looked after by these friends for about six months. During these periods, she rarely saw her father.

She contacted me for psychotherapy at age 38 following an unsatisfactory experience in a once weekly group with a colleague who had died suddenly. She was shocked but not saddened, perhaps even relieved because this gave her the chance to leave the group.

Among her presenting symptoms were shame of her history of periodic phases of bisexuality, an intense persistent monophobia of cancer which was virtually a hypochondriasis, leading her to seduce many doctors to perform various medical investigations, and abuse of alcohol and a number of other substances.

After one year of one session per week and seven years of five sessions per week, we agreed to reduce the number of sessions to four. Soon after, in June, she became aware of a perineal fistula, treated surgically in July with apparent success. In August we took a break. In September the analysis resumed.

In the very first session she introduced the image of Pandora's Box as a metaphor for her rigid, hard, muscular and bony body. She did not look that way to me. She was convinced that her Pandora's Box contained powerful insects such as bees, hornets, giant and stingy little creatures. They were all dangerous but she felt well protected because she could suffocate them with poisoned aerosol sprays. She felt that I would stop treatment if I knew how vulnerable I was to her inner dybbuks. Before the next session she dreamt that her disreputable gynecologist used a laser to remove a birthmark mole from her cheek, and another mole from her buttock. In her dream the mole on her face turned into a pseudo-pod that stepped into my stomach where it became rooted in such a way that if she had to leave me it would have to be ripped out like a tumor or insidious weed. She associated these moles to stigmata of punishment for stealing and eventually for killing the unborn babies of her mother.

We understood this material in terms of her recent fistula, the reparative surgery, separation and the loss of a session, and her fantasies about the other patient(s) who had taken her session, and who would soon fill the space that she had vacated. We also focused on her further fear that I had abandoned her and that her abandonment of me would soon lead to further cutting of her sessions. I thought she was experiencing an intense fusion and confusion of her traumatized infantile self with her early maternal object, and with me and her analysis itself. Paradoxically, I felt that it was time for Pandora to begin to reduce her sessions further, and that she might be ready to come into one of my twice-weekly groups.

MY THEORY OF INCOHESION: AGGREGATION/
MASSIFICATION OR (BA) I:A/M

I will now outline my theory of Incohesion: Aggregation/Massification or (ba) I:A/M. I will first remind you of Bion's theory of basic assumptions. Using a Kleinian model of the mind, Bion (1961) conceptualized three basic assumptions associated with specific kinds of anxieties and specific kinds of anxieties and roles: Dependency, associated with envy, idealization and the roles of omnipotence and grandiosity, on the one hand, and passive compliance, on the other; Fight/Flight, associated with envy, denigration and roles of attack, on the one hand, and retreat, on the other; and Pairing, associated with the use of sexuality as a manic defense against depressive position anxieties and the roles of romantic illusionaries, on the one hand, and messianic salvationists, on the other. All basic assumption processes are manifest in patterns of interaction, normation, communication, styles of thinking and feeling, and styles of leadership, followership and bystandership. People with particular patterns of anxiety are attracted to the roles of particular basic assumptions.

This theory is a remarkable contribution, although it is not without certain inconsistencies (Billow 2003; Kernberg 1998). However, using an alternative model of the mind associated with the Group of Independent Psychoanalysts of the British Psychoanalytical Society, and shared by sociology and group analysis, it is possible to conceptualize a fourth basic assumption of Incohesion. This model of the mind (Hopper 2003a) can be defined in terms of a set of axioms, as follows:

1   In the beginning there is no such thing as an infant but only a mother/infant couple; the mother/infant couple can be described as two bodies/one mind; moreover, the mother/infant couple or dyad always exists within a social context that includes the father/male partner and/or within a family set-up or arrangement within a wider community, etc. This can even be applied to the unique object of the mother/fetus couple. (It is curious that many analysts who are pleased to regard the womb and amniotic fluid as the baby's pre-birth environment do not continue to show the same interest in cultural orientations, language systems, power structures, family arrangements, etc.)

2   An original ego of adaptation precedes an emergent ego of agency, which is based on social relations mediated through communications, ultimately through language; although an infant may be born with an original ego of adaptation, or with a body-ego or a perceptual apparatus, this is hardly what we mean when we talk of an 'ego' or the 'self' as an 'I' with agency.

3   As a complement to body-ego, we need a concept of a society-ego or other-ego or what G. Klein (1976: 178) called a 'we-go'. However, the

body-ego and the 'society-ego' are equally primary, and develop in parallel and in interaction with one another.

4   Psychic facts are preceded by both social and organismic facts.

5   Psychic life begins with processes of internalization.

6   The first emotion is not innate malign envy based on the so-called 'death instinct', and the first psychic act is not a projection of the anxiety inherent in it. Although envy is ubiquitous, it should be understood as a defense against the fear of annihilation as a consequence of personal and social helplessness rather than as an expression of the anxiety inherent in the so-called 'death instinct'. Envy is a spoiling attack on people and their parts who are perceived as able to be of help but who will not.

7   Although external objects are impregnated with projections, they can be and often are internalized in their pristine form.

8   'Unintegration' precedes 'integration', but 'disintegration' follows trauma, especially breaks in attachments, and impingements to the safety shield.

9   Trauma and traumatogenic processes are central to the study and treatment of psychopathology, which is not to deny the importance of unconscious fantasies based on instinctual impulses.

10   Aggression is a function of frustration and aggressive feelings, and the normative orientations towards the expression of feelings generally and aggressive feelings specifically.

11   Helplessness and shame are closer to the heart of the human condition than are envy and guilt.

12   Persons and groups are open systems; thus, groups are always open to the personalities of their participants, and vice versa, from conception to death. Thus, people are affected profoundly by social, cultural and political facts and forces at all phases of their 'life trajectories'.

13   In clinical work the exercise of the transcendent imagination (or the development and maintenance of mature hope) is as essential as the analysis of the transference of past experience which may involve a sense of despair and the loss of hope.

Although these axioms are not self-explanatory, I hope that they convey that it is possible to be sensitive simultaneously and recursively to the constraints of body, mind and society, and to work within all the cells of the time/space paradigm. The 'complete interpretation' of processes within the 'Here and Now' should include the 'Here and Then' and the 'There and Now', or in other words, experience from the three cells of the Therapeutic Triangle. However, group analysts also work in the 'There and Then', the long ago and far away, that is, in all areas of the Therapeutic Square, without feeling that in doing so we are being defensive against the heat of the moment. (Some of us also work in the 'If and When' with respect to the exercise of the transcendent imagination.)

My theory of (ba) I:A/M is centered on two propositions. The first is that the fear of annihilation is caused by traumatic experience, which may be ubiquitous but is clearly a matter of degree. The second proposition is that the fear of annihilation is bipolar and characterized by oscillations between fission and fragmentation, and fusion and confusion, as outlined above. Hence, (ba) I:A/M involves an assertion of identity when identity is under threat – I:A/M is an acronym of 'I am'. When the fear of annihilation is prevalent, then, based on malignant forms of projective and introjective identification concerning intra-psychic fission and fragmentation, the group is likely to become an 'aggregate' through a process of 'aggregation'. The terms 'aggregate' and 'aggregation' are taken from early sociology and anthropology. A social aggregate is not quite a group, but nor is it merely a collection of people who have no consciousness of themselves as being part of a nascent social system. Among the metaphors for an aggregate are a collection of billiard balls or a handful of gravel. An aggregate is characterized by contra-groups rather than subgroups, who experience long periods of silence in which they do not relate to one another. Aggressive feelings are rampant, although they may not be expressed in actual aggression. (Turquet (1975: 103) referred to this state of affairs in terms of 'dissaroy', and Lawrence and his colleagues (1996: 29) in terms of 'me-ness'.)

As a defense against the anxieties associated with aggregation, the group becomes a mass through a process of massification, involving an hysterical idealization of the situation and the leader, and identification with him, leading to feelings of pseudo-morale and illusions of wellbeing. This defensive shift is based on malignant forms of projective and introjective identification of intra-psychic fusion and confusion. Among the metaphors for a mass are warm wet sponges squeezed together or a piece of feces. Some might prefer the icon of a nice piece of chopped fish. (Somewhat confusingly Freud (1921) originally referred to this state of affairs as a mass, but sometimes he referred to a horde, and sometimes to a mob, which are really very different from one another; unfortunately, Freud's mass has often been mistranslated as group, which is misleading; Turquet (1975) and others have conceptualized the group as a mass in terms of the concept of one-ness, which is the basis of Kernberg's (1998) later work on mass psychology.)

The development and maintenance of massification is based on a variety of complex patterns of aggression towards objects that are perceived to be obstacles to the process of massification, that is, the collective desire to merge with the idealized breast. No sounds, colors, textures, smells, etc. may be allowed to interrupt the hallucinated fusion with the idealized breast and its milk. In fact, during massification traumatized people are likely to seek the milk of the breast, possibly as an equivalent of amniotic fluid. In this sense even the skin of the breast is an obstacle. All of the aggression associated with aggregation is still present, but it is used in the service of marginalization, peripheralization, neutralization and even 'annihilation', because the desire to annihilate follows from the fear of annihilation. Typical patterns of aggression in the context of massification include severe and prejudiced moral judgments, anonymization, scapegoating, and assassination. Of course, character assassination occurs more often than actual assassination, but perhaps fantasies about assassination occur even more often than character assassination, especially in the political life of our professional organizations.

We must think in terms of processes. Although the first group-based defense against the anxieties associated with aggregation is a shift towards massification, the first group-based defense against the anxieties associated with massification is a shift back towards aggregation, thus precipitating the same anxieties that provoked the first defensive shift from aggregation towards massification in the first place. In other words, in the same way that a person who is overwhelmed by the fear of annihilation tends to oscillate between states of fission and fragmentation, on the one hand, and fusion and confusion, on the other, a group in which the fear of annihilation is prevalent is likely to be characterized by oscillation between aggregation and massification, the two bipolar forms of incohesion. However, such oscillations are rarely total and complete, and, therefore, at any one time vestiges of aggregation can be seen in states of massification, and vestiges of massification in states of aggregation. It is useful to think in terms of primary and secondary oscillations, and to take a historical perspective.

During these oscillations between aggregation and massification, typical roles emerge. For example, the 'lone wolf' is typical of aggregation, and the 'cheerleader', of massification. Difficult patients are highly vulnerable to the valences or suction of these particular roles, and, therefore, they tend to personify these roles, and to be experienced by others as doing so. Specifically, crustaceans are likely to personify aggregation processes, and amoeboids, massification processes.

In sum, not only are our most difficult patients likely to create the bipolar states and processes of aggregation and massification, they are also likely to personify the key roles associated with them. Having been exploited and scapegoated by their families (mainly in order for their families to minimize various anxieties and to prevent their own disintegration) difficult and traumatized patients feel compelled unconsciously to strive to recreate their early experiences within their later life, which is especially and painfully evident in their groups. This is the key to the application of my theory of the fourth basic assumption to our clinical work.

I would like to make two further points. First, the experience of psychotic anxieties within a group, and especially the experience of the fear of annihilation, may occur in several ways: the members of the group may regress to an early phase of life in which certain kinds of traumatic experience are virtually universal and ubiquitous; the members may share a history of specific kinds of trauma; and the group may itself become traumatized, possibly through management failures on the part of the group analyst, or by other events that break the boundaries of holding and containment causing the members of the group to feel profoundly unsafe. And second, it is important to take account of the phenomenon of equivalence, that is, traumatic experience in any one system may be recapitulated in either a higher or lower order system, for example, a group that meets for the purpose of psychotherapy may recapitulate the tensions of the wider society, both contemporaneously and historically.

A CLINICAL VIGNETTE FROM GROUP ANALYSIS

Some of the processes associated with Incohesion and its personification can be seen in the following vignette of sessions from a mature slow-open twice-weekly heterogeneous group. In it, I will also illustrate how I was helped by the group to be a more perceptive analyst; they allowed me the time and space in which I could consult myself about difficult, discordant countertransference processes. I will also indicate some constraints of the social unconscious in connection with gender identity and sibling rivalry, and the gradual emergence of a hopeful attitude associated with the development of the 'workgroup'.

Pandora will be at the center of our attention. She was in the second, group phase of her therapy, and had stopped seeing me individually. In this vignette she personifies massification by becoming a cheerleader. Not only was she sucked into the role, but also helped to create it. However, eventually, after much hard work, she came out of the role and showed a new capacity for insight and the integration of feeling and thought.

With respect to the group itself, I will focus on a sequence of aggregation in response to separation for the holiday break, followed by the emergence of massification as a defense against aggregation, and then by the recovery and continuing development of workgroup functioning. The central underlying dynamic was aggregation manifest in engendered contra-groups, that is, subgroups of men and women who began to define themselves in terms of not being members of the other subgroup even more than on the basis of being members of their own subgroup. This was stopped by the rapid fusion and confusion of these contra-groups with a lost and abandoning object that they held in common based on the sexualization of explosive rage. The group slowly regained its capacity to recognize and to accept differences and imperfections, eschewing the temptation to become a massification cult. This was connected with my own ability to resist the group's demands that I become a cult leader.

1. Aggregation based on impending separation caused by the forthcoming Xmas break

Pandora found it very difficult to share her new group with me, and to share me with the new group, especially with those people in it who had become her favorite rivals, her so-called 'sibling figures'. Although she had begun to settle, shortly before Xmas, when I would be taking a break for a couple of weeks, I sensed within the group levels of separation anxiety and annihilation anxiety that threatened their feeling that they could and would go-on-being. The group began to display patterns of gaze-avoidance; frequently many people talked at the same time; and subgroups carried on their own conversations. Also, the group sat in a pattern grouped in such a way as to represent splits and polarities with respect to at least nine variables: religion, clinical history, profession, sex, age, country of birth and marital status. I have rarely experienced a group that evinced so many subgroups and polarities simultaneously, and, therefore, potential contra-groups.

2. A shift towards massification personified by Pandora

Pandora began to generate an unauthentically cheerful, slightly manic atmosphere of pseudo-morale. She established patterns of interaction and of verbal and non-verbal communication that influenced the group to feel that they all ought to join one another in becoming more aware of their successes in life and of how they had been helped by their therapy. People started to agree that as a result of their participation in this particular group they had made marvelous achievements and had no need to fear the impending holiday break. These communications became a frenzied but almost rhythmical litany of idealization of the group and of me, coupled with the denigration of a few of my colleagues and their groups, giving me immense gratification, and confirming my own judgement.

There was an attempt to silence and split up a couple of patients who were a little less enthusiastic. When they attempted to talk about their fear of the holiday they were attacked. They retreated contemptuously into a silent, somewhat conspiratorial, partnership maintained through eye contact and the mutual raising of eyebrows.

3. Work group functioning: the group analyst and his interpretations

Pandora continued to express her adoration of me and contempt of my colleagues. This gave me enormous pleasure, in fact too much pleasure, the dawning awareness of which alerted me to the possibility that I was on the receiving end of projective identification in the service of sucking me into the illusion of perfection, based on idealization. I resisted this, and wondered aloud if the refusal to allow any differences of points of view, any expression of individuality, and the need to maintain a continuous pep-talk, were attempts to avoid the fear that we might all go our individual ways never to return, and, thus, that the group would dissolve and fall apart.

Pandora came to the forefront of my mind. On the basis of seemingly good advice, she had recently undergone yet more surgery. She had a mole removed from her lower lip, which actually I understood as yet another somatic expression of an encapsulation. I reminded her of her surgery for a fistula, which had also developed at a time of separation. I asked her if she might be a little more worried about the impending break than she was prepared to acknowledge.

> She replied that she had forgotten that last night she had a nightmare. She was standing outside a large house with many rooms and many windows, unable to get in. She began to throw rocks, but there was still no response. Finally, she threw one big rock that was somehow not really a rock but a very explosive strong weapon. There was a white light, not quite an explosion. She became very frightened. The rock bounced off the window and started to come back at her. Despite her terror, a transformation occurred. 'Mercifully,' she said. This so-called weapon-rock turned into a thousand tadpoles which became very slimy and tried to get into her mouth, her ears and her body, searching for what she called 'appropriate openings'.

4. Some countertransference considerations

I felt very frustrated. I wanted to be alone with Pandora in order to analyze the dream with her. Also, I assumed that I was involved in projective and introjective identification of Pandora's frustration and anger with her group rivals for my attention. I felt confused with her, and not at all clear as to who was who, and whose objects belonged to whom. However, I started to think about the work of Fairbairn (1952) in connection with his concept of the moral defense, and the work of Andre Green (1986) and his concepts in connection with the dead mother, in addition to the work of other intellectual fathers of Independent psychoanalysis.

Clearly, I was involved in a concordant transference/countertransference relationship (Racker 1968), feeling what Pandora was feeling, but whereas she was using amoeboid, merger-hungry defenses, I was using crustacean, contact-shunning defenses. However, I was aware that my feelings and defenses were also connected with my own more personal and 'discordant' countertransference to her. In other words, transference/countertransference relationship was not only a matter of communication, but was also co-constructed by Pandora and myself on the basis of our respective unconscious conflicts and preoccupations.

I remembered how determined Pandora was never to be blocked from a space in which she felt that she would be protected and looked after, and in which she would not have to communicate with words in a grown-up way. Her experience of maternal space, including the flat to which she had been taken when her mother was hospitalized, had been transferred to my body, my mind, the group and even to my consulting room. Nonetheless, I became more and more preoccupied with my own experiences of failed dependency both very early in life and more recently. In other words, I was both in touch with Pandora and not in touch with her, because more in touch with myself. I realized that my initial preoccupations were too intellectual, a sign of my own defensiveness against my emotions. Perhaps I was seeking some supervisory help with my maternal objects; certainly I was using theory in a defensive way, in order to protect myself from painful experience (Hirsch 2003). In any case, I decided to remain silent, and to let the group respond to Pandora and to allow the central group tension and the collective transference to develop more clearly. This was the right thing to do and the safest thing to do, because I needed to protect myself and the group from my sudden anxieties, and to clarify my countertransference and to try to analyze it (Hopper, in press).

5. The group as co-therapist

With considerable empathy, the group began to work. One patient talked to Pandora about her rage and pointed out that although it was reactive it was so quickly projected and re-introjected. Another said, 'That's sexy stuff Pandora. Clearly those tadpoles were sperms.' As hysterical as she was, Pandora was surprised that she had reported a sexy dream. It is likely that she felt sexually aroused. This was unusual for her.

Pandora then told us with feeling about her being alone and feeling empty. She described her despair as a female, and her envy of male creativity. She felt caught in a dilemma that as she came to accept herself more and more as a female she would not feel creative unless she had a baby, but if she felt herself to be female and had a baby, she would lose her sense of herself as a male, sacrifice other things in her career.

6. Work group functioning: the recovery of the group analyst

By this time I had regained my ability to think. The group had functioned as a good enough container for Pandora's destructive projections, tolerated her sexualization of her violent feelings, and communicated to her as equals who did not judge her strange and sexy thoughts and feelings. Although her dream was a gift of sorts, there was definitely the possibility that with further interpretation of the dream Pandora and the group could start to shift back towards an aggregate as symbolized in the dream by her pebbles and rocks, and by the pane of window glass as a traumatized and overly intellectual analyst/mother who would soon be separating from her. Before this occurred, however, I commented about retaliation from the house-mother, who did not let the weapon break into her. In fact, the weapon was rejected or repulsed, and transformed into a thousand tadpoles, which if they symbolized sperms might not be expected to come from her mother. In any case, aggression had been sexualized protectively. I wondered about her image of her father as a fertile man, and what sort of access she felt her mother had allowed them to each other. I had worked with her on this sort of material a thousand times, but somehow it all felt very fresh. I wondered about myself as a housemother and housefather, and about my being an amalgam of the two. I said maybe there was some confusion about her mother as a father and her father as a mother.

Another patient then said that the impending holiday was like a menstrual period. After another brief silence, which was not contemptuous of the remark, but involved an attempt to think, I spoke of the loss of perfection and the loss of hope, replaced by a wishful search for a protective inner circle and a compulsion to enter it. I also said that a menstrual period could be understood as a reference to the group's falling apart, but that a period is not the same as an abortion, and perhaps more like a holiday break.

In response Pandora spoke of her fantasy that during the holiday I would see one of the patients who was a training candidate at an event at the Institute of Group Analysis. I said that I understood that the group generally felt hurt and angry about the holiday break and also felt fright-ened both about their ability to function without too much anxiety and about their impulse to express such feelings to me, because they might hurt me and themselves. I also said that Pandora had transformed her fears about falling apart into a desire to make the group totally and absolutely whole and to put herself inside it, and to attach herself to the group and to me, as she felt the male training candidate would be able to do. I went on to imply, but not to spell out, that she had a fantasy that only a boy could really do this, or at any rate a girl with a penis, which she thought was the only creative sexual organ.

7. Work group functioning: deeper insights originating in the group rather than in the group analyst

Pandora acknowledged her conviction that only males could be creative in a general way. She then became a little angry with the male candidate and the group, which she had not been able to do before. Another member of the group said that it was obvious that she was treating this man as though he were her younger brother. Several members of the group then reminded her of her considerable achievements in the field of the arts. Pandora then asked one of the members of the two-person contra-group to tell more about their feelings of doubt. Imagine, this woman was inquiring as to the feelings of others with whom she might have been in competition. This led to some anger and sadness and memories of having been let down repeatedly during childhood, which was an experience shared by the entire group. The encapsulated contra-group began to dissolve. The group began to discuss in an authentic way Pandora's confusion concerning her sexual identity and her gender identity. Pandora showed some understanding that she could be her 'own' kind of woman who might even develop some of the same intellectual and emotional characteristics that she felt only men were entitled to display.

8. Some aspects of the social unconscious

When the group returned after the Xmas break, they reclaimed their sense of mature hope. They returned to Pandora's dream again and again. As spring approached, this dream became the basis for discussions of conflicts between Arabs and Jews in the Middle East, attempts to enter the Promised Land, the River Nile and the plagues, and the River Jordan.

It occurred to me that when a few months before I became defensively preoccupied with the work of Green on the dead mother, I was also attempting to work out tensions between green/envy and green/springtime and hopefulness. The group put frogs in my 'river', a symbol for mother, and, therefore, for the group and me, and this was a punishment for my enforced separations during holidays. Thus, Pandora's dream was a personal dream, as well as a dream dreamt for the group.

Following my interpretations of the 'river' as a symbol for mother and her body, ethnic group rivalry and sibling rivalry became the central focus of the group. A consensus was reached that in a way younger siblings were always both 'chosen' and 'little brothers', especially when they really were. In other words, the group began to consider the possibility that their preoccupations with sibling rivalry and gender identity reflected both their idiosyncratic concerns and personal histories, and the unconscious constraints of various social, cultural and political factors, not only in the 'Now and There', but also in the 'There and Then'. This was reflected in the connections that they made between how they had been influenced by World War II, and were now affected by the events in the Middle East.

Several members of the group wanted to discuss whether I was a Jew and what this meant in the group. For example, several members of the group acknowledged that when they were involved in scapegoating the small contra-group who tried to express their reservations about me as a group analyst and about the efficacy of group analysis in general, they had also experienced some anti-Semitic feelings. At this moment the contra-group were experienced as Jews, although it was known that I was myself a Jew. This was explored in terms of sibling rivalry and ambivalence towards rebellious sons, but slowly and eventually we came to feel that unconsciously the group was also enacting their perceptions of what had happened to Jews in Germany. It was accepted that following World War I, Germany experienced intensive and extensive aggregation based on various kinds of social insecurities, and as Germany shifted towards massification, various forms of aggression were directed at Jews and others who were described in terms of attacks on the mother-tongue, blackness, strange hair, bad smells, etc. Obviously, they had to be eliminated in order for massification to develop and offer its transient and illusionary sense of safety.

9. Summary

In this group vignette a patient with pronounced borderline disturbances personified a specific massification role as a defense against the anxieties associated with aggregation following an experience of failed dependency in connection with the holiday break. This enabled Pandora to become the focus of therapeutic attention in such a way that we could see how together we colluded in setting up situations that were potentially destructive based on the unconscious attempts to avoid anxieties of a particularly painful kind, as had happened very often in her own daily life in a particularly pathogenic family and during other phases of her life. The group helped me to have the space that I needed to understand my countertransference to Pandora. Several individuals were able to make connections between their own present functioning in the group and their previous experiences. Although Pandora had experienced a long period of psychoanalysis, and psychoanalytic psychotherapy, the quality of her experiences within the group was new, providing both an affect-laden experience of unconscious role creation and enactment, and a space for reflection. Reciprocity and complementarity were the basis for the development of the optimal cohesion of the therapeutic workgroup.

Eventually, Pandora left the group. I still see her occasionally. Many of her symptoms have abated. She has never established a relationship with one partner for more than a few months at a time, and she has not had a child. She has established a career, and has an active social life, perhaps too much so.

CONCLUDING COMMENTS

In this chapter I have outlined my theory of (ba) I:A/M, and have illustrated these processes with clinical data concerning the treatment of a particularly difficult and highly traumatized patient. I have also showed how a group can help the group analyst with troublesome countertransference processes, especially those that resonate to a predominant basic assumption. I have tried at least to indicate how the social unconscious is of continuing and constant relevance in clinical work.

It is incumbent upon the group analyst to do his very best to keep in mind the group as a whole, and to support the development of a mature work group whose members can see how they tend to collude with one another in the recreation of their respective traumatic experience. The group analyst must also keep himself in mind. Nonetheless, although very often the best policy is to contain and to hold, containment and holding are not always sufficient for the maintenance of the therapeutic process. It is also necessary to engage in interpretive analytical work, that is, both to stay with affects and to keep alive the reflective process.

Within relatively closed institutional settings such work can become almost impossible, mainly because the unconscious material is more highly amplified. Relationships among colleagues – nurses, doctors and managers, perhaps between people within the hospital and people within the referral system – are all affected by the projection of encapsulated fears of annihilation and related phenomena. Whatever the setting, it is essential to maintain a kind of mental and organizational hygiene in the face of this impossible work. I have in mind a hygiene in which the good, the resilient, the optimistic, the hopeful, the transcendent and the hardy prevail over the bad, the despondent, the pessimistic, and the despairing in connection with our inevitable failures to realize our highest aspirations for our patients and ourselves in our work.

REFERENCES

Alonso, A. and Rutan, J. S. (1990) 'Common Dilemmas in Combined Individual and Group Treatment', *Group*, 14: 5–12.

Billow, R. M. (2003) *Relational Group Psychotherapy: From Basic Assumptions to Passion*, London: Jessica Kingsley.

Bion, W. R. (1961) *Experiences in Groups and Other Papers*, London: Tavistock.

Caligor, J., Fieldsteel, N. D. and Brock, A. J. (1993) *Combining Individual and Group Therapy*, Northvale, NJ: Jason Aronson.

Fairbairn, W. R. (1952) *Psycho-Analytic Studies of the Personality*, London: Tavistock.

Freud. S. (1921) 'Group Psychology and the Analysis of the Ego', *Standard Edition*, 18: 67–144, London: Hogarth Press, 1964.

Gans, J. and Alonso, A. (1998) 'Difficult Patients: Their Construction in Group Therapy', *International Journal of Group Psychotherapy*, 48: 311–326.

Green, A. (1986) *On Private Madness*, London: Hogarth Press and The Institute of Psycho-Analysis.

Hirsch, I. (2003) 'Theory as Countertransference', *Journal of the American Psychoanalytic Association*, 51(Supplement): 181–202.

Hopper, E. (2003a) *The Social Unconscious: Selected Papers*, London: Jessica Kingsley.

Hopper, E. (2003b) *Traumatic Experience in the Unconscious Life of Groups*, London: Jessica Kingsley.

Hopper, E. (in press) 'Countertransference in the Treatment of Traumatized and Difficult Patients in Psychoanalysis Followed by Group Analysis: A Theoretical and Clinical Study of the Personification on Incohesion or (ba) I:A/M in the Unconscious Life of Groups', *The International Journal of Group Psychotherapy*.

Kauff, P. (1991) 'The Unique Contributions of Analytic Group Therapy to the Treatment of Preoedipal Character Pathology', in S. Tuttman (ed.), *Psychoanalytic Group Theory and Therapy*, Madison, CT: International Universities Press.

Kernberg, O. (1998) *Ideology, Conflict and Leadership in Groups and Organizations*, New Haven: Yale University Press.

Klein, G. S. (1976) *Psychoanalytic Theory: An Exploration of Essentials*, New York: International Universities Press.

Lawrence, W. G., Bain, A. and Gould, L. J. (1996) 'The Fifth Basic Assumption', *Free Associations*, 6, 37: 28–55 (reprinted in *Tongued with Fire: Groups in Experience*, London: Karnac Books, 2000).

Racker, H. (1968) *Transference and Countertransference*, New York: International Universities Press.

Turquet, P. (1975) 'Threats to Identity in the Large Group', in L. Kreeger (ed.), *The Large Group: Dynamics and Therapy*, London: Constable (reprinted in 1994, London: Karnac Books, pp. 87–144).

Chapter 8

Telephone, psychotherapy and the 21st century

Sharon Zalusky

Rebecca, a young analysand whom I have been seeing four times a week for seven years marries. Her commute to my office triples in time. Coming in four days a week, three hours on the road, a demanding job and a new marriage seems torturous. She doesn't want to cut down, but she cannot spend her whole life in a car. We agree to see each other three times a week in the office and once a week on the phone.

Annie applies to graduate school. She is placed on a wait list and is told that it is unlikely that she will be accepted this year. At the last minute, a space opens and she has an opportunity to pursue a dream. She doesn't want to leave her analysis yet she wants to pursue her career.

Ray, an unknown actor, lands a leading part in a movie that is filming outside of Los Angeles. He wants to continue his analysis on the telephone to help keep him grounded during this important, though stressful time in his life.

Diana because of serious complications during pregnancy is required to stay in bed. She feels she is in crisis. She wants to continue her analysis.

John, now 22 and away at college in Australia is a young man whom I first started treating when he was 14. Each developmental step has been met with reluctance. Recently, unexpectedly, I turn on my computer to find an e-mail from him. He tells me he loves going to school abroad, but finds himself fantasizing about one of his male friends. He does not know what to make of it. He finds it both exciting and terrifying. He wants to know if we can communicate via e-mail. I recommend the old-fashioned way, sessions via the telephone until he returns.

(Zalusky 2003)

It is obvious we are living in a rapidly changing world where advances in telecommunications, travel, and biotechnology are changing the way our patients and we live, travel, and communicate with each other. Technologies expand our boundaries by creating an extension of our bodies and/or our physical presence (Rifkin 1998). The world, as we know it, is getting smaller and closer, and in the process we are becoming more interconnected and interrelated. Technologies are impacting almost every aspect of society, including our relationship to our self and to others. It is no wonder in this changing world that psychoanalysis and psychoanalytic psychotherapy have overwhelming shifted their focus from a one-person psychology to a relational psychology (Friedman 2004). Being wired is being connected, albeit in new and interesting ways.

Over the years I have pondered the use of the telephone and its meaning in clinical practice both for the patient and the therapist. Our first connection with our patients and theirs with us, more often than not, takes place either on the telephone or on voicemail. The telephone is ubiquitous. It has become an essential part of our clinical life. We use the telephone as an extension of our office and our self.

The telephone itself has become mobile and unwired. With global satellite technology we can take our telephone along with us wherever we are in the world. It no longer needs to be situated in our office, but can literally go where we go. In practical terms you call my unique number and I have the potential of responding, if I desire, whether I am in Los Angeles, New York, London, Paris, Rome, or Beijing, or whether you are. With this fact our notion of availability expands. Our ability to simulate ourselves in different forms (telephone, e-mail, videoconferencing) at different times opens up the field in which we, as therapists or patients, can and do operate.

As the technology changes, our attitudes about the telephone also change. For example, when I started my analytic training, almost everyone had an answering service. Today such a practice would be anachronistic. It would feel intrusive to have a third person, a stranger, respond to the need of our patients. We would question confidentiality, the propriety of it all. But twenty years ago it was common practice.

By now we have grown accustomed to our voicemail. Not only is voicemail used for messages, but also some patients call us knowing that we will not answer. They do not need to talk to us directly, nor might they even want us to know that they called. They need only to hear our simulated voices in order to assure themselves that we continue to exist in our shared absence. Our patients may use our voicemail in an effort to self-soothe. We may never learn directly about that need, or the way in which a particular patient gratifies it, but that does not stop the fact that a form of technology, may be used as transitional space (Aronson 2000) and has the potential of helping certain patients manage their own anxiety during times of separation. As clinicians we have grown to appreciate voicemail's potential auxiliary function in the psychotherapeutic treatment. As we incorporate it into our practice, we also integrate it into our theory of change. I believe for some patients voicemail may be used to reinforce a budding inner representation of the available (soothing) therapist.

At times technology is accepted by one element of society before it has truly been incorporated into the social consciousness of the whole of society. E-mail is a good example. At first I was taken aback when I would turn on my computer and find e-mails from any number of my younger patients requesting scheduling changes. Initially I saw their e-mails as a resistance to intimacy until I realized that e-mail is our young patients' mode of quick information exchange. E-mail to them is like voicemail is to me and the answering service was to my older colleagues. Society changes and our mode of communication changes and with it expectations change.

As my experience working on the telephone has increased and I have seen positive results with a number of patients, my attitude about the telephone in psychoanalysis and psychotherapy has significantly loosened. Originally when I started writing about the use of the telephone in psychoanalysis, I did so in an apologetic manner (Zalusky 1998). At that time there had only been one article written about its use in psychoanalysis (Lindon 1988). I underlined the conflictual nature of telephone analysis, because it almost always represented a therapeutic compromise. In the land of the ideal, continuing on the telephone would never be the treatment of choice. However, we rarely live in the land of the ideal. Treatments are inherently complex and messy. Certain patients have special life histories that require special adjustment in technique. When treatments are long, life often intervenes in our work and we need to come up with flexible and creative solutions.

Up until recently, there seemed to have been a don't ask, don't tell policy about analysts' use of the telephone in clinical practice.[1] Privately one would hear as an aside, 'I have to go now, I am about to do a phone session with a patient.' However, that seemed to be the extent to which this matter was ever discussed. It was as if telephone sessions were to be revealed, if at all, only to one's closest friends and colleagues. The subject of the telephone in analytic practice was not brought up in seminars. Nor was it ever written about in case studies. It was clear that our past traditions and prejudices were preventing many analysts from openly considering telephone analysis as a potentially viable treatment option at the right time with the right patient for the right reasons.

The topic of the telephone in psychotherapy and psychoanalysis has recently moved out from behind the closed booth into the open. As of today there have been several articles (Leffert 2003; Zalusky 1998, 2003), an

---

1 It may be true that analysts have been reluctant to talk about almost any deviation from the traditional psychoanalytic frame.

edited book, *Use of the Telephone in Psychotherapy* (Aronson 2000), and a dialogue written in *International Psychoanalysis* (2003), the official news-letter of the International Psychoanalytical Association, on the topic of telephone analysis. There have been panels, and there have been presen-tations at both the meeting of the American Psychoanalytic Association and Division 39 of the American Psychological Association, as well as at a number of local societies.

I believe we have come to the point where many clinicians would agree that the telephone can be an important and effective tool in psychotherapy and psychoanalysis, even though the majority of our work still takes place in the traditional venue of our office. The loudest of the critics against using the telephone in clinical practice admit to never having tried it. Their arguments are often based solely on abstract theoretical concerns. Though their concerns may be interesting, they do not seem to take into account the contemporary world in which we live.

THE PROCESS: SIMILARITIES AND DIFFERENCES

Many of the authors who have written about telephone analysis (Lindon 1988; Leffert 2003) have stressed the similarities, without adequately discussing the differences between the process that takes place in the office and the process that takes place over the telephone. I believe that is because these pioneers were concerned with demonstrating effectiveness and felt that was the best way to put forth their argument. I take a different tack. I believe, embedded in patient and analyst communications is often a recog-nition, conscious or unconscious, of what each gains and loses, the feelings evoked and the meanings attributed by doing analysis with only data from the verbal realm available. By being sensitive to what we are losing, we help our patients be more open about their own feelings of loss. We find that by analyzing the differences, the loss, that often they lead us, as we might expect, into the internal world of our patients and by doing so we add to our therapeutic effectiveness.

The two forms of treatment, though very similar, could never be the same. Because we do not have the physical presence of the other available, each participant of the psychotherapeutic dyad has to create and sustain mental representations of the other in fantasy. Because the work takes place without the visual presence of the other, something interesting has the potential of happening. The transference, rather than being diluted as many have suggested, may instead be intensified, because it develops without the benefit of reality interfering with the transference (and I add counter-transference) distortion. The analyst in fantasy and the patient in fantasy are never the same as those two that have met in the office. On the telephone we create a new analytic dyad. Along with it, a new analytic process emerges. If, as Freud (1913) suggests, the couch induces a regression in which the analyst as a person does not interfere with development of the transference, then the telephone should be a vehicle par excellence in this regard. Without the visual interference the transference is allowed to ripen. It is not until we see each other again that these fantasy distortions actually stand out. In order to take advantage of this phenomenon I have found it important to schedule occasional office visits. Elsewhere (Zalusky 2003) I reported the following example:

> It had been 8 months since I last saw Rebecca. During this time, Rebecca openly explored her feelings about me in the transference. She dealt frequently with her experience of not being in the room with me, and her great loss of not having me literally there to see her. Rebecca would ask, 'How can I know if you are paying attention to me. If I was in the room with you, I could turn around and see you looking at me.' Reliving these feelings in the transference, allowed her to remember her childhood experience of believing her parents, though physically present, never really saw her. During this time, we both felt we were doing productive analytic work. And we were. Yet, it was not until we actually laid eyes on each other during an office visit that it became clear that another powerful aspect of the transference remained hidden from both of us. Upon seeing me, I noticed Rebecca was visibly disturbed and I asked her about it. 'You look so different. You aren't my analyst who's with me on the telephone,' Rebecca stated. 'In my mind you are so much older than you really are. *My analyst* is old and frumpy. You are neither.' We were able to use this opportunity to understand why she needed to create me in that manner. She revealed to herself and to me how she doubted her own attractiveness. Instead of feeling competitive, she turned the tables in her mind. It was much less painful, Rebecca imagined, than dealing with her own sense of inadequacy. That evening she dreamt that I took her shopping for bras. She associated to how her mother used to cut her hair short when she was young. People often confused her for a boy. In fact, her mother hid her own femininity to the world. Secretly, she wished I could teach her how to be a woman.

(Zalusky 2003: 15)

As we worked together again in the office, Rebecca and I were struck by the poignancy of our physical reconnection. Rebecca could literally see how she created me in fantasy. She did not need me to interpret her transference. It stood out for her in bas-relief. She and I both were curious to understand the reasons behind her desire to keep me in fantasy the way she did.

Another interesting aspect of telephone work is that in many ways therapy taking place on the telephone focuses, concretizes, and condenses such basic analytic issues as separation, loss, availability, the needs of both patient and analyst and the analytic frame and deviations from it. The patient does not need to wonder whether or not you will remember them when they are not with you. Each time they talk to you on the phone, they remember that you remember. Hearing the voice of the other, repeatedly over time, while there and not there, helps to create a mental representation of the caring other. The telephone serves as transitional space. It may very well function for some patients who are in the process of developing object constancy as an adaptive defense against separation anxiety.

There are obviously some problems working on the telephone. One that requires special attention for some patients who have difficulty taking care of themselves is helping them provide a safe environment to do the work on the telephone (a quiet private room where they can be free to say whatever is on their mind). We are used to providing that for our patients. Recently I have had patients call me from their car. Just as I would not knowingly allow a patient to come to session drunk, I will not have sessions while a patient is driving. It is certainly not safe and definitely not therapeutic. One difficult, angry patient of mine who does not regularly have phone sessions called me from the car when it was clear he would not be able to make it to the office on time. Instead of falling apart and disintegrating which he often did when he feared that he was going to miss time with me, I suggested to him, 'Why not do something different? Call me when you get home (which was a few minutes away) and we can do a phone session.' He did, but initially could not let go of his anxiety. When I asked him about it, in an outburst he yelled at me that he did not want to dirty up his house with our work. Naturally his remark became grist for the mill and also helped me to understand why some disturbed patients cannot tolerate working on the phone.

Clearly working on the telephone is not for everybody. I believe it is most appropriate for patients whose intense or regressed transferences make it impossible to terminate or transfer without causing some degree of harm. It may also be extremely important to patients whose early life was characterized by inconsistent and emotionally unavailable caregivers. To have one special person witnessing one's life through disappointments and victories can be extremely meaningful. The ability to maintain consistent emotional contact with the same analyst, rather than interrupting or terminating treatment, has the potential of creating an analytic space where the patient's transference could be analyzed and worked through. As more than one patient has told me, you are not interchangeable. Therapists are not like goldfish.

One of the benefits having done telephone analysis is that I feel comfortable using the telephone with certain patients who have a difficult time with self-regulation and ultimately intimacy. Many of these patients have had extremely complicated and traumatic early life experiences and losses.

For these severely traumatized people the telephone may allow a necessary space in which they can begin to tackle the fears associated with intimacy.

I was referred Margie, 25, from a colleague in another city who warned me that though Margie is a delightful young woman, she rarely came to sessions. In the first session, I meet Margie, this bright, vibrant, adorable person who gives me a history that is packed with death, illness much pain and anguish. As a child Margie suffered from early deprivation at the hands of very nice parents who were struggling with their own extraordinary grief and illnesses. They certainly did not mean not to be there for their baby daughter, but people cannot help the cards they were dealt.

Margie and I arranged to see each other three times a week. For many months Margie's treatment was mostly an analytic game of hide-and-seek. Margie would disappear and I would call and try to find her. She would be happy to be found and would tell me that she meant to come to session, but she was sleeping. No matter what hour of the day or afternoon, she could and usually did sleep through our appointment. Then one day I tried to engage her on the telephone. She spoke to me of her difficulty taking care of herself. She explained she slept when people were up and was up when the rest of the world slept. She did not eat normally. She smoked cigarettes and self-medicated. Nothing about her was regulated. At the end of her telephone session I told her that I would really like to see her in person. She agreed to come to the next session. Though extremely late, she arrived nonetheless. For many more years, I had to live with the uncertainty. Sometimes Margie came to sessions (always late). Other times she slept through them. And still other times Margie, from her point of view, had more pressing matters that kept her away from me, her therapist. I would interpret to her that I thought she was doing to me what had been done to her. She never knew when her parents would be available either emotionally or physically. I too would wait for her not knowing if today was the day Margie would come to her therapy session or not. The interpretation seemed to have a far greater impact on me than on her. It seemed to help me be accepting of her.

At some point when I became more important to Margie, she would call after her missed sessions, usually at two or three in the morning, to apologize for not being there. I would return the call later and leave her a message letting her know that I hoped to see her at our next session. As time went on and her affection for me grew, she would leave me messages before her missed session, apologizing in advance for not being able to make our appointment. At some point we would always reconnect: at times on the phone, at times in the office. Then Margie began to call me at the exact hour of her session. We would have a telephone session.

After having sessions with her on the telephone for a period of time, I could feel our connection was deepening. Margie was very attached to me both in her absence and her presence. One day she called and I took it as an opportunity to up the ante. Instead of having a telephone session, I told her I thought she should probably come to session today in person. She stated the obvious, 'By the time I get there I will only have five minutes.' I replied, 'Five minutes in person, I think it would be worth it.' Margie did not complain, instead she got in her car and drove to my office. She arrived with a smile on her face. It was obvious Margie was happy to see me, but also pleased that I wanted to see her. Sometimes she would use her sessions to tell me about what was happening in her life. Intermittently we would do some very deep painful work and predictably Margie would then disappear again. For a while she was coming to her sessions three times a week, but for many reasons, some of them internal others external, she would become overwhelmed and the process would have to start over again – with the hide-and-seek, telephone calls, short sessions. Recently, she went through a serious crisis in which she disappeared as she had in the beginning. We now schedule sessions for five days a week. Margie says that helps because when she leaves she does not feel so abandoned by me. Interestingly enough, with the security of the five-days-a-week treatment, she has dared to express her anger and her disappointment in me.

I report this vignette, because I cannot imagine how one could treat Margie, or many of our patients like Margie, without the telephone. Without the telephone her self-imposed separations most likely would have been experienced as my total abandonment of her. The telephone allowed me to seek her out, which was for her a necessary condition to do the work. The telephone allows her to know that I continue to exist, even in her absence, and, more important to her, that I continue to care about her as a person, not just as a patient. The telephone is used as a way in which Margie can control and modulate a level of connectedness that she is able to tolerate. When the office sessions become too much, she can talk on the telephone. When the telephone sessions are too much, we can touch base. When she hides, I can find her. With the telephone we are able to reach out and touch each other metaphorically.

CONCLUSION

Initially many analysts, like myself, were apologetic about the use of the telephone in clinical practice. Our past traditions and prejudices were preventing many of our colleagues from openly discussing deviations from the traditional frame. Because we never exposed our more creative approaches to our disapproving colleagues, we were unable to evaluate the effectiveness of our approaches or the limits from which we could generalize from one patient to the next. However, times really are changing. Gabbard and Westin (2003) wisely conclude in their article in *the International Journal of Psychoanalysis*, 'Rethinking Therapeutic Action', that analysts must stop asking whether something is analytic, but rather whether it is therapeutic. Reviewing the literature on therapeutic action, they conclude what most sensitive clinicians already know, that there is not one type of therapeutic action, no matter how complex the theory, but many.

Today the telephone is viewed by many as an important tool in our therapeutic armamentarium. Depending on the need of the client (and sometimes the need of the analyst) the telephone has the potential of both creating and removing space.

We are living in the era of technology. Rapid changes in the way we communicate are having enormous rippling effects throughout society. As therapists we have the opportunity of using advances in communication to help people we might not have been able to reach before. If we take as a given the premise that we therapists are interested in helping our patients deal with their suffering and lead more meaningful lives, then I believe we must be open to unusual circumstances. Originally, I could not have imagined how a therapist could ever do telephone work with a patient he or she has never met. Then I read a paper (Gelman 2001) in which an analyst was contacted by a person living in Asia, where there were no therapists who spoke English. The patient was in crisis but was not moving to Los Angeles for another three months. Gelman decided that the best option was for them to begin a treatment over the telephone, even though they never had met, and when the patient moved, they would, if it seemed to be the right decision, continue in person in the office – unusual; yet it worked.

For me psychoanalysis remains a transformative experience for the patient, for the analyst, and for culture in general. It goes without saying that when we transform our patients, we are transformed in the process. The aim of analysis or any psychoanalytic psychotherapy concerns itself with new ways of relating to oneself, to others and most broadly to the world in general. It begins often with new ways of relating within the analytic relationship. To help our patients adapt to a changing world, we too need to take advantage of what that world can offer us. How can our theory be the only thing that stays static?

REFERENCES

Aronson, J. (2000) 'Use of the Telephone as a Transitional Space', in J. Aronson (ed.), *Use of the Telephone in Psychotherapy*, Northvale, NJ: Jason Aronson, pp. 129–150.

Aronson, J. (2000) *Use of the Telephone in Psychotherapy*, Northvale, NJ: Jason Aronson.

Freud, S. (1913) 'On Beginning the Treatment', *Standard Edition*, 12: 123–144, London: Hogarth Press, 1964.

Friedman, H. J. (2004) 'Transference in Relational Psychoanalysis: Defeating the

Legacy of Drive Theory', presented at the International Psychoanalytic Association meetings in New Orleans, March 13, 2004.

Gabbard, G. and Westin, D. (2003) 'Rethinking Therapeutic Action', *International Journal of Psychoanalysis*, 84(4): 823–841.

Gelman, M. H. (2001) 'The Use of the Telephone in Analysis: Therapeutic Compromise or Primary Modality of Treatment', presented at the Sandor Ferenzi Conference in Budapest Hungary, February 23, 2001.

Leffert, M. (2003) 'Analysis and Psychotherapy by Telephone: Twenty Years of Clinical Experience', *Journal of the American Psychoanalytic Association*, 51: 101–130.

Lindon, J. A. (1988) 'Psychoanalysis by Telephone', *Bulletin of the Menninger Clinic*, 52: 521–528.

Rifkin, J. (1998) *The Biotech Century: Harnessing the Gene and Remaking the World*, New York: Tarcher/Putnam.

Zalusky, S. (1998) 'Telephone Analysis: Out of Sight But Not Out of Mind', *Journal of the American Psychoanalytic Association*, 46: 1221–1242.

Zalusky, S. (2003) 'Dialogue: Telephone Analysis', *International Psychoanalysis, Newsletter of the IPA*, 11(2): 13–17.

Chapter 9

Conquering geographic space: teaching psychoanalytic psychotherapy and infant observation by video link

David E. Scharff

This chapter reports on a project teaching students in psychoanalytic psychotherapy who are at a significant geographic remove from each other and from the teachers from whom they wish to learn. I will report on the establishment of a videoconference capacity in four centers, discuss briefly some of the technical challenges the equipment and technology pose, the opportunities and challenges to in-depth communication, and some of the dynamics that have emerged in our early experience with the technology. Examples illustrate some dynamics of teaching through this medium to overcome the barriers of geographic separation with large and small group seminars, and in long-term group supervision.

Many students want to learn psychoanalysis and psychoanalytic psychotherapy but live and work at a prohibitive distance from the centers of training. The barrier of geographic space has historically posed a major obstacle to the teaching and learning of psychoanalytic theory and therapy for those areas without analysts. Students in such areas have either been precluded from training, or have only been able to train by dint of great personal sacrifice. In addition, some of the teachers or schools of analysis, and some specialized analytic skills exist only in certain centers, making access to those teachers difficult and available only by special, often expensive, arrangement. Modern technology offers to change many aspects of this situation, and perhaps ultimately to alter the landscape of training. There have already been reports of psychoanalyses and psychotherapies conducted by telephone, and occasionally by video link (Aronson 2000; see also Zalusky, Chapter 8 in this volume). There are also reports of supervision by video link (Arlene Richards, personal communication) and of online discussion groups and courses that offer a chance for students to communicate with teachers and other students at great distance (Sebek, 2001). Perhaps none of this is surprising in our era of information technology and of rapidly expanding communication. However, to our knowledge, there is no report of training in psychoanalysis or psychoanalytic psychotherapy that experiments with the use of the most advanced methodologies in face-to-face communication in real time across large distances.

Part of the wonder of using the technology of live point-to-point video communication is how rapidly it allows participants to feel that they know each other even when they have never been in the room together. Many of us have now had the experience of meeting for the first time after participating in videoconference seminars, and have discovered that we feel we do know each other in a way that holds up over time. If anything, the video link seems to heighten and intensify experience in the way that a special and highly anticipated learning experience can also do. For many of us, such conditions serve to hone attention and amplify ordinary situations, serving perhaps to idealize opportunities that might seem ordinary in ordinary circumstances. With time and experience, the situation tends to normalize, but has so far retained a special residue that helps participants to tolerate the technical complications and occasional disappointments that attend the process.

ESTABLISHING THE VIDEOCONFERENCE TECHNOLOGY

After more than two years of deliberation and pilot tests, the training organization of which I am co-director agreed to invest in equipment that would let us make regular contact with our programs in Salt Lake City, Long Island and Panama City, Republic of Panama. We had also been in negotiation with the Tavistock Clinic in London, where the Chief Executive Officer had bought video equipment to support the clinic's role as an international training institution. The work reported below is taken principally from varying uses of these sites, supported by working partnerships with faculty of our own programs and of the Tavistock Clinic.

I do not want to suggest that one can walk into using this medium without any difficulty. There are technical difficulties and adjustments in the use of this equipment. We had early frustrations requiring tolerance and help from faculty, students and staff. A running-in period allowed us to become comfortable with the equipment, and we needed initial adjustments that were made fairly easily by the training provided in live-time by the vendor, and by the help desk that was always available. In undertaking this kind of venture, the technical difficulties should not be ignored. In our experience they can be dealt and lived with, but participants should be forewarned and ready to put up with some degree of difficulty, more during the early adjustment phase than later. The intrinsic value of the project needs to be sufficient to compensate for initial annoyances and interruptions. Our students' strong support of this way of working has gotten us through.

The first project I will use in illustration was a seminar in infant observation run by an experienced child psychotherapist at the Tavistock Clinic in London, Jeanne Magagna. This method of observing infants in their families has been a mainstay of psychoanalytic and analytic psychotherapy training in Britain for many years (Miller *et al.* 1989). Let me give two vignettes from this seminar with the lessons we have learned from early in the process.

The first comes from the initial meeting of the seminar, in which Ms Magagna introduced the methods of infant observation as developed in London and especially at the Tavistock Clinic. In this method of studying infant development, the student makes weekly hour-long naturalistic observations of an infant at home, after which the student writes up the observation from memory, including personal reactions to the baby, the family, and the experience. There is no intervention, except in cases of extreme need, neglect or abuse. This exercise in observation and reflection without action provides first-hand data for learning about child development including the influence of parents and family. It also focuses on the use of the self as an observing and experiencing instrument in the presence of the infant mental state, a valuable preparation for working with countertransference in the conduct of psychotherapy and psychoanalysis.

In this first meeting of the seminar, Ms Magagna reviewed the methodology of conducting infant observation that the students had already read about (Miller *et al.* 1989), and then surveyed the anxieties of students as they contemplated recruiting and interviewing families. In order to detoxify anticipatory anxiety, she used role play to rehearse the first interview with the family. She had often done this before in small seminars, but this was her first experience at using it to overcome the barriers of spatial separation between seminar participants. She made time for hearing the participants' worries and ambivalence about asking families to let observers view their babies – babies that have usually not yet been born at the time the student approaches the mother. In order to get used to communicating across a distance of five thousand miles, the teacher in a room in London suggested that the student who would role-play the potential observer should be in Washington, and those playing the potential parents be in Salt Lake. Then she asked the other seminar members to report on their impression of the feelings of each role-playing participant, rather like the 'double' in psycho-drama who speaks for the inner thoughts of a participant. While this method may seem contrived to the psychoanalytic therapist, on this occa-sion it served two purposes admirably. First, it let the group members put themselves in the shoes of all participants of an observation, the observer and the parents. (In this case, the baby had not been born yet. Presumably, in another case, someone could have also role-played a baby.) But more importantly for our purposes in convening a seminar by video link, it placed students at sites that were geographically remote from each other in an intimate exchange as they conjectured about the psychology of the unfamiliar infant observation situation. The role play was helpful practice for the new venture, to be sure, but it was even more effective in providing a bond for the learning project between students not in the same room. They found they were able to talk across the distance, use each other's empathy, correct each other's perceptions that seemed inaccurate, and enjoy the relief of finding shared anxieties.

In the next meeting, one student reported her first observation, as she would have done in an ordinary infant observation seminar with all students in the same room. Other students had not yet found babies to observe. This focus on one infant let that group also secure their bond, and learn about beginnings together. Each week, before that first student in Washington reported, Ms Magagna asked a student in Salt Lake to be ready to review the observations from the prior meeting of the seminar and give her own understanding of issues. This innovation provided for active participation at both sites. From this point, Ms Magagna worked with the students in Salt Lake to support their recruitment of families for observation, and when they soon found a first one, they felt a new sense of balance between the two sites. Soon there were infants being observed in both sites, and the two subgroups came to feel like equal participants in the shared project.

At this point, the story of the seminar becomes more or less the story of an ordinary seminar teaching this particular psychoanalytic method, including any usual use of group dynamic interpretation to facilitate the study task. My second vignette concerns the study of that first baby, a girl I'll call Michele, who was born into a family where her mother's attention was at first distracted because of the rivalrous importunities of the 2-year-old brother. The seminar participants in both sites experienced the drama of Michele's fight for room to come to life in a family that was ambivalent about giving her space. It was difficult for the group to tolerate hearing reports of the inattention of a mother preoccupied with her demanding older boy, who at times seemed to them to be the villain of the piece. Nevertheless, the liveliness of the entire family and of the student who conducted the observation infused the group with energy and carried their hopes not only for the infant's development, but for their own progress and learning as well. This led to some idealization of the process. Soon baby Michele settled in to secure her place with her mother by competing quietly but competently with her brother, who then seemed less like a giant and imposing ogre, and more like a healthy and slightly anxious 2-year-old.

In a parallel way, the Salt Lake seminar group felt like a second child who did not have her own space. At first they did not have a baby of their own to observe, and so they had to fight for space to relate to Jeanne Magagna. There were more students in Washington, and I was there with my own previous experience of infant observation, while the faculty member in Salt Lake, although skilled and enthusiastic, was inexperienced in the teaching of infant observation. Even though Ms Magagna adroitly gave Salt Lake its turn and paid kind and dutiful attention to students there, they were younger and lesser sibs. It was only as they began to present their own observations that they came into their own. I could see the parallel to the way baby Michele claimed a space with her mother, and the relief and pleasure the mother took in making a more secure bond with the infant, just as now Ms Magagna and the Salt Lake students made a more robust working bond for which I could now see that the entire group had been saving space.

In many ways, the dynamics of this seminar divided by 5000 miles closely resembled the dynamics of any group containing subgroups, of any such seminar teaching psychoanalytic concepts and method. The difference is that the use of the videoconference technology and the existence of two subgroups amplify certain aspects both of the group's dynamics and of the case or situation being examined. These can be understood and worked with using the same internal monitoring processes that an experienced teacher uses in ordinary teaching of a seminar.

USING VIDEOCONFERENCE FOR A SEMINAR IN FOUR CITIES

The next example of the use of videoconference equipment to teach psychoanalysis and analytic psychotherapy comes from a lecture/workshop given in February, 2001, by Anne Alvarez of the Tavistock Clinic, a renowned teacher of work with autistic, developmentally delayed and severely disturbed children, as described in her classic book, *Live Company* (1993). Teaching from London she was linked by video with approximately 30 students gathered in Washington, DC, Salt Lake City, Utah, and Panama City, Panama. It began at 2 p.m. in London, which was 9 a.m. in Washington and Panama, and 7 a.m. in Salt Lake City.

For the first hour, Mrs Alvarez gave a lecture on a conceptual scheme for differentiating levels of interpretive intervention in patients with differing levels of illness. Drawn from her work with autistic and developmentally delayed children, this lecture sketched an innovative framework for kinds of interventions that promote self-observation, psychic integration, transferential interpretation and genetic reconstruction. During and after the lecture, students interacted with her through questions and comments.

In the second hour, a student presented a case of a mildly autistic boy in analytic therapy. The student had the case in weekly supervision with Mrs Alvarez by telephone, but they had never met face-to-face. Their way of working in the video group supervision demonstrated the rapport they had already established, and their pleasure in seeing each other for the first time was obvious. The boy was articulate with that brand of exaggerated and awkward insight not unusual in some mildly autistic children who arrive at ordinary insight with an intelligence that astounds their therapists. The therapist's process notes therefore provided moments of high entertainment. For instance, at one point the boy, who had come into the session with his fly open, talked about his father's pride in his 22–foot-long car, exclaiming that there was no way that car could be that long. The therapist said to him that perhaps he was thinking of other things that might be longer than someone would expect. The boy agreed, astonished that she would know that, but was unable to bring himself to say the word. After waiting, the therapist said, 'Like penises?' 'That's it,' said the boy, 'but don't worry. I won't tell anyone you said that word.'

When the therapist read this part, the group at her site in Washington immediately burst into laughter, and on the screen, one could see the other sites begin laughing a split second later. The pleasure and responsiveness among all four sites was obvious on the screen. At the end of the session, after the therapist had made another interpretation that met with the boy's approval, she announced it was time to stop. 'OK,' he said. 'I'll see you next time. And I want to congratulate you on your psychic powers today.' Again the three groups and the teacher burst into laughter a split second apart, and the mood of delight sparked by a wonderful session, the kind that brightens a child therapist's heart, was palpable across the vast space – 5000 miles of live communication. Then discussion of the case resumed, and Mrs Alvarez discussed the boy's situation and the therapist's handling of his internal issues and particularly his transference to her.

In this situation, we were able to demonstrate that intense learning and sharing can take place across sites, producing a teaching experience that is in many ways indistinguishable from ordinary analytic case conferences. Students can communicate the intricacies of analytic process, carry on discussion that is rich in affect as well as intellectual understanding, and can profit from a teacher who would otherwise be unavailable to them. While this particular group supervision was entertaining, what is most notable about it for our interest here is the ordinary aspects – the ease of students' communication with each other and the teacher, and the satisfaction the teacher felt with the teaching and learning situation.

TEACHING ABOUT VIDEOCONFERENCING ACROSS GEOGRAPHIC SEPARATION

We had occasion to travel to the Tavistock Clinic to present this work. While the Tavistock had the equipment, few of their staff had so far been able to bring themselves to use it. To dramatize the live quality of the medium, we asked some of our students in Washington to join us live. Sitting in our conference room in Washington beginning at 6:30 in the morning, they joined us live throughout the presentation in London that began at 11:30

a.m. there. The Washington students were able to see for the first time the edited video we showed in London at the same time the group in London saw it, a video that showed the examples I have described above. The London group expressed some interest and enthusiasm, commented on their own resistance as being typically British and in the nature of an analytic conservatism. They also spoke helpfully of an idealization of the process that seems to energize it in ways that analytic process can also be idealized, and that should be taken into account in its use. The most dramatic moment occurred when a member of the London audience said that she felt there was a kind of unreality to the medium, a way in which people on the video screen felt to her as if they weren't quite there. 'I think I resent that,' one of the Washington students spoke up. 'I feel very much that I'm here!' The suddenness of the response caught the woman in London and the entire group off guard, and made the point that real people experienced themselves in direct communication with us as immediately as if in the room.

AN EXAMPLE FROM GROUP SUPERVISION

For two years, a group of six therapists from one our institute's 'satellite programs' in a geographically distant city had been meeting with me for twice-monthly supervision by video link. Each meeting was two and a half hours. Each participant had an hour for the group to discuss their case once every six weeks, and that left thirty minutes of general group discussion, which usually included time for the group to work with their own process in the mode of the affective learning groups developed at our institute (Scharff and Scharff 2000). They were close colleagues before the supervision, and so from the beginning they had been able to share relevant personal material in the group in order to explore the resonance of such material with the supervised cases. Such events were shared occasionally during the case presentations, or in the group affective process usually held during last part of the meetings.

On this day, it was Sherry's turn to present. She began by telling a dream she thought pertained to supervision. 'I was sitting with you (DES) on the patio of a restaurant with your wife and 7-year-old granddaughter. You had stitches on your face and forehead, and your wife also had stitches and obvious recent scars on her face. I wondered if I should bring it up with you. Finally I asked, and you said, "A month ago there was a terrible accident, but we're recovering." It seemed OK to discuss, but I felt badly as we went on. Behind me someone leaned over a balcony, smiling at me, like "Have a nice dinner." I thought that person was you too, but it couldn't have been. Then I was awakened by thunder.'

Sherry said she has a patient who was hit by a train. The accident had scarred her face. She also thought the dream pertained to the fact that because she had missed the previous supervision, she had gone a month without meeting with me and the group. She missed the group, and thought that it had been also a longer time since all members of the group were present at the same time. One of the members, Julia, had twins recently, and she had paid her a visit, but worried that this new mother wouldn't have time to continue the group supervision. Another member said he also wondered if Julia would rejoin the group, and Julia acknowledged the internal debate she had experienced about rejoining. Her life had changed altogether – dramatically like the train wreck connected to Sherry's dream, only in a positive way. Sherry said the dream also made her aware of wanting grandchildren herself, but, she said with humor, 'My own children aren't ready to oblige me just yet.' Another member, Kathy, said that this group supervision is where we discuss scars, and where she often also wonders about the safety of revealing herself here. Sherry agreed that she also shared the quandary about whether to present a case that had not gone particularly well, exposing her own scars to the group and to me. She said, 'I felt I needed the help with that patient and I didn't know how to get it safely.'

This discussion had taken about fifteen minutes, when Sherry now proceeded to present her continuing case. He is a man with significant trauma history, much improved. The wife has areas of difficulty, too, but generally hides behind the husband and acts as though all the problems are his. Sherry sees the man individually weekly and meets with him and his wife every other week. We have discussed this arrangement, which the group and I support given the needs of the case. Sherry apologized profusely for not having prepared an individual session. 'All I have is a rather ordinary, not very interesting couple session. Nothing earth-shattering.'

The session opened with the patient saying he felt deflated because he had been unable to surprise his wife as he had wished. He had ordered a satellite dish for her, hoping it would be installed in time for a special annual program not carried on regular channels, but this week he had to tell her about the surprise as she was making plans to watch the program at her mother's house. The wife said, 'I really like that program and want to watch it every year. We haven't had cable installed in our new house, but once he told me about his gift, I was fine planning to watch it at home.' The man said he did have an ulterior motive. He also wanted to help his wife be less bound to her mother and be with him more. She said that was fine with her.

Sherry paused in her presentation for group discussion. Members of the group noted the positive change in quality of this couple's work, from a time when the couple's material was shot through with effects of the husband's early trauma. This so-called ordinary material seemed to them to reflect both the individual's and couple's progress. In this material, he had expected her to be disappointed and angry, while she had been able gently to hold him psychologically. The scars had faded for him and for them, like the scars in Sherry's own opening dream. They noted the resonance of Sherry's dream with the treatment. The couple is expecting their own first child, a kind of therapeutic grandchild for Sherry, when she is still attuned to their scars. They liked the way this 'ordinary' material from the opening of the session demonstrated individual, couple and family growth, a fading of the scars on every level.

Sherry resumed. In the session, the man now began to reflect on his wife's TV watching. She will watch anything, when much of the time he would like her to do things with him. He feels defeated when she seems to disappear into the TV. The wife is a bit defensive, saying she thought her TV-watching had been better lately. The husband started to cry when Sherry asked if he would be able to negotiate with his wife about watching TV. Sherry asked, 'Are you afraid the relationship won't survive if you ask her to watch less TV, that she won't love you enough to give it up?' The man said that's true, that he didn't feel he could negotiate at all about TV. The wife now said, 'Of course you can ask me, and I'll turn it off. There's only one show a week that's important to me, and I can give up all the others. But I know there are other things you do for me that are about your fear I won't love you. Like when we're out for dinner, you save the last good bite of your food for me, or push dessert on me even if I don't want it.'

A member of the supervision group interrupted Sherry here to remember the wife's eating disorder, noting that the husband was doing a mild version of what the wife's mother had done to her chronically, pushing unwanted food on her. Sherry hadn't noticed that echo, and thanked him for calling her attention to the link. After brief discussion, she returned to the session. She had asked the husband why he offered his wife the 'best food' in that way. He said, 'I want her to feel that she loves me.' The wife answered, 'You're very generous with me. I want to do things for you, too.' The couple went on to discuss the way his mother was so awful to both of them, that they could see this would lead to his worry that the wife would treat him badly. The wife said, 'Your mother dismisses you and me, too.' The man grew openly sad and wiped tears from his eyes. The session was almost over. He began to write Sherry a check, noting he had not paid her in some time, and said, 'This isn't much, but there's more coming soon.' Sherry said in summary, 'It felt good! They talked about the core of his fear, and she was gentle and responsive.'

The group noted the continuation of the trusting feeling in the session leading to the linking of the husband's fear of loss of love and the relationship with his mother. This session was calmer than earlier ones, even though it moved rather smoothly into the core issue for the couple of the husband's fear that the wife would not love him if he asked her to give anything up, and the way the wife took care of this fearful residue of his trauma in a loving way. They then turned to a more extensive discussion of the wife's way of turning attention away from her own issues, and that this brief mention of his pushing food on her was a small inroad to the struggle over food with her own intrusive mother, which she avoids discussing. She has turned down Sherry's suggestion for individual therapy several times, so the only therapy she can allow is these couple sessions. Then a member of the group said, 'Well the satellite *dish* he wants to give her is unconsciously related to food too, so his gift is a displaced, symbolic offer of food that comes from him instead of her mother. He's afraid she won't take it from him. In a hidden way, he's dealing with her eating disorder and the way it has tied her to her mother.' The group discussed the way the husband tries to get her to accept his care of her, and how she vigorously avoids an awareness of her own needs and fears by solicitous discussion of his situation instead of her own buried hurts.

As the group carried on the discussion, I noticed how well they were working as a group, making thematic discoveries without much less input from me than usual. I felt a little left out, superfluous, in resonance perhaps with the husband's feeling left out by his wife's connection to her mother rather than to him. In a way, I wanted them to connect to my satellite TV, to be fed more by my 'satellite dish'. It was getting close to the end of the time for discussing Sherry's case, when Kathy said, 'I just thought: David is watching our TV channel. It's like he's on the balcony, watching and smiling at us.' The group now began to discuss the way they felt I was tuned into them and providing a holding environment, one in which they could face their patients' scars. I said as I now thought about Sherry's dream, I saw the way the group often saw the reflection of their own scars in me, like the way their patients often felt their scars reflected by the therapist's face, painful but also holding out hope for change. Sherry's hope for grandchildren was a countertransference to the couple's expectation of a child, the fertility of the treatment, and at the same time, the members' own hopes for growth of themselves as therapists. In resonance with the case, they use TV at a 'satellite' location, ergo 'a satellite dish' to get professional feeding and repair, for opportunities to lessen their connection to old ways of doing things through a strengthened connection to me across a significant geographic separation. I now felt better about the 'dish' I could provide in standing by as they were able to feed themselves. In later reflection, I also realized that Sherry's dream contained some residue from reactions to facial cosmetic surgery I had about the time the group began meeting with me, and with previous surgeries my wife had and about which they might well have known. The dream resonated with the feeling of need for repair at all levels, for individual patients, couple, therapist, and in the supervisory relationship with me.

The dynamic resonance of this session of group supervision demonstrates the parallel processes found in ordinary group supervision, unimpeded by the use of the distance-learning video technology. In this particular session, the group was able to identify ways that the television technology itself became part of the theme that tied together experience echoing up and down the line from patient, to couple, therapy, and to supervisory relationships. The technology, far from interfering in the process, instead became part of it.

CONCLUSION

The use of the new videoconference technology enables us to link groups that would otherwise not be able to join in analytic study. With improving technology and decreasing cost, it is now feasible to join colleagues, students and teachers at several sites across any distance in real-time teaching and supervision. In our experience, the technical and personal adjustments to the use of this technology are surmountable, and the opportunities then open up to allow the sharing of analytic ideas and clinical experience in a way that we are only beginning to explore.

REFERENCES

Alvarez, A. (1993) *Live Company: Psychoanalytic Psychotherapy with Autistic, Borderline, and Deprived and Abused Children*, London: Routledge.

Aronson, J. (ed.) (2000) *Use of the Telephone in Psychotherapy*, Northvale, NJ: Jason Aronson.

Miller, L., Rustin, M. and Shuttleworth, J. (1989) *Closely Observed Infants*, London: Duckworth.

Scharff, J. S. and Scharff, D. E. (2000) *Tuning the Therapeutic Instrument: The Affective Learning of Psychotherapy*, Northvale, NJ: Jason Aronson.

Sebek, M. (2001) 'Internet Discussion Review: Varieties of Long-Term Outcome among Patients in Psychoanalysis and Psychotherapy: A Review of Findings on the Stockholm Outcome of Psychoanalysis and Psychotherapy Project (STOPP), by Rolf Sandell *et al.*', *International Journal of Psycho-Analysis*, 82: 205–210.

Chapter 10

Exploring space in workgroups

Susan E. Barbour

INTRODUCTION

The concept of psychological space in workgroups is not widely discussed in the psychoanalytic literature. There has been especially little discussion concerning how a leader or consultant might understand and utilize space to facilitate group cohesion. A. Kenneth Rice and Eric Miller used the Tavistock model, a convergence of psychoanalysis and social science in the study of group relations (Obholzer and Roberts 1994). The A. K. Rice Institute adapted the model in the United States (Colman and Bexton 1975; Colman and Geller 1985) to consider authority and social systems. Neither, though, discusses space in relation to their concepts.

In this chapter I focus on space in a small workgroup (ten members or less) and define the elements that facilitate group cohesion. I review theory relevant to the creation of workgroup space including: group mentality and the basic assumption group, primary task, the concept of the group-as-a-whole, workgroup boundary and the mechanism of projective identification within groups. My example illustrates, first, the different ways that leaders conceptualize their roles and, then, with or without the group's involvement, delineate the primary task and manage the workgroup boundary. Second, I examine how leaders might structure workgroup communication and think about workgroup relationships in ways more conducive to cohesion and productivity.

SPACE APPLIED TO WORKGROUPS

I had begun a consultation to a small workgroup when I had a dream about space. I dreamt that I was a therapist in a mental hospital. I was in a group room where psychotic or otherwise disturbed folk shuffled in and out. I was trying to bring some cohesion to the group. Tables formed a square in the middle of the room with an inaccessible open space in the center of the tables. I was inviting one person and then another to take a seat at the table where they could talk to each other, but my effort was useless, and the patients would shuffle out of the room. I felt that my efforts were ineffective and futile. There was no group per se, and no group cohesion. Everyone was lost in their own world.

The inaccessible space struck me. The tables, where the group might gather together, served to block, rather than to facilitate space. The world of the individual took precedent over the interaction of the group. Upon awakening, I thought of Ogden's (1997) concept of reverie in relation to therapeutic space. Object relations theory considers the internal (intrapsychic) world as a space into which affects (associated with various identifications with people, groups, etc.) can be taken in or expelled. Reverie has to do with the containment of those affects within a shared frame, one that allows meaning to gradually evolve, and become crystallized, cognitively known and later articulated in the experience between analyst and patient. Reverie is a state of being, being with, and being in. Reverie presumes internal space, as well as an interpersonal space made possible first by the analyst's receptivity and then via the maintenance of the therapeutic frame. The idea is similar to Winnicott's concept of 'potential space' (Winnicott 1971: 41, 107) in which the analyst, like a mother, maintains an 'unconscious receptivity to being made use of' (Ogden 1997: 9). Ogden describes several ingredients fundamental to reverie: the analyst's creation of internal space that gradually fosters the possibility of space between analyst and patient, reflection in lieu of action or reaction, and an attitude that there is 'time to waste' (Ogden 1997: 161). An unhurried atmosphere allows meaning to emerge in an integrative way and is qualitatively quite different from speedy action prone to concretize and produce results.

Connected to beginning the organizational consultation, my dream communicated my resonance with those from this workgroup who felt incompetent and ineffective. Similarly, Ogden describes the analyst's 'emotional tumult of reverie' (Ogden 1997: 162) as the feelings of uncertainty, confusion and incompetence experienced when sitting with a patient. Identifying with Ogden's comments, I began to think about staff members' discomfort as a venue to understanding this workgroup. The other members of the workgroup, while concerned for their colleagues, felt confident. However, almost all staff members felt less like members in a group than isolated individuals. The dream conveyed the affective disconnect of a crazy ward where preoccupied individuals came and went in their own world. The essence of their shared subjectivities, the cohesion of the 'group-as-a whole' had shattered (Wells 1985: 109).

GROUP STRUCTURE AND CONTAINMENT

Groups operate on two levels, according to Bion (1961): (1) the workgroup, which is reality-oriented and carries out the task, and (2) the basic assumption group or group mentality. The workgroup's primary task is its mission or that which is most central to the survival of the workgroup (Miller and Rice 1975). However, task completion in and of itself is only one aspect of workgroup life.

> The internal world of a group is made up then, first of the contributions of its members to its purpose and, second, of the feeling and attitudes the members develop about each other and about the group, both internally and in relation to its environment.
>
> (Miller and Rice 1975: 55–56)

Members pair with each other as they resonate with each other's conscious and unconscious interests, needs, values, and convictions. Wells, basing his ideas in part on Bion's (1961) concepts of dependence, pairing and/or fight–flight, describes the internal world of a group as the network of relationships that form through the 'lattice of projective identifications shared among group members' (Wells, 1985: 116). These pairings may result in scapegoating or marginalizing some members of the group.

Organizational changes can have dramatic effects on the internal life of a workgroup. I shall refer to two in particular. When there is a change of leadership and/or when there is a shift in the primary task, the unconscious life of the workgroup shifts. A change in the primary task may arouse anxiety and affect conscious and unconscious pairings between individuals which in turn, may heighten the 'irrationality' (Shapiro 1985: 354) of the workgroup. The cultivation of shared potential space, on the other hand, may contain the anxiety of the basic assumption group and allay counterproductive forces that otherwise impede group cohesion and task completion. Just as the potential space between mother and infant provides a receptive holding environment that modulates the infant's anxiety, so too, shared potential space becomes the 'third area of human living', (Winnicott 1971: 110) made up of the shared subjectivities of workgroup members and may provide a holding environment in which group members relate to and accomplish the workgroup task.

Klein first considered the phenomenon that occurs between mother and child in the intersubjectivity of potential space (Klein 1946 (in Scharff 1996)) and introduced the concept of projective identification, now recognized as occurring in relationships throughout our lives. In projective identification, disliked, undesired or indigestible aspects of one's self are unconsciously projected onto someone else. Projective identification is also active in groups and is both an intra-psychic mechanism and an interpersonal transaction that affects individuals in unspoken ways. Individuals' perceptions, reactions, thoughts and feelings may be impacted, leading to a transformation in behavior (Horwitz 1985: 22). Wells comments that group life cultivates 'strong, conflicting, ambivalent feelings of love and hate' in its members and that individuals in groups bond together in unconscious tacit agreements that express the 'group Gestalt' as they respond to the 'group-as-mother' in ways that parallel the 'infant-in-relation-to-mother' (Wells 1985: 114–117). Therefore, anxiety is generated by group life and how the good-enough leader and the good-enough organizational structure contain and manage that anxiety is of utmost importance in forming a more cohesive workgroup.

While Wells describes multiple levels of organizational life, for the purpose of this discussion on space I focus on his concept of the group-as-a-whole, or the supra-personal level of organizational life and the inter-organizational level of relations between institutions and the environment in which they exist (Wells 1985). Individuals and sometimes entire subgroups within organizations share an unconscious consensus. Subgroups blame other subgroups as they unwittingly distance themselves from their disliked projections and in so doing, exacerbate defensive posturing that ricochets back and forth between subgroups through blame and rebuttal (Halton 1994). Splitting occurs in groups as it does intrapsychically and members identify with and become receptacles for each other's projections as a result of the splitting used to manage anxiety. Shared patterns of projective identification lead to repetitive behaviors and predictable responses between subgroups.

Wells names some of the most common dichotomies that form in workgroups around defensive positions: 'affective vs. cognitive, hero vs. villain, process concerns vs. task concerns, fight vs. flight, hope vs. despair, competence vs. incompetence' (Wells 1985: 120). In health organizations, we commonly find dichotomies such as: medical vs. psychological, administrative vs. applied, scientist vs. practitioner, doctor vs. nurse, etc. As a consultant, I too became a receptacle for the split-off aspects of the workgroup's unconscious and through reflection (psychological space) on my dream I could begin to define the meaning of the communication from and about the disruptions in this workgroup's cohesion.

Furthermore, a workgroup is an 'open system' that survives by 'exchanging materials' with its environment like a 'biological organism' (Miller and Rice 1975: 43). It has a region of regulation around the activities of the system and this region has two boundaries, an inner boundary between the internal activities of the system and the region of regulation and an outer boundary that separates the region of regulation from the activities of other groups or from the organization (Miller and Rice 1975). The inner boundary has to do with how the workgroup perceives and manages its activities and the outer boundary with how the environment perceives the workgroup's activities. Regulation involves modulating what comes into and goes from the workgroup and distinguishes the workgroup's distinctive tasks and contributions. Those outside the workgroup perceive the roles and functions of the workgroup in one way, and the workgroup may perceive its roles and functions in another, thus the region that is most functional is the shared frame of reference. Without the shared frame of reference, communication, expectations and the relationship itself can break down (Szmidla and Khaleelee 1975).

A workgroup is continually negotiating its role in systemic relationships; projections are continually put into the group and accepted or expelled by the group across the semi-permeable boundary area. The leader is primarily responsible for the definition and negotiation of 'boundary control functions' within and from outside of the group based on the definition of the workgroup's primary task (Miller and Rice 1975: 47). Boundary regulation is a continuing process and offsets the unconscious migration of workgroup roles that can occur through the non-verbal impact of projective identification described earlier. Turquet points out, therefore, that structure and primary task are intricately and dynamically related and that the boundary control is key. 'Only by drawing clear boundaries between conflicting primary tasks can a group resolve tensions and confusions' (Turquet 1985: 72).

Therefore, workgroups need ways to talk about complex or conflictual issues. A workgroup benefits from a framework for communication – regular forums for meetings on different topics. Like the environmental mother (Winnicott 1963) who holds the infant, the leader creates a structure for the group to come together as a whole. A network of relationships forms and may become a holding environment for the workgroup, one in which staff members feel safe. Heifetz and Linsky describe the workgroup holding environment as follows:

> A holding environment is a space formed by a network of relationships within which people can tackle tough, sometimes, divisive questions without flying apart. Creating a holding environment enables you to direct creative energy toward working the conflicts and containing passions that could easily boil over.
>
> (Heifetz and Linsky 2002: 102)

Within the communication structure, consideration of the more deeply embedded patterns of shared identifications facilitates group cohesion. Groups benefit from the perspective that they exist as an entity, a 'radical view' (Wells 1985: 124) for leaders to hold. If there is a problem in the group, leaders typically focus on the individual who expresses the problem, rather than considering how the group is putting something into the individual via projective identification and by 'shared splitting'. A group-as-a-whole perspective assumes that 'when a person speaks, he/she does so not only for themselves, but in part, speaks via the unconscious of the group' (Wells 1985: 124). At times, an individual's expression may in fact be an accumulation of unconscious forces from the workgroup.

Cognizant of these interpersonal forces, a leader may begin by considering how these forces impact the leadership role, what feelings are stirred up, what the group is doing and 'how he feels the group inside himself' (Turquet 1985: 73). A leader's receptivity cultivates an atmosphere in which group members can also explore their experience in relation to the workgroup. Thoughtful reflection of one's experience creates space for speculation, a playful yet purposeful arena facilitated by the leader and made possible within the holding environmental structure. In addition, staff members need to feel that there is 'time-to-waste' for some period, without pressure to concretize the reflection into decisions. I illustrate in the next section.

CREATING THE SPACE FOR WORKGROUP CHANGE: WHAT A LEADER CAN DO

A leader can cultivate space in a workgroup in four interrelated ways: (1) delineation and maintenance of the workgroup's task and boundary, (2) establishment of a consistent structure for workgroup discussions, (3) creation of a precedent for reflection and engagement, and (4) implementation of a perspective that considers the group-as-a-whole. In the first two, the leader and workgroup structure the holding environment, the third has to do with the leader's thoughtful role management, and the fourth with a focus on the group rather than on disparate individuals. The latter two also involve the leader's capacity for psychological containment of the group. To address the group-as-a-whole, Wells proposes that a leader ask the following questions:

> (1) What have the group members been asked to carry on behalf of the group, (2) what may be being deposited into each member on behalf of the others, and, (3) is a group member who is identified as incompetent, inept, too aggressive, or too passive merely unconsciously being asked to carry these projected split-off parts and attributes for the group-as-a-whole?
>
> (Wells 1985: 125)

Case illustration – background

The ten-person, mostly male, health clinic staff group had held a long, stable and positive reputation in the community. The clinic operated independently providing outpatient services, but was affiliated with a research and teaching hospital. The staff had worked and aged together for many years and then experienced a number of retirements. Agreeing that diversification of the staff was beneficial, as positions became available, the openings were filled with younger female physicians. Two women were hired over a several-year period, but within a couple of years, first one, then the other, left. Their vacancies were also filled with women. A year later, a young man was hired, became unsettled but ultimately did not leave his position. New staff members said that they had difficulty feeling part of the established workgroup. Tensions increased when the Medical Director, Robert, retired after many years in his position and was replaced by a younger man, Kevin. I shall discuss each Medical Director's role vis-à-vis the four areas instrumental in forming space in a workgroup.

Delineation and maintenance of the workgroup boundary

Robert and the workgroup developed together over many years. They focused on providing direct patient care as the clinic's primary service and as their medical expertise. The Medical Director and the workgroup considered requests from the community for other services (e.g. emergency, public health services) on a situation-by-situation basis. By so doing they defined and negotiated the workgroup's priorities. When they believed outside constituents held perceptions of their work contrary to their views, they defined the pressures they experienced and addressed them through education about the importance of direct patient care and the value of their service to the larger organization and to the community. At times, they initiated reports about their services, written in an experience-near way to explain what they offered and its value. While at times they provided other services, for instance they ran an immunization program for a period of time, the prioritization of services was clear to staff members and was consistently maintained.

Kevin came to the Medical Director's position with a model of providing health care based on efficiency and outcome; a conception that differed from Robert's. He believed that the clinic's image was passé and that they needed to provide a wider range of services and better demonstrate its usefulness to the affiliated hospital and to the public. His view was breadth for many versus depth for a few. Initially, Kevin engaged the workgroup in a discussion about the clinic's primary mission but was met with a mixed response. The discussion was inconclusive and Kevin moved forward without consensus. Energetic, in a way the former director was not, Kevin roused staff to expand community programs, delegated assignments to staff members and set a precedent for services he thought would raise the visibility of primary care health interventions. To offset a potential threat of layoffs and reduced staffing, he wanted to reshape clinic services to conform to what the community most needed and valued. He encouraged grant writing as a way to subsidize the clinic. Demands on patient care time increased as some staff members' time was applied to research coordinator roles, affecting tasks that Robert and the older members of the group would not have considered central either to the clinic's mission or to its members' expertise. Gradually, the workplace atmosphere shifted from one that was more contemplative to a more proactive culture. Kevin, philosophically speaking, defined patient care in terms of efficacy, a perspective new for the clinic.

In contrast to Robert, Kevin's vision of the workgroup's activities, the inner boundary of the region of regulation, became more closely aligned with how constituencies perceived the clinic's services and in so doing he won external favor. The boundary around workgroup activities shifted, as did the prioritization of tasks, to accommodate what Kevin understood as the needs of external constituents, but the shift occurred without the engagement of the group. As the primary task changed, confusion in the workgroup increased, and the possibility to think about change and to discuss it, was replaced by frenetic activity and resistance.

Structure of workgroup discussions

Robert wanted to promote ways for the staff to interact. He had maintained a regularly scheduled formal and informal meeting structure: administrative meetings, medical case conferences, in-service training and a once-monthly leaderless staff group meeting to discuss issues related to work raised by staff members. The informal leaderless group offered a reflective opportunity for staff to talk about their work and sometimes about workgroup relationships. Robert participated in this group in the role of staff member, not as medical director. Newer staff members were uncomfortable and wary of conflict that did occur at times. In addition, staff gathered informally for morning coffee although new staff members were uncomfortable about these gatherings as well. They believed that they should get to work and were not appreciative of the way story-telling about the clinic's history was a way of passing on the torch.

Believing that discussion tends to expand to consume the time available, Kevin revamped the meeting structure. Consistent with his utilitarian focus, he increased staff meeting time to discuss business items and eliminated medical case conferences until staff members spoke up. He also discontinued the informal leaderless staff meetings because newer staff members were uncomfortable. There was no space for the uncomfortable affects to be discussed and, interestingly, it was a number of these same staff members who left their positions. The informal coffee gatherings became infrequent, sporadic, and then ceased altogether.

Creating a precedent for reflection and similarly engaging staff involvement

Robert modeled quiet thoughtfulness and engaged others in joint problem solving and program building. His reflective, exploratory and engaging style, as well as his punctuality, dependability and consistency, framed a reliable holding environment for workgroup communication. He was receptive, curious about staff members' lives, supportive and grateful for their ideas and contributions. He invited consultation and collaborative work. He confronted others when they did not consider their own contribution to a problem, warning them not to impugn motives. He encouraged more experienced staff to mentor, teach and support new staff, and he did so as well. He welcomed feedback and adjusted his actions accordingly. Some believed Robert was too laid back. Others experienced him as receptive and felt empowered by him. While the group struggled to retain new staff members, he was able to open the door for change and renewal.

Kevin also supported staff members but in a different way. He attempted to engage and rally staff members' enthusiasm by making suggestions and encouraging action. Some were responsive; others felt intruded upon. He took time to listen to individuals and often responded with an action-focused reply, rather than a reflective comment. Good-natured and proactive he maintained a fraction of the patient load of his predecessor or other physicians. Admittedly extroverted, he spent long periods of time outside the office responding to situations as they occurred, thinking on his feet and doing it well. However, group members sometimes wondered where he was and felt uninformed about the clinic's projects and issues. Staff joked that he was manic, and Kevin in turn, experienced the group as brittle and reactionary, aware that friction during group meetings seemed to have little to do with the topic at hand. His focus on the efficient utilization of time preempted reflection to address the underlying discord and ambiguities.

Group-as-a-whole

What was interesting about the evolution of this group is that, while Robert's personable management of the system's structure facilitated a predominately cohesive workgroup, that cohesion broke down as the group changed. Newcomers felt marginalized by the intense group loyalty and by comments that the group was a 'family'. Robert created a warm and conversational holding environment, but newcomers' discontent was not understood as symptomatic of the group-as-a-whole. Newcomers carried the despair of the dying group and the younger females felt ineffectual and intimidated as a counterbalance to the sense of sufficiency possessed by the men in the group that had been around a long time. Ultimately, the impact of these pressures led them to depart. Kevin, like Robert, viewed problems as individual ones, and group members' insecurities were further exacerbated with an implicit change in the primary task and, even more so, by the absence of a forum to discuss what was happening. Both Robert and

Kevin, in their different ways, brought noteworthy competencies to their jobs as leaders. However, it was striking that they both focused on individual staff members' tasks and issues and were not mindful of the perspective of the group-as-a-whole level of functioning. There was little space in them or in the workgroup to process at that level.

CONCLUSION: WORKGROUP SPACE

In this example, a once-cohesive workgroup was dramatically affected by staff turnover and leadership change. In spite of a clearly defined primary task, a reliable framework for communication and Robert's warm, supportive style, group anxiety was roused by change. While the holding environment helped the group communicate, group members did not consider what the group-as-a-whole was asking new staff members to contain for the group. Aspects of the group experience were projected into new staff members who became uncomfortable and left their positions, only for the process to begin anew.

The group's anxiety was further roused by the change in leadership and staff members' shifting identifications with the leader, by the new leader's different vision of the group's tasks, by the workgroup's lack of involvement with the development of this new vision, and by the dismantling of the structure for communication. As anxiety intensified the group fragmented and two camps solidified. Competition and envy intensified as individuals withdrew into solipsistic work patterns, represented in my dream as the patients shuffling in and out across the boundary of the room. Some in the workgroup rationalized that their colleagues had left because they had better offers elsewhere. Others reflected on how these staff members felt double-bound, ineffectual, and depleted and were unhappy about the change in leadership. No one attributed staff members' discomfort to the atmosphere of the group-as-a-whole. This workgroup was similar to workgroups of any kind that experience staff turnover or business failures, or that eventually seek organizational consultation.

The concept of a holding environment and the psychological space for containment of anxiety is central to object relations theory. The mother's empathy or the analyst's reverie make it possible for the infant or patient respectively to integrate unrealized aspects of oneself. The mother and infant are both affected in the shared experience of the potential space as they adapt to each other's change, vulnerable and different, but attuned. The mother's/analyst's holding and containing make it possible for the infant/patient to manage anxiety and find better ways of interacting with the world. The leader in organizations serves a similar function for workgroups.

The application of the concept of space to workgroups is inherently complicated, if for no other reason, then because of the number of personalities involved and the exponentially larger number of ways that people resonate with each other and, through projective identification, impact each other. Workgroups that lack an adequate way to manage the ubiquitous experience of a group's underlying anxiety, form defensive patterns to that anxiety that may ultimately and unknowingly impede task completion. The group atmosphere becomes brittle and symptomatic through, for instance, the potential for accidents, absenteeism, staff turnover, scapegoating, reduced productivity or lower morale.

Groups benefit from a way to reflect on their patterns of interaction. The creation and maintenance of space naturally implies the utilization of an internal structure of relationships that links group mentality to task completion. Winnicott points out that with overwhelming anxiety, an individual becomes 'cluttered up with persecutory elements of which he has no way of ridding himself' (Winnicott 1971: 103). Such is the case in group-life as well; a workgroup must have some way of ridding itself of the clutter of persecutory elements that are projected into members or into its environment. Otherwise entrenched repetitive patterns can lead to fragmentation, traumatic interaction and individuals' withdrawal.

My dream was about the lack of potential space in this workgroup. When an organization is in such a state of mind, a consultant can help the leader and the workgroup in a variety of ways. First, the consultant can work with the leader and/or the workgroup to consider the frame, group communication structure and address ambiguities in the primary task. Second, the consultant can, in part through the use of self, work with the leader to create a space in which to examine the structure of conscious and unconscious communication in the group. In so doing, a consultant can introduce the perspective of the group-as-a-whole. Third, and most importantly, the consultant can help the leader think about his or her experience with the group as a communication from the group-as-a-whole and help the workgroup explore individuals' valencies (Bion 1961) for what they contain for the group. All of these interventions can be carried out by the consultant leading meetings with the individual leader, with the workgroup or, frequently with a combination of such meetings.

From a psychological perspective, the consultant performing the above tasks provides holding and containing for the leader and workgroup as well as space for thinking about the experience of the group-as-a-whole. My reflection on my dream as a communication from the workgroup was the beginning of a space in and for this workgroup and for this leader. By understanding the group-as-a-whole a consultant can help workgroups cultivate space, evaluate their strengths and vulnerabilities, and form a more cohesive system able to respond to the competitive demands of a changing world.

REFERENCES

Bion, W. R. (1961) *Experiences in Groups*, London: Tavistock.

Colman, A. D. and Bexton, W. H. (eds.) (1975) *Group Relations: Reader 1*, Washington, DC: A. K. Rice Institute.

Colman, A. D. and Geller, M. H. (eds.) (1985) *Group Relations: Reader 2*, Washington, DC: A. K. Rice Institute.

Halton, W. (1994) 'Some Unconscious Aspects of Organizational Life', in A. Obholzer and V. Z. Roberts (eds.), *The Unconscious at Work: Individual and Organizational Stress in the Human Services*, London: Routledge, pp. 11–18.

Heifetz, R. and Linsky, M. (2002) *Leadership on the Line: Staying Alive through the Dangers of Leading*, Boston, MA: Harvard Business School Press.

Horwitz, L. (1985) 'Projective Identification in Dyads and Groups', in A. D. Colman and M. H. Geller (eds.), *Group Relations: Reader 2*, Washington, DC: A. K. Rice Institute, pp. 21–37.

Klein, M. (1946) 'Notes on Some Schizoid Mechanisms', in D. E. Scharff (ed.) (1996) *Object Relations Theory and Practice*, Northvale, NJ: Jason Aronson, pp. 136–155.

Miller, E. J. and Rice, A. K. (1975) 'Selections from: Systems of Organizations', in A. D. Colman and W. H. Bexton (eds.), *Group Relations: Reader 1*, Washington, DC: A. K. Rice Institute, pp. 13–68.

Obholzer, A. and Roberts, V. Z. (eds.) (1994) *The Unconscious at Work: Individual and Organizational Stress in the Human Services*, London: Routledge.

Ogden, T. (1997) *Reverie and Interpretation*, Northvale, NJ: Jason Aronson.

Shapiro, E. R. (1985) 'Unconscious Process in an Organization', in A. D. Colman and M. H. Geller (eds.), *Group Relations: Reader 2*, Washington, DC: A. K. Rice Institute, pp. 353–363.

Smidla, A. and Khaleelee, O. (1975) Unpublished memorandum, cited in 'The Politics of Involvement' by E. J. Miller (1978), *Journal of Personality and Social Systems*, 1: 37–50.

Turquet, P. (1985) 'Leadership: The Individual and the Group', in A. D Colman and M. H. Geller (eds.), *Group Relations: Reader 2*, Washington, DC: A. K. Rice Institute, pp. 71–87.

Wells, L. (1985) 'The Group-as-a-Whole Perspective and its Theoretical Roots', in A. D. Colman and M. H. Geller (eds.), *Group Relations: Reader 2*, Washington, DC: A. K. Rice Institute, pp. 109–126.

Winnicott, D. W. (1963) 'The Development of the Capacity for Concern', in *The Maturational Processes and the Facilitating Environment* (1965), New York: International Universities Press, pp. 73–82.

Winnicott, D. W. (1971) *Playing and Reality*, London: Tavistock.

Part III

Number

Numbers in mind, numbers in motion: an introduction

David E. Scharff and Michael Stadter

Numbers and mathematics can be viewed as an obvious part of everyday clinical practice. Here are a few examples: the number of patients in the room or in a group, members in a family, patients in our day, in our practice; the fees we receive; the numbers of sessions in a therapy; the frequency of sessions; the number of major transference complexes; the multiple fragmentations we come to know of a patient's psyche.

However, it is only recently that number has become an important point of reference in psychoanalytic theory. Most of Freud's writing focused on the individual, sometimes expanded to the threesome he found in his discovery of the Oedipus situation. He focused only occasionally on the twosome of the mother and infant. Analytic writing has more often focused on the two of the analytic pair, but Freud himself did not think consciously of the number two. He had focused on time and space, especially in his description of how dreams handled these elements, but not of the flux of internal objects. His discovery of the internalization of objects in the experience of loss and in the oedipal phase led to his description of structural theory as an evolving and interacting psychic formation, but one that tended toward a self-contained system rather than a dynamic organization in open interaction with the environment.

The physics of Freud's day – and especially of his scientific youth in which the early models were formed – did not deal with the complex dynamics of interacting entities. Even Einstein's theory of relativity, which became available in Freud's maturity, did not influence his developing models. Twentieth-century physics did not become available as a metaphor for psychological interaction until Fairbairn (Scharff and Birtles 1994) applied the theory of relativity to the interdependence of mental structure and content in the 1950s. Dynamic thinking about mental function and the interactions of transference and countertransference were already in evolution, but Fairbairn's application gave a new model from the physical sciences to that emerging understanding.

A comparable shift of paradigm is currently occurring. New models of science, derived from physics and mathematics in the study of chaos and string theories, give new ways of seeing complexity and uncertainty in the physical universe and in the psychological realm. As clinicians become newly aware of the role of complex and almost indefinable subtlety of interaction, there is a need for new models of mind and of minds in interaction.

The chapters in Part III explore several aspects of the way close examination of number expands our understanding of intrapsychic dynamics. We begin with James Poulton's study of the paradox of one-person and two-person psychology. Working with the ideas of Bollas, Loewald and Lacan, he argues there is greater richness in meaning if the paradox is maintained rather than being resolved in favor of one side or the other. We are simultaneously a single autonomous entity, and are constituted through relation to the other, a two-in-one and a one-in-two. Carl Bagnini's chapter on supervision expands our vision to the number three, not in the ordinary oedipal use of the number three, but in the clinical supervisory relationship. He first notes the important, frequently examined, aspects of the supervisee/ therapist's difficult role conflict and the parallel process often enacted between the two pairs of patient–therapist and supervisee–supervisor. Bagnini then maintains that attention to group process and 'the triadic field' of supervision provides a richer level for understanding the complex dynamics involved. His extended vignette demonstrates triadic influences including the impact of the patient's internal world on that of the supervisor and the supervisor's 'presence' in the therapy.

Christopher Bollas's chapter on the number four expands our vision to the realm of the family. His use of numbers to indicate levels expands the use of mathematics to indicate a level of magnitude, not only about the interaction indicated by the number, but also about the level of complexity the individual psyche has to compute in considering object relations in the family. Interestingly, in his chapter Bollas writes, 'It will be seen, naturally, that a psychoanalytic numerology bears no relation to mathematics proper.' In the context of Scharff and Scharff's Chapter 16 on chaos theory, and Scharff and Cooper's Chapters 14 and 15 on numbers we can see that an advanced conception of numbers does actually allow Bollas's sophisticated psychoanalytic theorizing to become compatible with modern mathematics, both through the application of complex numbers, and through the view of dynamic strange attractors that explains how several states of mind relate simultaneously to each other.

Finally, Hope Cooper and I (DES) offer a pair of chapters that deal with numbers in a wholly new way. Chapter 14 describes a system of notation that abstracts object relations to their numerical qualities in order to study the internal dynamics in a simpler way, to observe the dynamics of internal object relations stripped of their idiosyncrasies. While this takes away the richness of the particulars of the objects, it adds to our capacity to see the objects in direct and fluctuating relation to each other. Chapter 15 extends this thinking in two ways. First, we explore the mind's capacity to hold numbers greater than six or seven dynamically in mind, drawing on the work of Bion and Matte-Blanco to describe a model of the reduction of psychic understanding of large numbers to smaller ones more easily held in mind. Second, we propose that internal numbers are always in a kind of motion that represents the mind's continuous process of dynamic transformation. As this ongoing transformation takes place, it forms a geometry of inner space and time that represents dimensions beyond the four usual ones of three spatial dimensions plus time. Time and space, we contend, are frequently represented in dreams and other 'primary process' psychic productions, but in ways that represent higher, more complex dimensions of psychic organization. In this way, this part closes by drawing together the themes of time, space and number as fundamentally interrelated, and paves the way to Part IV's application of these themes to understanding normal and pathological states of mind that unfold in the treatment process.

The chapters in this section on number, taken together, demonstrate that mathematics offers a fruitful vehicle for the study of some of the most complex organizations and dynamics both of the individual psyche and of minds in interaction – of mutual influence, of dynamic oscillation between complex organizations of mind, and of psychological interaction in families and groups and in therapy.

REFERENCES

Scharff, D. E. and Birtles, E. F. (eds.) (1994) *From Instinct to Self: Selected Papers of W. R. D. Fairbairn*, vols. I and II, Northvale, NJ: Jason Aronson.

Chapter 11

Number theory, intersubjectivity and schizoid phenomena

James L. Poulton

ONE, TWO AND THREE

The concept of number, as it applies both to metapsychology and to technique in psychoanalysis, has been receiving increased attention in recent years from theorists representing various perspectives. One reason for this interest has been the upsurge of intersubjective concepts in analytic theory, which have functioned to blur the distinctions between such traditional notions as one-person vs. two-person psychologies, or independence vs. interdependence. In consequence, theorists have been prompted to rethink what these concepts might mean, and whether it still makes sense to speak of the traditional *one* of the individual subject (i.e., the analysand or the analyst, taken individually) or even the *two* of analysand and analyst in interaction with each other.

Thomas Ogden's concept of the analytic third is a case in point. Ogden (1994) describes the analytic third as the 'analytical subject', jointly created by the analyst and analysand's individual subjectivities and by their intersubjective interdependence. Involved in this process are the analyst and analysand as *both* separate entities *and* as interdependent. As separate entities, they are 'subject' and 'object' to each other. In the mode of inter-dependence, however, they form a third subjectivity, the analytic third, which represents an intermediate ground of shared subjectivity that exerts its own influence on their separate subjectivities. The analytic process, then, is conceived by Ogden to be the outgrowth of a dialectical interplay between *three* 'subjectivities': analyst, analysand, and the analytic third.

As a result of theoretical advances like Ogden's, the old concepts of the one and the two have become questionable. They have, in a word, become infected by the intersubjective, in that the one (of either analysand or analyst) is no longer simply one, but also contributes to a *third* that is essentially another (though quite different) *one* formed by the fusion of the *two*. In this chapter these confusing concepts will be explored, particularly as they have been transformed by the infusion of the intersubjective. The chapter will have two primary goals. First, theories pertaining to the one, the two, and the intersubjective will be critically examined, and a particular view of the intersubjective, that it participates in an oscillation between individual independence and the interdependence of shared subjectivity, will be suggested. Second, the idea of oscillation will be illustrated through a case study of an analysis of a schizoid character.

THEORIES OF THE ONE, THE TWO, AND THE INTERSUBJECTIVE

In his chapter entitled 'One, Two . . . Seven' in *The Mystery of Things*, Christopher Bollas (1999) discusses the one of one-person, and the two of two-person, psychologies (also see Bollas, Chapter 13 in this volume for his additional thinking on number). One-person psychology, he says, is the proper domain of 'the self in relative isolation – quintessentially in the dream, but also in daydreams, unconscious fantasies, passing mental fragments, affects, instinctual derivatives and so forth' (Bollas 1999: 52). Two-person psychology, on the other hand, 'receives the work of the self in relation to the other' (1999: 52), in that it involves real interactions with others in which each are called upon to reveal their subjectivity. When analysands explore their one-person psychology, they use the analyst 'as an object of thought for an elaboration of the analysand's state of mind' (1999: 53). To force the interaction toward relationality at this moment, i.e., to attempt to interpret the one as evidence of the two, would be 'remedial', a 'category error' (1999: 53), and would undermine the essential work of analysis. When the two is predominant, however, the analysand 'both acts upon and talks to the analyst, and the analyst feels his otherness called into interpersonal engagement' (1999: 55). Here mutuality truly occurs, in which the subjectivity of each participant transforms and modifies that of the other.

With these definitions in hand, Bollas questions whether concepts of intersubjectivity add any value to our understanding of the analytic process. To his question, 'where does the intersubjective operate in the analytic pair?' (1999: 51), he gives two responses, both of which underscore the concept's apparent lack of utility. First, he says that the intersubjective 'must' operate in the analyst's and analysand's unconscious, but if it is unconscious, then it is 'fundamentally unknowable' (1999: 52) and any effort to identify it 'bears the strain of the rationalized' (1999: 52). Second, he wonders if the intersubjective could exist in 'some mutually constructed interpersonal area, equidistant from the participants?' (1999: 55). Since this image is absurd (picture the intersubjective hovering like a hummingbird in the space between the two), he has no difficulty shooting it down. Of course that isn't where the two-person exists, he says. *'For after all, the two shall always be registered in the one.* . . . . In the end, all relations between two people are collapsed into the labile immateriality of the individual psyche' (1999: 55, emphasis added).

Bollas thus appears to reduce the intersubjective to merely that which registers in the individual psyche. From this perspective, the intersubjective has the same epistemological standing as any other content of consciousness: we experience and think about it, but always in the privacy of our own individualistic theater. In this view, the other appears to the independent and isolated subject only contingently, in the form of an interaction between essentially separate psyches.

It is telling, however, that Bollas, having gone so far as to assert such an isolated subject, then retracts some of the sharper edges of this view. Near the end of his article, he states, quite enigmatically, that the unconscious, 'that strange object of our endopsychic awareness, is substantially derived from what Laplanche terms the "enigmatic signifier": the mother's unconscious seduces us into psychic life. . . . Thus the very zone of the deconstructed – what we term the primary process – derives in the very first place out of a relation' (1999: 56).

The contradictions in Bollas's work are not unfamiliar to those who investigate the intersubjective. The confusion arises from the fact that analytic theory encompasses two sets of inconsistent, yet equally grounded intuitions: that experience is a product of social construction and that each individual lives alone in a private inner world. Most theories have tended to resolve this confusion by making one intuition foundational and demoting the other to being derivative. There have been theories, however, that refer to both the individual and the intersubjective as *aspects* of experience, a theoretical move that paves the way for a resolution of what first appeared to be a contradiction between the two. Instead of requiring that one intuition be privileged over the other, these theories assert that human experience should be viewed from different perspectives, one that contains the individual and the other the intersubjective. In these theories the themes of dialectic and oscillation are predominant, implying a self that is divided by its participation in the intersubjective, but which nevertheless functions as a unity, i.e., as a one and two at the same time.

Loewald (1980), for example, argued that the self can legitimately be seen as separate and independent *from one perspective*, but that some of its experiences, or aspects thereof, are also organized by an intersubjective that begins in the fusion between mother and infant and continues throughout life (Mitchell 2000). Loewald goes so far as to argue that from the intersubjective perspective, traditional dualities such as self vs. other, internal vs. external, and even reality vs. illusion, are dissolved.

It is from this perspective, incidentally, that the inadequacy of Bollas's use of a spatial metaphor to undermine the intersubjective becomes most apparent. For if the intersubjective is as Loewald conceives it, it resides in a separate realm from any considerations of spatiality, or of inner and outer which form the foundations of concepts of space. To reject the intersubjective, then, because it cannot be located in the space between two individuals is akin to arguing that a tree cannot exist because it can't be found in the spaces between its leaves.

Jacques Lacan (1946) adds another elaboration to the theory of an oscillation, or dialectic, between the individual and the intersubjective. Lacan asserts that an individual subject only arises when in the act of speaking, but since language is a system whose rules are established by a community of speakers, the subject's separateness is eroded in the instant it arises. Rudolph Bernet puts this point succinctly: 'The experience of self in speaking is necessarily connected to the experience that the significance of everything that I say about myself has its origin simultaneously and undecidably both inside and outside myself' (Bernet 1996: 176).

The theories of Loewald, Lacan and others all point in a single direction: that the confusions inherent in the one, the two and the three can only be resolved if both the intersubjective and the individual are considered to be aspects of experience, and if neither are considered to ground the self exclusively. As aspects of experience, the intersubjective and the individual interact in a dialectical or an oscillatory relationship, in such a way that the self, both in isolation and in interaction, sometimes is in one and sometimes the other. Understanding intersubjectivity's role in this way, in the economy of a self characterized by differential aspects, helps to illuminate two very different forms of the intersubjective.

On one hand is the view that the intersubjective appears when two individuals share their subjectivities so that each is aware of the other's thoughts, emotions, desires, etc. This might be labeled the 'experiential intersubjective', since it requires the experienced recognition in each person of the other's subjectivity. The experiential intersubjective appears in the work of Bollas (1999) as well as many others (Benjamin 1998). The other view advances a more comprehensive theory that the intersubjective is an essential aspect of the construction of human experience, and that it does not require that the individual experience any particular conscious content. This view, which can be called the 'radical intersubjective' (Crossley 1996), has two primary forms: the familiar form, from developmental theory, which asserts that the sequential construction of selves requires the essential influence of the other, and that in early infancy self and other are indistinguishable; and the less common form that asserts that the self, even in adulthood, is inextricably embedded in the social. It is the radical intersubjective, particularly in its adult form, that forces consideration of an oscillatory relationship between aspects of experience, neither of which are privileged (i.e., have more epistemological priority) over the other. The radical intersubjective also was what moved Stephen Mitchell to exclaim: 'an individual mind is an oxymoron' (Mitchell 2000: 57).

The simple numbers of one and two, which have long undergirded psychoanalytic theory, have been rendered substantially more complex by the intrusion of the intersubjective. While the simple, traditional *one* can still be seen in individual subjectivity, and even the *two* in experiential intersubjectivity, these are a one and a two that have undergone sweeping transformations through their relationship to the radical intersubjective, which has constructed a *third* out of both the one and two, comprising the fusion between self and other. While numerous analysts have argued that the one persists in analysands' most self-contained moments, in dream states, for example, or the reporting of dreams, they are only partially correct. For the radical intersubjective, in both forms, already occupies the dream, since clinical experience convinces us that elements of figures internalized from developmental periods, as well as elements of the internalized analyst in the real-time relationship, appear with surprising frequency (Poulton 2002; Wallis and Poulton 2001). Indeed, David Scharff (1992) has argued that not only should analysands' dreams be regarded as interpersonal communications, but they may also be socially constructed, either by a couple, or by a family, or by entire social organizations. Even in the analysand's 'self-contained' moments, then, the other can be found to be present, and it only depends on the contingencies of the analytic relationship whether the individual or the intersubjective becomes the focus of the conversation.

Analysands seem to be more or less capable of utilizing the dialectic between the individual and the intersubjective. Perhaps a mark of healthier patients would be that they are capable of light-footed oscillation, considering first one then the other perspective without being overwhelmed by either. Less healthy patients, however, favor one over the other: for some, the intersubjective, with its implications of fusion, is sought as a haven against the anxieties of individuation; for others, the intersubjective is experienced as dangerous territory that instigates rigid defenses designed to bolster the isolated self. See also Hopper, Chapter 7 in this volume.

THE REFUSAL TO BE TWO

In the case of schizoid personality organization, the intersubjective in both forms creates a profound irritant against which an array of aggressive and isolative defenses is employed. The schizoid hates the intersubjective, first and foremost, because the other is characterized via internalized objects as life-eliminating, and because the other's presence signals the onset of toxic affective responses rooted in past experience. Additionally, the schizoid can be seen to *hate the very construction of self*, since it the self's essential nature that introduces the intersubjective as an ineluctable aspect of experience. The schizoid personality, then, may be profitably conceived not simply as a consequence of internalized bad objects, but also as an existential disorder, arising from hypersensitivity to the realities of a self divided by the presence of the other. In consequence, the schizoid continuously attempts to isolate, not only from their bad objects, but also from their core intersubjectivity, and thereby to establish a protective enclave characterized only by the single, removed and individual self. The schizoid's primary purpose, then, is to attack the two, in terms of both the experiential and the radical inter-subjective, and to reside solely in the separate and radically individual one.

The schizoid is often quite successful in attacking the experiential intersubjective. Analysts are familiar with the manifold ways in which their own subjectivity is denied – from refusing recognition of the analyst's own life, to treating the analyst's subjectivity as irrelevant to the analysand's projections and transferences. The radical intersubjective, however, presents the schizoid with a more substantial challenge. For how does the schizoid eliminate the other when the other is an indissoluble aspect of the self? The dilemma faced by the schizoid at this juncture is encountered in analysis more often than is usually recognized.

Mr T, a 44-year-old single professional in thrice-weekly analytic psycho-therapy, exhibited both schizoid and narcissistic characteristics. He com-monly stated that he preferred not to have relationships because they were too frustrating, and he utilized contempt and devaluation of others as a means of achieving protective isolation. Despite these rigid defenses, Mr T would at times consider using me as an intimate in order to explore his interpersonal process. After these flirtations with the intersubjective, how-ever, he would reject me, either through a deadening attack on the liveliness of our interactions, or through contemptuous dismissal and a grandiose reassertion of his desire to live without anyone.

These ambivalent patterns were especially apparent in two sessions from the third year of therapy. Mr T began the first session by complaining that he felt imposed upon by other people's desires and expectations. He wanted to make them leave him alone. He said the only thing that would make him take his girlfriend back (from their recent breakup) was 'my fantasy of her, not the reality since I can't really tolerate being with her.' I said that when he excludes other people because their expectations intrude upon him, all that is left is his fantasy, which seems to make him quite lonely. In response Mr T silently stared out the window. I felt his silence to be an exclusion of me also, perhaps another retreat to fantasy, so after ten minutes I said, 'Maybe you feel that I'm intrusive too. When I try to understand, you exclude me through silence.'

Mr T responded angrily, 'It's interesting that you take my silence as excluding you, when in my silence I was actually thinking hard about what we have been talking about.' I said that my interpretation appeared to have broken his sense of a connection with me, but he explained that he felt overwhelmed by other people sometimes, and he knows he withdraws.

The next session began with a brief silence. Mr T then described his plans to spend the weekend with a woman he met recently. 'On the one hand I'm quite frightened, and on the other I'm excited.' He wasn't sure what his motivation was to see this woman, or whether his plans would be successful. He associated to a friend who died of a heart attack while riding his bicycle. 'You know,' he said, 'this guy's troubles are over. He's dead, on the side of the road. It'd be nice to have no troubles, to be dead and to not want anything anymore . . . The dead have no desires. I want to go to Mexico, to live on a beach, to live a freer life. I want to have nothing I have to do, nothing I want, nothing anyone else wants from me.' I said he seemed to be considering both death and fantasy as solutions to his distrust of people and their presence to, or in, him, since he believed that if he made a move toward recognizing them, he would somehow be damaged.

He became silent for a long time, which seemed to be both a test of whether I would still tolerate silence as his mode of connecting to me, and a way of telling me that his relationship with me scared him, and that he preferred the isolation of either fantasy or death to that kind of fear. In the prior session, I believe he had felt connected to me, in a certain sense, and that I had enacted what he feared: at the point that he was trying to tolerate and even preserve the connection in his silence, I had misunderstood this paradox and failed to appreciate the dilemma hidden in his discussion of how intolerable it was for him to interact with any but a fantasy image of his girlfriend (and me by extension). The true irony of this interaction was that Mr T was connecting with me by talking about his desire to not connect with anyone. My misreading of this mobilized his defensive attack on my presence. We can thus see that the entire interaction was charac- terized by his oscillation between two modes of being – the individual subjective, which he sought in anger and defense, and the intersubjective, with which he was flirting in hidden and timid ways. In the current session Mr T seemed to be operating again in terms of this oscillation. This was why his second silence felt like a test: he was once again undertaking his experiment in intersubjectivity, to see if it could be trusted.

Mr T broke the silence to say he knew he needed approval from people, and that he always felt that he was losing it. He then said: 'I don't feel like I have all the freedom I want. I feel like I've constructed a world where approval is still necessary.'

These brief words highlight the terrible dilemma the schizoid patient faces. On the one hand, Mr T's image of the beach in Mexico reveals his desire to retreat from the experiential and the radical intersubjective, since that image is of the single, individual subject unrelated to anything or anyone else. On the other hand, no matter how much of others' presence he tries to eliminate, Mr T still wants to be connected with them, to get their approval. That is to say: although he claims he wants freedom from his own and others' desires, he continues to discover others within him, at the foundation of his being, and their presence is revealed through his spontaneous desire. His relationship with desire is the microcosm that illustrates the oscillation between the individual and the intersubjective: his desire refers to the trace of the other that is already present in his self, and through his faith in the individual *one* he attempts to eliminate, through fantasy, death or Mexico, his desire.

Mr T continued by describing a supervisor who acted as though 'I would do everything he wanted just so I could have his approval . . . I don't want his approval and I don't need it.' I suggested he was talking about our last session, when I had misunderstood his silence, and I wondered if he felt I had been disapproving. He responded angrily, 'It wasn't just that I *felt* you were disapproving. You *weren't* approving.' I said that his anger meant that he also had wanted my approval, and since this frightened him, he had pushed me away and told himself he'd rather be dead or in a fantasy. He answered by saying, 'Well, first I gave you the opportunity to redeem yourself, and fortunately you latched onto it and understood what I was saying.'

I believe Mr T meant by this that I had saved myself from the death to which he at times consigns me. This, then, was a moment when his refusal of the intersubjective was mollified by his calmer acceptance of the presence of, and his desire for, the other. The session ended in a reflective mood, in which he recognized that the same fearful attack on the intersubjective had occurred with his ex-girlfriend. 'If you think about it,' he said, 'that's what happened to my girlfriend. I simply stopped talking about her, and I tried to stop thinking about her. It was as though I made her die.'

THE RETURN OF THE INTERSUBJECTIVE

Because the schizoid character hates the intersubjective, in the forms both of the other's actual presence, and of the deep structure of a self that is already embedded in the social, they are doomed to a repeating pattern of ejection and rediscovery of the other's influence. For Mr T, this pattern appeared as an oscillation between desiring the other, which reveals the other within himself, and a concerted attack, grounded in his faith in his individuality, to rid himself of any of the other's traces. Mr T didn't want to just eliminate the other as a content of consciousness. He also wanted to void the self that contains the other in the form of desire. His ultimate anti-intersubjective goal was to finally achieve the one of the purely subjective individual self. To do so, both the two of experiential intersubjectivity, and the two-in-one of radical intersubjectivity had to be eliminated. This left him facing his torturous dilemma: by eliminating the other's presence in the original unity from which he himself also arises, he eliminates himself. The only self that remains after the other departs is an empty container. His images of being in Mexico, without others or himself, are haunting illustrations of this emptiness.

The origin of the self lies in the two, both in terms of its developmental path and also in its moment-to-moment experience in the presence of others. But the two of radical intersubjectivity is also interpenetrated by the one of individual subjectivity. This dialectic leads the schizoid into excruciating territory, since the boundaries between self and other are no longer clearly delineated. The schizoid protests against this basic structure of self, since their desire is to eliminate the other *as the second*, under the logic that if there are two, then taking one away will leave the narcissistically cathected one that will finally be comfortable with no needs and no uncontrolled desire for the other. The schizoid's defensive structure, then, rests primarily on the belief that the core of human experience is the two from which one can be eliminated. The impossibility of accomplishing this explains the schizoid's characteristic repeating pattern of oscillation between the one and the two.

CONCLUSION AND FURTHER THOUGHTS

If the most appropriate way to describe human experience is, first, that it is grounded both in the individual and the intersubjective, and second that any person, either alone or in interaction, oscillates between the two positions, then it is possible that some conceptions both of pathology and of analytic technique will require reconceptualization. Viewing the schizoid character from the standpoint of such oscillation enriches our understanding both of the existential dilemmas they face and of the fact that the very structure of self can be experienced as traumatic. We neglect these dilemmas at the cost – to our patients and ourselves – of failing to conceive of human life in all its dimensions. To forget the intersubjective in our patients' and our own lives is to fail to recognize that the one, the two, and the three are essential aspects of experience, and negotiating among them is not an easy task.

REFERENCES

Benjamin, J. (1998) *Shadow of the Other: Intersubjectivity and Gender in Psychoanalysis*, New York: Routledge.

Bernet, R. (1996) 'The Other in Myself', in S. Critchley and P. Dews (eds.), *Deconstructive Subjectivities*, New York: State University of New York Press, pp. 169–184.

Bollas, C. (1999) *The Mystery of Things*, London: Routledge.

Crossley, N. (1996) *Intersubjectivity: The Fabric of Social Becoming*, London: Sage.

Lacan, J. (1946) 'Logical Time and the Assertion of Anticipated Certainty', trans. B. Fink and M. Silver, *Newsletter of the Freudian Field*, 2: 4–22, (1988).

Loewald, H. (1980) *Papers on Psychoanalysis*, New Haven: Yale University Press.

Mitchell, S. A. (2000) *Relationality: From Attachment to Intersubjectivity*, Hillsdale, NJ: The Analytic Press.

Ogden, T. (1994) *Subjects of Analysis*, Northvale, NJ: Jason Aronson.

Poulton, J. (2002) 'A New Look at Freud's Dream of Irma's Injection', presented to a conference of the International Psychotherapy Institute, Washington, DC.

Scharff, D. (1992) *Refinding the Object and Reclaiming the Self*, Northvale, NJ: Jason Aronson.

Wallis, K. and Poulton, J. (2001) *Internalization: The Origins and Construction of Internal Reality*, Buckingham: Open University Press.

Chapter 12

Super-vision or space invader?
Two's company and three makes
for paranoid tendencies

Carl Bagnini

INTRODUCTION

The transference dimension of supervision has been widely discussed in psychoanalytic literature, but attention to the supervisor–supervisee–patient triad has been narrowly focused on two of the three participants, mainly through the patient's transference to the therapist, and the therapist's countertransference to the patient. Fiscalini (1997) found that the triadic implications of the transference–countertransference between supervisor-supervisee, and supervisee–patient were neglected. Berman (2000) has pointed out that little attention had been paid to how patient–supervisee-supervisor unconscious processes influence the learning of psychotherapy.

Stimmel (1995) refers to the patient–supervisee transference which may parallel the supervisor–supervisee relationship; however, focusing on one parallel process or another leaves out the supervisor's countertransferences to the supervisee and his patient. Traditional supervision studies the unconscious relationship in the supervisee–patient dyad, and then feeds it back to the supervisee to facilitate learning (Teitelbaum 1990). Some supervisors limit their study to supervisee countertransferences to patients: a 'treat' vs. 'train' approach (Rosbrow 1993). Broader use of interpretive efforts in psychoanalytic supervision merits more investigation (Gorman 2001). To fully research supervision we have to study the entire field of unconscious realities involving the complex triad of patient–supervisee-supervisor. Treat or train is a narrow and false dichotomy. Using the perspective of 'an intersubjective matrix' (Brown and Miller 2002), super-vision research can be expanded to triadic influences. This chapter discusses the triadic field of supervision, and a vignette illustrates its impact on the teaching and learning of psychotherapy.

GROUP PROCESS AND SUPERVISION

My interest in expanding supervision theory stems from many years of teaching psychotherapy from a group affective learning model (Scharff and

Scharff 2000) that focuses on the effects of projective identification on the therapist's use of self. In discussions with colleagues who practice group analysis, I further noted the importance of working with multiple transferences, and how group process concepts are underutilized in supervision. Application of group process can aid in understanding the triad.

For instance, triadic transferences include the subtle or indirect transferences of the patient to the therapist resulting from the supervisor's influence on the treatment relationship. Another example is the impact of the therapy process on the supervisor's inner world.

A ROLE PARADOX FOR THE THERAPIST AND SUPERVISOR

Significant role paradoxes influence the supervisee in the triad. One aspect of the paradox concerns the therapist as 'expert', and the patient as 'learner'. In supervision, however, the supervisor is the 'expert' and the supervisee the 'learner'. Ambiguities are inherent in the shifting from expert to learner. Therapists work with dependency–autonomy issues of patients, and at the same time deal with their subordinate role in the supervision space, which can overlap, or merge with the role of the patient. The object relations operating in the triad profoundly affect each participant's conscious and unconscious interpretation of their roles.

I propose that the supervisor struggle with a similar paradox and be a 'learner' about the interactive field (Szecsody 2000). Supervisor and supervisee need to examine how supervision presses into the treatment in ways that interfere with the supervisee's freedom to be alone with the patient. Dependency in supervisory sessions may foster 'accommodative' learning (Szecsody 1994) rather than 'assimilative' learning. Assimilative learning is subtle, as it adds to what is already known. Accommodative learning is superimposed on pre-existing cognitive style and replaces what is known. When the supervisor is geared toward interpreting the case, rather than distinguishing the supervisee's ideas and theories, rationales and potentials, the result is accommodative learning. The study of triadic object relations can facilitate assimilative learning.

THE PRESS OF TRIADIC OBJECTS ON THE SUPERVISEE

Whose objects are present during the therapeutic encounter? The therapy dyad includes the objects of the patient and of the therapist in readiness for use by each other. The patient's objects also influence the supervisor's unconscious. What must be added to the menu, as though the cafeteria of objects is not complex enough, are the supervisor's objects. The triad functions as a circular feedback loop, containing mutual unconscious influences.

A paradox exists in trying to be alone with one's patient (one dyad) in light of the tensions of being scrutinized and evaluated outside the setting. The therapist working with the patient must deal with the 'presence' of the supervisor *in* the analytic setting. Depending on projective processes the supervisor's presence may be experienced as sharp or subtle, kindly or carnivorous. Whose patient is it? How is the supervisor's influence utilized and therapist creativity promoted? As therapists pursue the requisite knowledge and skills for practice, they attempt to remain personally and uniquely individuals. Supervisees need help with negotiating the authority–dependency supervisory relationship and its reversal in the therapy situation. This intensifies and promotes projective process, blurring boundaries, and leads to a natural paranoid tendency. Supervisees may feel they are on their own, but are they?

I view countertransference analysis as the major tool in egalitarian super-vision (Rock 1997), as it can provide the supervisor with a detailed view of triadic mental space. Egalitarian supervision refers to a co-constructed and less authoritarian approach to the learning process. Supervisor self-monitoring through countertransference analysis expands the landscape of supervision by accessing everyone's transferences. When warranted, the supervisor leading a frank discussion of all participants' narcissistic sensitivities may actually improve the supervisee's confidence.

FROM EGO IDEAL TO PARANOID TENDENCIES

The process of supervision inevitably changes, beginning, for example, with the supervisee's view of the supervisor as ego ideal, and leading to the supervisor as a critical superego figure. There may be instances in which the supervisee expects disappointment or is already in a state of mistrust. The role of learner/less knowledgeable therapist can foster superego-dominated passivity.

Compliance, in particular, is a negative transference response in super-vision, and when not identified, it can promote an inauthentic imitative therapeutic approach. The companion, if not parallel process, is the supervisor's initial appreciation of, and high expectancies that a new supervisee will prove to be a satisfying investment. Initially invested with positive feelings, the supervisee seeks out the supervisor's support and approval, takes in what the mentor says, whether as theoretical points, clinical insights, transference analysis, or discussions of the frame. Armed with notes and inspiration, the therapist models the therapy after the learned mentor.

Developmentally, some infantile dependencies are natural and adaptive in supervision. Moving up the developmental line there are attendant overlays of childhood needs for nurturing and support, adolescent autonomous strivings against authority, with suspicions, or ambivalence, and the more adult equality pursuits. The supervisee who occasionally gets stuck at the lower end of the developmental continuum needs an acknowledgement of normative regression. The supervisory process can inhibit the proper surfacing of conflict over autonomy and dependency within the dual roles of therapist and supervisee. Inevitably, there are oscillations between paranoid/schizoid and depressive reactions throughout the treatment (Klein 1946) that surface in the supervision.

UNDERSTANDING ENACTMENTS IN THE TRIAD

Supervisory intervention in a patient crisis requires awareness and judgment in helping the therapist contain the patient. The supervisor can take into account the supervisee's potential for blurring self with other when there are infantile, or pre-oedipal issues involved in treatment. If the supervisor quickly assuages the supervisee's anxieties, instead of taking the multiple transferences into account, supervision will temporarily shore up therapist uncertainty, while omitting the supervisor's anxieties as mutually useful information.

How else can supervision impair learning? In early treatment there is a crucial period of trial identification with the patient (Casement 1997). This is when the patient is understood from inside their own experience, in order for the therapist to locate important aspects of the transference. Restraint in interpreting is required in this initial period. The supervisee may reflect: How does the patient view the process, the relationship, and me? If the supervisee studies the patient's issues around dependency needs *and* autonomous strivings, interpretive attempts will be better tailored to both tendencies. What if the autonomy of the supervisee is jeopardized owing to the supervisor's over-identification with the patient's ambivalence or caution? Learning is sacrificed if the supervisor's impatience prevents the supervisee's gradual discovery of the patient's internal world.

Another negative potential is the supervisor who reinterprets the therapist's interpretations before sufficient time has elapsed for the patient to absorb them. The prescribed approach is for patience in offering reinterpretive comments, allowing the patient to communicate reactions to the supervisee; and if the supervisee does not report the patient's responses, an inquiry can be made as to what is missing in the case reporting.

I now present a vignette to illustrate triadic dimensions of supervision. I offer my understanding of the various transferences, and share my countertransference to demonstrate its efficacy in grounding the teaching and learning process.

VIGNETTE OF A SUPERVISEE WHO FELT GUILTY

Kathy, 56, in private practice for nine years, sought supervision for a difficult case. Kathy had been seeing Kim, age 17, for one year in weekly analytic psychotherapy and had not been in supervision during that time. Kim was sixteen when she sought help with cutting school and academic underachievement, rebellion at home, inability to make friends with male peers, feelings of inadequacy, and unwillingness to date. Kathy described Kim as a feisty young woman, a good talker, and full of potential.

Kathy reported a central traumatic situation that provided crucial understanding of Kim's difficulties. During the eighth month of treatment Kim revealed her one-year-older brother had sexually molested her from age ten to age twelve. There was no intercourse and no evidence of intimidation or force. Kathy encouraged Kim to bring up the incestuous experiences to her parents. Over a period of two months they discussed the consequences of telling her parents. Kim alternated between fear her parents would do nothing and hope they would hear her and understand why she had so many problems. Kathy championed family sessions with mom, dad, and Kim. Two family sessions were held and Kathy actively helped Kim talk about the brother–sister incest. The parents listened, and father responded with sympathy, and a 'what can you do now?' attitude. Mother sat slumped and withdrawn, mostly silent, a customary complaint Kim had raised before. Kathy believed Kim's progress in treatment and in life would depend on the parents confronting their son, who was now living away as a college freshman. This did not occur.

Subsequently, Kim changed in physical appearance and communication. Kim's shift consisted of a series of 'I don't knows' as Kathy posed questions that Kim usually raised on her own. Affect was generally blunted, with shoulder shrugging, and a diminished interest in talking. She wore bland colors, less feminine in style, and she slumped in her chair, making less eye contact. Once she showed an uncustomary irritability by exclaiming, 'You're the therapist, you figure it out.' Kathy believed the basis for Kim's withdrawal and uncooperative attitude was the disappointment with her parents from the family sessions. Kim's response was that she now had her first boyfriend, and he made her feel loved, so what did it matter about her parents? There was, Kathy thought, both a triumphant feeling behind having her first boyfriend and a contemptuous tone that Kathy believed glossed over the parents' indifference. Kathy related in supervision that she felt anger at Kim's parents for not supporting their daughter and the efforts to bring out the incest experience.

As Kim's sessions continued Kathy felt that having the new boyfriend might mean Kim was ready to wind down the therapy. Without planning to, Kathy said those very words during a particularly tedious session when Kim was lethargic and uninterested. Kim did not react when Kathy mentioned that summer was coming, and perhaps Kim would want a break, given that her social life and first love were encouraging.

Kim canceled her next session, and in the following session reported there was a strain in the boyfriend–girlfriend relationship. He wanted to date other girls but stay with Kim. Kathy had offered Kim a way to take a break from therapy but was now confused. Much more had occurred than she had understood. She felt guilty, and decided to seek supervision.

The supervisor's impressions

Kathy was visibly upset as she spoke about the case. She had little insight about Kim's sullen and silent behavior and was therefore not able to interpret. Kathy worried she had lost the patient by suggesting the break in treatment. She had concluded that the patient's problems stemmed fundamentally from the incest, and focused on that. Kathy did not report how the molestation specifically impaired Kim's functioning, or how the sexual contacts between the siblings became central in her thinking. Kathy over-identified with the sexual component so that family sessions seemed a correct move. Kathy's decision-making process concerned me, especially the choice of brother–sister incest as a 'trauma' to focus on. She used that term in advocating family sessions. I believed the incest was important, but trauma was reductionistic. I thought she had made an inaccurate assessment of Kim's emotional difficulties and had essentially missed all of the transference issues. This stemmed from unconscious countertransference inducing Kathy to provide direct and unambiguous mothering to contain Kim's many problems. She had reacted to the incest with personal horror rather than with measured thinking.

Had she examined the individual and family psychodynamics more carefully, several hypotheses might have emerged. Incest can be a flight into sibling pleasure as a defense against neglect and depressive anxieties, and if so, Kathy might work with Kim's recent rejection of Kathy as a projection of rejecting or apathetic parents. Sexual over-stimulation by the parents was another possibility in Kim's childhood, and I wondered whether Kim could have perceived Kathy's zealousness as over-stimulation, if not a promise that Kathy would repair the family deficits. Kathy's countertransference had limited her receptivity and locked her into a one-dimensional clinical approach by only seeing Kim's problems as caused by the combination of a depressed mother–daughter relationship and incest. I surmised that Kathy was influenced by her earlier work with Kim on the long-term mother–

daughter estrangement and that she over-identified with these nurturing deficiencies.

Kathy was burdened by a combination of her own relational vulnerabilities (Rock 1997) and needed a frame for rethinking so she might discover the personal basis for overzealous application of her conclusions. The two participants in the therapeutic process had been enacting without understanding the implications of transference and countertransference. Kathy, like the mother and daughter, was in a 'slump'.

My task consisted of how to offer a frame for discovery without humiliating Kathy. The issue in supervision partially paralleled the treatment dilemma, in which Kathy attempted to offer the patient a wholesale plan for feeling better as her advocate, but there had been a lack of patient self-discovery. Kim was not currently respectful of Kathy. It was clear that Kathy did not comprehend Kim's reactions to her, labeling them as resistance (unanalyzed) with no historical or relational basis. I took a more instruction-oriented approach at first, emphasizing what she had already accomplished with Kim. At that time I did not fully realize I carried triadic transferences related to criticizing, fearing criticism, and disappointments in unreliable dependency. Building the supervisor–supervisee relationship requires an appreciation of role confusion. The therapist is expected to contain personal fantasies and feelings while with the patient. Supervision (Konig 1995) promotes a different role. The supervisee is called upon to offer ambiguity through the expression of personal feelings and fantasies about the patient to expand self-awareness. This appears to run counter to the therapeutic role in doing treatment, but supervision necessitates a free sharing of all factors that may affect therapy, including use of self.

I found it important to mention the tensions in the different roles so that Kathy might become comfortable discussing their ambiguities. Trusting me with her feelings about the patient required that she tolerate bad feelings along with good ones, and I felt that this could be accomplished by taking a matter-of-fact approach to role ambiguity as a tool of supervision.

The supervisee initially idealizes the supervisor

Idealization of me occurred early and helped establish rapport. I believed this was due to her desperate need for immediate help, temporarily reducing anxiety all around; but the honeymoon was short, as most are.

My usual style is to raise unconscious transference–countertransference enactments when there is an impasse or rift in the therapist–patient collaboration. I also ask for associations to widen the scope of thinking. While I do not initially know about the supervisee's life, it often turns out that what is salient there finds its way into supervision. As I get to know the supervisee's personal valences we make a start in self-discovery that I hope will lead to re-connecting with the patient.

I addressed Kathy's unconscious slip in telling Kim to take the summer off, introduced examples of projective identification, starting with Kim's idealized reports of boyfriend bliss, followed by troubled couple relating, and suggested we look for other paired difficulties. Kathy listened to my references to paired relating and its parallels with the current troubled treatment process. She visibly relaxed, as though a great burden was lifted. Empowered by newfound knowledge to turn the tide in the case, she bypassed feelings associated with inadequacy, or lack of confidence. She did grasp the sequence of dynamic events: Kathy failed to make restitution between Kim and her parents, Kim became sullen and uncooperative, and Kathy rejected her. I pointed to a parallel group process in the failure of the parents to fulfill Kathy and Kim's desires for restitution, and the unconscious similar feelings of rejection that Kathy and Kim had not discussed. A small glimmer of countertransference awareness accompanied Kathy to her upcoming sessions with Kim.

A learning issue remained on my mind: had I indirectly prevented her from comprehending unconscious processes by filling in the missing 'information' through substitute analysis? If so, would Kathy take a smaller dose of learning from me than I would have preferred? I took comfort that Kathy used what she could at the time. My helping her in a concrete way, rather than exploring the anxiety areas, was motivated by concern that Kathy recover her therapeutic position.

De-idealization and 'paranoid tendencies'

The process of learning psychotherapy from a supervisor is complicated by the regressive–progressive pulls back and forth across the two boundaries, supervisee–supervisor, and therapist–patient. In Kathy's situation, examples of paranoid tendencies took the form of incomplete reporting or withholding of case material. On one occasion she announced at the beginning of supervision she had left her notes in the office. At that time I recall responding that her dog hadn't eaten her homework, but close! Another example had to do with partial or selective relating of sessions. The parts left out included moments following an intervention on Kathy's part, with no reference to Kim's responses. Opposite recording gaps focused on Kim with no references to Kathy. In each situation one of them was left out of Kathy's written work, or in her discussion of the session.

The unconscious withholding of material indicated that Kathy was splitting the relationship between Kim and herself, in favor of a pairing with me that left out a third person. In systems theory a weak dyad usually leads to confiscation of another to promote a triangle. The triangle functions as a defense draining off conflict in the dyad. I felt Kathy was alternating who was to be included in the dyad. It was either Kim with me, or Kathy and me, but not the two together with me. I felt this as displaced anxieties having to do with conflicted pairings in a triangle. Kathy's defensive case reporting was an example of 'paranoid tendencies'.

Example of triadic transference–countertransference

Learning about the supervisor's influences on the therapist can occur through the patient's transference to the *supervisor* through the therapist. Several examples of triadic transference–countertransference are in order. One consisted of the patient seeking a boyfriend after the family sessions failed, partly as an age-appropriate developmental step. However, Kim's timing of the relationship was an unconscious flight from disappointments in Kathy. Kim's seeking a boyfriend was not mere coincidence, nor was Kathy's seeking out a male supervisor, to restore hurt parts of her therapeutic self. Kathy's initial idealized dependency in supervision resembled that of Kim's earlier dependency on Kathy. The second element in the triadic transference–countertransference was that I installed myself between Kathy and her patient, supplying Kathy, so I thought, with the needed linkages for a re-pairing (*repairing*). My countertransference reaction stemmed from my family of origin and my earliest role as the middle child, the only male sandwiched between a younger and an older sister. I often over-functioned in the role of male parental go-between in the family.

The above personal awareness allowed discovery of a third feature of the triadic transference–countertransference. I had been affectively taken over by a powerfully charged triadic projection process that related to Kim's admonition to Kathy: '*You're the therapist, you figure it out.*' Kathy's impasse led her to me to unconsciously bail her out, and, in the role of supervisor-as-over-functioning child, I was taken in by the projective identification. I experienced a slight twinge of painful enlightenment, as the triadic projection process became clear: the patient needed the therapist, and the therapist needed the supervisor to understand something together that was not previously known, so it might become available in the work. My awareness of my childhood memories shed light on Kathy and her patient's projections. Discovery had taken place for use in future supervision sessions with Kathy. I realized 'paranoid tendencies' were symmetrical with my childhood role as protector, projected as the tendency to over-function as Kathy's and her patient's 'rescuer'.

I decided to discuss with Kathy how the patient was affecting me and the circular process I sensed in the case and in supervision. I did not share my childhood insights when approaching the material in supervision, although they were valuable to me in opening a new supervisory space. In two supervision sessions I asked about idealization, guilt, and identification in the supervision, and raised the parallels in Kim's early treatment relationship. I shared my honest frustration about the patient's withdrawal and how I was talking a good deal in supervision. My countertransference reenacted Kim and Kathy's impasse. Kathy and I were over-functioning. Kathy was able to think about her early idealization of me, and the patient's idealization of her. She further explained that she had not recognized how she had worked so hard to keep Kim's faith in her. She went on to explain her need to follow my lead, and this did not initially allow for expansive thinking about the relationship from an unconscious standpoint. By being a follower, she was not yet able to work with the whole experience. Similarly, Kim had withdrawn from the whole experience of the therapy, was less invested in the work, and let Kathy do the talking, withholding important disappointments she felt in Kathy. In later supervision Kathy offered that fear of being a disappointment was a core issue during her childhood and adolescence. She was embarrassed but relieved, paving the way for more openness in her work with Kim and in supervision.

I later learned an important lesson from Kathy, that in early supervision she felt I had spoken with such certainty about the case that she elected to take what was given as 'gospel'. She shared that my teaching had allowed her to put the issue of responsibility for the case in my hands, rather than between us as a collaborative effort. I appreciated the frankness in her depiction. The discussion resulted in fewer directives by me and a more attentive stance by Kathy to what was *not* being said in Kim's sessions. She enquired if Kim had been reluctant to take on the issue of Kathy's letting her down with the parents. A discussion ensued that brought out Kim's disgust with her parents, as well as her fears of hurting Kathy. Kathy later reported that Kim knew Kathy was pushing the meetings with her parents, and she had passively followed her lead in making the incest the only issue.

Kathy realized that winding down treatment with Kim stemmed from the de-idealization and unconscious disgust Kathy felt for failing Kim, projected as Kim's not needing to come anymore. Kathy made use of the supervision to de-repress therapeutic blockages and restore her working treatment relationship.

CONCLUSIONS

This chapter expanded psychoanalytic supervision to the study of triadic object relations with emphasis on the supervisor's use of self. The supervision vignette demonstrated triadic transferences in the case and in supervision by illustrating how patient, supervisee, and supervisor are an interactive field, susceptible to the interpenetration of projective material.

Two questions were raised earlier. Does the supervisor claim any *super*-vision and can the supervisee remain alone with the patient. Yes and no. Yes, the supervisor has the potential for developing a super-transference or vision of the total situation (Teitelbaum 2001). No, the therapist cannot be truly alone with the patient, any more than the patient and therapist can completely rid themselves of all of their internal objects.

Supervisors and therapists are subject to having personal issues exposed and their technical skills tested. Humility is a useful ethic in this regard. The supervisor and professional colleague are best served by examining their complex and different roles. The more that role paradoxes are openly discussed the better the dialogue, reducing hierarchical restraints. Subjective forces are also at work in the choices therapists make in selecting a supervisor. One's feelings, as well as word of mouth in the therapy community about who is good to learn from, govern the choice. Unconscious and conscious fantasies and motives ought to be part of the eventual supervision dialogue. I find that supervisees who freely choose supervisors for help with cases tend to respond favorably to offers that they share their mistakes in a non-judgmental atmosphere. This may not be the case in training institutions, given the greater evaluative component.

Group process theory can assist in providing requisite knowledge for supervision practice. However, as the panorama of objects to study expands, complexity can add distress for supervisor and therapist. As mentor and mentee discover the internal and external affective landscape, normative paranoid tendencies can initially reduce therapeutic efficacy.

The analysis offered in this study may also prove useful to those practicing group supervision, an activity with additional levels of richness and complexity. Whether in group or individual supervision, supervisees are well informed to expect complementary relational configurations. As noted, supervision causes regressions (Frawley-O'Dea and Sarnat 2001; Roberts 2001) and progressions in the service of improving analytic skills and empathic responsiveness. The study of triadic mental space offers a more complete canvas on which to base supervisory interventions.

REFERENCES

Berman, E. (2000) 'Psychoanalytic Supervision: The Intersubjective Development', *International Journal of Psycho-Analysis*, 81: 273–290.

Brown, L. and Miller, M. (2002) 'The Triadic Intersubjective Matrix in Supervision', *International Journal of Psycho-Analysis*, 83: 811–823.

Casement, P. (1997) 'Towards Autonomy: Some Thoughts on Psychoanalytic Supervision', in M. H. Rock (ed.), *Psychodynamic Supervision: Perspectives of the Supervisor and the Supervisee*, Northvale, NJ: Jason Aronson, pp. 263–282.

Fiscalini, J. (1997) 'On Supervision Parataxis and Dialogue', in M. H. Rock (ed.), *Psychodynamic Supervision: Perspectives of the Supervisor and the Supervisee*, Northvale, NJ: Jason Aronson, pp. 29–58.

Frawley O-Dea, M. G. and Sarnat, J. (2001) *The Supervisory Relationship: A Contemporary Psychodynamic Approach*, New York: Guilford.

Gorman, H. E. (2001) 'Interpreting Transference in Supervision', in S. Gill (ed.),

The Supervisory Alliance: Facilitating the Psychotherapist's Learning Experience, Northvale: NJ: Jason Aronson, pp. 181–199.

Klein, M. (1946) 'Notes on Some Schizoid Mechanisms', *International Journal of Psycho-Analysis*, 27: 99–110.

Konig, K. (1995) *The Practice of Psychoanalytic Therapy*, Northvale, NJ: Jason Aronson.

Roberts, J. L. (2001) 'Stage Fright in the Supervisory Process', in S. Gill (ed.), *The Supervisory Alliance: Facilitating the Psychotherapist's Learning Experience*, Northvale, NJ: Jason Aronson, pp. 81–91.

Rock, M. H. (1997) 'Effective Supervision', in M. H. Rock (ed.), *Psychodynamic Supervision: Perspectives of the Supervisor and the Supervisee*, Northvale, NJ: Jason Aronson, pp. 107–132.

Rosbrow T. (1993) 'Significance of the Unconscious Plan for Psychoanalytic Theory', *Psychoanalytic Psychology*, 10(4): 515–532.

Scharff, D. E. and Scharff, J. S. (2000) *Tuning the Therapeutic Instrument: Affective Learning in Psychotherapy*, Northvale, NJ: Jason Aronson.

Stimmel, B. (1995) 'Resistance to the Awareness of the Supervisor's Transference with Special Reference to Parallel Process', *International Journal of Psycho-Analysis*, 76: 609–618.

Szecsody, I (1994) 'Supervision: A Complex Tool for Psychoanalytic Training', *Scandinavian Psychoanalytic Review*, 17: 119–129.

Szecsody, I (2000) 'Berman's Psychoanalytic Supervision: The Intersubjective Development', *International Journal of Psycho-Analysis*, 81: 1223–1225.

Teitelbaum, S. H. (1990) 'Supertransference: The Role of the Supervisor's Blind Spots', *Psychoanalytic Psychology*, 7: 243–258.

Teitelbaum, S. H. (2001) 'The Changing Scene in Supervision', in S. Gill (ed.), *The Supervisory Alliance: Facilitating the Psychotherapist's Learning Experience*, Northvale, NJ: Jason Aronson, pp. 3–18.

Chapter 13

Four: on adding up to a family

Christopher Bollas

There is something to be said now and then for refusing to take anything for granted, a Cartesian act that suspends assumed knowledge.

For example, we have all had a father, and while we may imagine the way he appeared, or we may recall some particular moment with him, or think of him through the sound of his name, or just sense him as part of ordinary unconscious contemplation, yet all these thinkings will be rendered under the generic concept of 'father'. But what exactly is that, we may ask, what is a father? Simply because we have one, can remember moments with him and can name him does not suggest that we know what he is.

To some extent psychoanalysis over the last forty years, especially in the work of Jacques Lacan, has been asking that question. Part of the Lacanian answer is that 'a father' is more a name than a person, associated with lawmaking, interdiction, and judgement. Lacan elaborates Freud's definition that earlier identified the father as the figure who would castrate the son if he were to defy him and as the figure who announces the presence of the sexual relation to the mother, which dispossesses the self of any illusion of divine, immaculate, conception.

Yet of course, each of us does have our own individual father – along with the functions held in his name – and it is psychologically impossible not to mix – or mesh – our individual experience with the integrity of the object. Whatever 'father' is as a set of functions personified in this name, the father we actually have in our own life is a composition of many differing impressions derived from many differing types of experience: in reality and dream life.

We may also ask, what is a mother? – a puzzle that preoccupied Winnicott (1965) in some ways, although by concentrating on 'the good enough mother' he might appear to have over localised his question in a domestic soap opera. But he wrote about the 'holding environment', 'the facilitating environment' and about the intelligent care mothers provide when they assist their infant's 'going on being', and when he wrote about the 'essential aloneness' in all of us, a memory of sorts, of our transition from pre-birth to birth, and further back, from the inorganic to the organic; this essential aloneness seemed to form something of the core of the self's 'capacity to be alone' which was always paradoxically dependent on the presence of the other. And it would always really be on the presence of the mother. He once wrote that 'there is no such thing as a baby' and then he paused long enough to create an aperture of surprise before he said 'without a mother'. But he demonstrated this in his prose, because when writing about the self's aloneness, capacity to be alone, its true self gestures, and its need for continuity in being, he was also always talking about the presence and the work of the other, of the mother who holds these elements of the infant's life in her psyche-soma. The mother is everywhere in Winnicott's writing. The challenge still remains, however, to think what we mean by the thought of a mother and the fact that we all had one and that we all refer to one actually rather disables us from considering the mother-idea.

To think this idea, we would have to fashion a potential space out of the work of constructed ignorance; we would have to assume that we know nothing of her and by not knowing what mother meant, we inhabit a mental space that allows us to create her anew and thus to rethink the mother-idea.

John Rickman's (1950) seminal paper, 'The Factors of Numbers in Individual and Group Dynamics', set both Michael Balint and Winnicott to work on a psychoanalytic numerology. These days we may safely assume that the number one refers to the self alone, the number two refers to the infant–mother relation, and the number three refers to the self's relation to the mother and the father (see also Poulton, Chapter 11 in this volume). Each of these numbers suggests in the minds of many psychoanalysts different psychologies: i.e. one-body psychology, two-body psychology, and three-body psychology. It could be argued that the clinical usefulness of this numerology is that in thinking about which number is prevailing at any one moment in time the psychoanalyst knows whether he is engaged with a one-body presentation, a two-body presentation, or a three-body presentation. In terms of a psychoanalytic numerology he is working either with the number 1, the number 2, or the number 3.

Counting on this distinction means that the analyst presumably knows which sorts of interpretations to make. If the analysand, for example, is talking to the analyst about his wife it might be presumed that the analyst is listening to the patient's work with the number 2. In fact, as we know from object relations theory, the patient may in fact be talking to a part of himself by projection into the wife; the patient is working with the number 1, or more aptly, indicating that there is something about being one of 1 that he cannot bear well, so he resorts to creating a false second. Alternatively, a patient might be talking about a particular character dimension, such as his inability to think properly about what he regards as the more important issues of his life. In time, however, the analyst might discover that in fact this point of view is the death work of the other: that it reflects the projective identification of one of the parents. Thus what looks like the patient's work in the area of the number 1 in fact is work with the number 2.

Assisting the psychoanalyst in the development of a psychoanalytic numerate *sense* will be the countertransference. The patient talking about this deficiency nonetheless calls upon the psychoanalyst's inner sense that what the patient assumes to be his own creations feels to be the nature of oppression. The patient's affective turmoil surrounding this topic, including his hesitations, his sudden grammatical breakdowns, and so forth, seem to be the work of an 'interject': that is, an internal object that has been projected into the self by the other. The interject reflects the unconscious work of the other and sits inside the self subject to very little unconscious elaboration, as it never constituted the desire of the subject in the first place. After a while and shaped by the form of the analysand's transference, the psychoanalyst can sense whether this object addressed by the patient is work in the area of 1 or 2.

Our numerology is further complicated by psychic striation. A segment of time within a session may express work in all three numbers at the same time, segregated only by psychic function, not by temporality. So a patient might be talking to a part of himself – 1 – while simultaneously undertaking a dialogue with the mother and also engaging in some conflict with the father. Which of these numbers, to ask a Freudian question, bears the highest 'psychical value'? We might say that at any moment in time the entire numerology is present and engaged in some form of work, but from moment to moment does one number intensify in relation to the others? A patient talking about a wife may one moment be discussing his own femininity, another moment his unconscious attitude toward his mother's disposition towards him, another moment the object of his father's desire. All three numbers, like all three structures, are always present, but it is a matter of which number is the most active in any moment in time.

It will be seen, naturally, that a psychoanalytic numerology bears no relation to mathematics proper.

For example, from a psychoanalytical mathematic, $1 + 1 = 3$. In psychic life there is one event which psychoanalysis must count in this way. For when the mother and the father copulate and the mother bears a child $1 + 1 = 3$: mother plus father create a baby. That is, if the family were counting, it would now add up to three. Matters are almost infinitely more complex than this, for as Lacan and others have argued, at any sexual moment there are six people present: each partner's parents. So in this respect, intercourse counts as follows: $1 + 1 = 6$.

If the family were counting.

But how could we assign a numerate function to an immaterial entity? Let us say that I can count, my father can count, and the rest of the members of my family could count, but on what basis would we be able to say that the family-in-itself could count? Perhaps we mean that we could assemble the family and then ask them to count together out loud all at once. But I have just said in the addition $1 + 1 = 3$ that the family is counting and we know at that point that the infant cannot count. And if the family does not exist until the number 4 – which is what I shall be shortly arguing – then how could we say that the family is counting when in fact it is not yet there in a position to count?

This is quite a problem.

I shall hedge by saying 'if' the family could count, it would make the above addition, but presuming *psychic numeracy*, any couple could contain the number 4 within them, and it would be from this numerate function that 'the family' – as an internal object – could make the addition.

We know, for example, that a couple on the verge of having their first child are beginning to assemble in their respective minds what it means to be *forming a family*. It takes many forms. The couple search for the child's name. They outfit the baby's room and buy its first objects. In many countries they sign it up for a private school before its birth. They arrange in some way for visits to come of differing members of their respective families of origin and they shall receive gifts from family and friends in anticipation of the infant's birth. In the system unconscious much more work is taking place than this as the partners find thing-presentations gathering in the unconscious around the number 4. They also begin a very long and complicated effort to construct a shared number 4, and in psychoanalytic numerology this would be a case where $1 + 1$ cannot $= 4$ (it could only establish the number 2), but bearing in mind that in intercourse we said that six people were present, is this a case of $1 + 1$ equalling 6: one partner plus two parents and another partner plus two parents? But that does not add up to 4, it is 6? All along, the idea of there being four people present is based on the number 1 thinking this. That is, in the psyche of one individual participant in intercourse there are four objects present: the self, the sexual other, and the self's parents: i.e. 4. But if we think of this from the future family point of view – that is from the future number 4 back to this $1 + 1$, then as all members must count . . . as is the case with family life, then we must include both participants' parental couples of origin, in which case there are at least six objects in some form of intercourse. (It will be obvious to some that I am also leaving out other objects that would make for a higher number, the most important being any couple's imaginary or actual children who are also part of the primal scene.)

From a psychoanalytic perspective we may find a psychic numerology that not only does not add up, but multiplies in difficulty each time one attempts such adding up.

We can see that the problem with the above is the fecund effect of sexuality upon psychic numeracy, as $1 + 1$ in the sexual addition does not add up to 2, but actually makes 3 and creates the possibility for 4.

To come more directly to the point – and I hope in the nick of time as I am very very far from the world of mathematics – I shall be counting on the number 4 to count for the family. If 1 stands for the self, if 2 stands for self and other, if 3 stands for the after-effects of sexual intercourse, then 4 stands for the family.

But wouldn't 3 be the family? And isn't it an odd way to describe the birth of a child as 'the after-effects of intercourse'?

When a couple copulate and the after-effect is a child we cannot assume there is the presence of a family. For the family to 'arrive', further addition is necessary. There are many more contributing elements to the family than simply the arrival of the prospective family members.

For example, to take the failure to count to 4, Isobel and James have intercourse and the after-effect is Jill. Isobel never loved James and after her birth Jill is given up for adoption. Isobel gave James his marching orders before the birth of Jill, and although the child was born, the family was not.

Harry and Jessica are childhood sweethearts having grown up on the same street only yards from one another. Harry's father committed suicide when he was five and his mother – left with three young children – became severely depressed, took to drinking spirits, and by Harry's age 9 she was hospitalized for the first of many admissions. Harry was looked after by his mother's brother, but his uncle hated him and subjected him to severe beatings until he reached mid-adolescence. Jessica's mother had been married twice before and had six children before Jessica was born. A born-again Christian she was extremely exacting and devout in a misguided way, demanding that the children 'do without'. When Jessica was eleven the mother began to have visions of Jesus visiting the home and one day heard him say that she must strip naked and walk the middle lane of the street as a form of prayer for him to come to her. This she did although she was hit by a car and severely disabled, a shock to her life that she met with stony silence and a refusal to do anything but weave quilts for a Christian Aid store in the small town where they lived. Harry and Jessica seemed to constantly run across one another during these years. They didn't so much play together as they spent blank time in one another's presence. When Harry's uncle ran off and Harry's mother was put into care, Harry dropped out of high school and lived in another neighbour's garage. Jessica helped him get some of the things he needed and one day that seemed to be Jessica and they fell deeply in love when they were both seventeen. They moved into a large Chevrolet Impala where they slept, had meals together (from the local fast food merchants) and tried to put a life together. They eventually moved from their 'home' town and travelled to California where each took up differing jobs, although problems began to arise in their relationships. They seemed to have little ability to tolerate the other's imperfections, such as they were, and they could not talk it through. Both had psychotic episodes, one turned to crack cocaine, and although they lived together, for all intents and purposes they were no longer a couple. They *had* talked about having a family. It *had* served as an important *object* of conversation, but to the counsellor who eventually saw them – in their late twenties – it was very clear that the fourth object in this was an aspiration considered from –1.

Minus-1 I shall use in this situation to identify a position within psychoanalytic numerology that would follow Bion's (1962) concept of –K. Where K stands for knowledge, –K would therefore stand for a mental state organised to rid the self of what it knows. Anyone counting on his future from –1 will only add to further losses. –1 + –1 = –2. The more that Harry and Jessica talked about their life and their future the more they added to their own subtraction. In five years they were so full of psychic losses, each attempted addition only adding to their woes, that they had accumulated a numeric imbalance. There were too many losses. They had to give up on each other – as Harry was to say 'we must cut our losses' – in order to start again.

We may conjecture that the concept of –1 in psychic numeracy identifies a position in which any self is less than 1. To be less than 1 – or to use Bret Ellis's title even *Less than Zero* (1985) – is to have so many parts of the self missing that the self does not add up. In this case, it does not add up to 1. Such is the fate of the psychotic individual and in thinking of Harry and Jessica, both of whom were parented by psychotic parents, and each of whom was divested of important parts of the self by the work of their own psychotic methods, we may see how psychic losses can lead to a form of adding up that only makes further losses inevitable. For if the mind cannot add in the first place, then any attempted addition will ultimately subtract from the solution, and the self will be left with a never-ending loss.

We could think of many situations in which intercourse and the after-effects do not create a family, just as we can think of many situations in which a couple thinking of a family are not actually counting up to 4.

To count to 4 in psychoanalysis, one must make the following addition. After 1 + 1 = 3, there is further addition. Out of these three people another object is formed. It is the first interpersonally constructed vital shared object that serves the function of opening lines of communication between its participants in order that the family may be created. If one partner in the couple cannot count to 4, then even if the other partner can, and even if they go on to have many children, we can say that they have not been able to construct the fourth object: they will not, then, have become a family.

Another way of considering this numerate distinction – between 3 and 4 – is that 3 counts for the family of origin and 4 for the family of one's own creation. Each of us is an after-effect of 1 + 1 and we are part of 3 that we take to be a family of origin, but as I shall argue shortly, we may be overly presumptuous to argue that this group of three is in fact a family. A child born as a result of the mother's rape by a stranger is part of 3, but not part of a family of origin.

Family work, whether in family therapy, in group therapy with couples, or even in individual psychoanalysis with the patient's transference of the family reveals deeply painful failures of groups of people who cannot count to 4. Of course, with a Harry and a Jessica – as with many psychotic couples – it is very clear that no family can be created and we bear witness to a different type of pain, to the awful realisation that psychosis only subtracts from life. They might try false additions, but in time their losses will show up on some psychic accounts sheet.

But the more common anguish psychotherapists face is the group of three or four or six or eight who have in one way or another struggled mightily to form a family and have failed.

Jim is in analysis and he has almost no memories before the age of thirteen. He is thoughtful and relatively insightful and his initial seeming amnesia was puzzling. He was not at a loss for trying to tell himself about his mother, his father, and his three sisters in my presence. He could do this. But he was describing individuals who were part of a group but who had never formed a family. So 'family memories' were, paradoxically enough, recollections of the group, but not remembrances of the family.

The group of people brought together through the after-effects of intercourse are not the same as a family.

So what then *is* a family? What is that additional integer that makes 3 into 4? I answer solipsistically. It is the number 4 that has already added itself up.

It is the integer that arrives only when the group has *created* the space for the fourth object to show up, a psychic object that serves the thing-presentation called 'my family' that will, in itself, act as a form of intelligence in the unconscious communications between the members of the group.

A family, then, is a special evolution in the history of the unconscious.

Indeed the history of the word 'family' reflects this evolution. According to the *Bloomsbury Dictionary of Word Origins* the word for family is from the Latin *famulus* which meant servant. From this was derived *familia* which referred only to the domestic servants in a household and their employers. It was introduced into English in its original Latin sense and so it survived until the end of the eighteenth century, but by the seventeenth century it widened in its usage to mean the whole household. Finally it narrowed to 'group of familiar people.'

So we come to *familiar*. Bloomsbury writes that familiar originally meant 'of the family' and intriguingly its most common usage referred to a familiar enemy or familiar foe, that is, an enemy within one's own household or family. It then broadened to mean 'intimately associated' and finally to 'well-known from constant association' (218).

From this etymology we can see a progression: from a collection of people who form a group, to a group of people who become 'intimately associated' with one another: that is, who become familiar with one another. An intermediate meaning seems to have been – familiar enemy – an enemy within the group. (We may keep this as a question. Does the fourth object have something to do with facing an enemy in a group, an encounter which *adds* to one's psychic economy?)

The Oxford English Dictionary's fifth definition of family is 'the group of people consisting of one set of parents and their children, whether living together or not; any group of people connected by blood or other relationship' (913). If the *blood* connection is intrinsic to the creation of family we see here the after-effects of sexuality. A family will be created out of the blood link between mother and father, giving rise to the potency of the statement 'he or she is blood', meaning in contemporary usage: family. The OED also informs us that in the sixteenth and seventeenth centuries in England there was a sect called 'Family of Love' which had many followers – called 'familists' – who 'stressed the importance of love and held that absolute obedience was due to all governments' (913).

Interesting, isn't it?

Let us imagine that stressing love was a key psychic act in the formation of a family *in order to* establish a type of mentality that could process conflict with one's family enemies. For the OED then provides us with the following meanings:

> *happy families, family see* HAPPY a. *Holy Family*: see HOLY a. **in a family way** in a domestic manner; informally. **in the family way** *colloq.* pregnant. **of (good family)** descended from noble or worthy ancestors. *start a family*: see START *v* ! **the family** *slang* the criminal community.
> (OED 913)

The OED gives us a kind of free association which is of use to us. In the effort to solve the problem of rivalry within the household, then especially within the family proper, love is stressed in order to create a good family.

And the Mafia family, the criminal community? Here then we have family not as an act of love, as such, but bonded together by *blood*. He is 'blood'. Indeed the Mafia family engages in war with other families and directs hate existent within its own household into the outside world. Under no circumstances must anyone within the family betray the blood relation that forms the group. In the 'happy family' the law is that one must *love* one another and a high ideal – the holy family – is invoked as an exemplar of sacrificial love that forms a divine family.

We come to a crossroads in family life. One group can only go so far as blood relations, admittedly a step on the road to forming a family. But the next step is to find in the concept of 'love within the family' a principle that will confront enemies within the group in a way that does not necessarily lead to projecting the murderousness outside the group.

The OED tells us that *familiar* also means 'informal, unceremonious' and 'known from long or close association, recognised by memory' (913). So a family is a group who become intimate and informal and whose long associations together are 'recognised by memory'. That's an interesting way to word it. But let us imagine that memory now seems to do the recognising – memory as a slightly split off part of the self, so that it seems to recognise the family, while the self is a bit behind.

This would allow us to insert the Freudian concept of the unconscious as memory. So our unconscious life recognises family even if we do not quite do so in ourselves. Perhaps this is why Freud played on the German word *unheimlich* which means both familiar and uncanny. In his essay on the uncanny, Freud (1919) found that the uncanny is actually the familiar. But it is the self's arrival in a situation which is unconsciously known without being consciously comprehended.

When we think, then, of the group's construction of the number 4, we may come to an intermediate conclusion (a subtotal), that a group of people come together, face the common enemies intrinsic to group life by belief in the power of love as a form of law, which intermixes with the everydayness of this group to effect a type of informal intimacy with one another. This informal intimacy – the many shared moments together – evolves out of this law of love and becomes a type of psychic structure that serves as the group's memory. A set is established in the system unconscious, in other words, that we could condense into the following word-cluster: group–sex–blood–rivalry–love-law–informality–intimacy–memory.

'Time and intercourse have made us familiar' wrote Samuel Johnson (OED 913). In the Freudian order, we should have it in reverse: sex and time have made a group familiar. The after-effects of sexuality: blood, rivalry, love-law, intimacy, and the structure is in place.

Of course the meaning of this cluster has behind its evolution the entire dramaturgy of the family imagined in Aeschlyus and Sophocles and before that, in the imagining of the Old Testament. There one finds the group seeking to propagate itself yet torn by envy, rivalry, and the forces of the death instinct, seeking to impose a new law – the law of love – that would serve as the eroticism of the group as a whole.

Love-law is a vital part of the fourth object. The law that says 'thou shalt love thy neighbour as thyself' is an edict issued a very long time ago which we may now look back upon as part of the history of the unconscious, an early stage in the formation of what we know as family.

Part of the structure of these dramas – whether Old Testament, Greek, or, looking ahead a bit, Shakespearean – is the decisive moment, whether it is a follower deciding to sacrifice his son to his God, whether it is a father deciding between his daughter's survival and his duty as King, or even whether it is the decision to travel to a city on a certain day that one's father takes to the road. This structure is intrinsic to the formation of family, even if these examples seem so tragic and fated. We may say the structure is *the moment of decision* when the self must choose between two opposing elements, when in the extreme the self is torn between deep loyalties; in the terms of this essay, this would be the moment when two people come together to *decide* to form a family. Why should this decision seem so ominous?

We are arguing that the formation of a family means to create a group that will unleash powerful internal forces that may tear it apart, unless a powerful law – the law of love – can impose itself sufficiently upon the group to see it safely through to the development of a new psychic structure, a memory-set, composed of good enough lived experience together.

But each couple presuming to form its own family does so in unconscious murder of the families of origin: blood is on the hands of the new couple. Out of this ordinary matricide and patricide, the new children assume themselves to sleep in the space of propagation; not the space of copulation, but the place from which the new family is to emerge and the symbolic fact of this murder is of course ritualised in the differing marital ceremonies, with the parents giving away the children to one another. The unconscious sense in each couple that in marrying they have murdered their parents is, of course, yet another of the many after-effects of the Oedipus complex.

But it is merely a foretaste of many things to come. For this *decisive moment*, when each partner must make an impossible choice – one that results in the death of a loved object – is only the first of many murders at the crossroads. Each partner brings with him and with her the myths, legends, historical facts, laws, visions, and aesthetic drives of the family of origin. Some of these elements will be conscious and can be discussed, but all of them will also be deeply rooted in the self's unconscious life, forming a thing-presentation that we would see as the self's unconscious relation to its fourth object. (From this point forward for a while I shall assume that this object has been constituted within the self and is there ready for marriage.)

Each partner in the couple brings, then, entirely differing sets of elements constituting fourth objects within. They feel that in marrying they are killing the family of origin. In fact, this murdering as it were is a deeply essential act of destruction, as both participants dismantle prior fourth object structures in order to recombine a new fourth object, a psychic intercourse between family elements that is essential to fourth object reconstruction.

The homicidal element, then, that pervades the notion of family life is not simply the effort of the group to process rivalries emerging from its own actual formation, it is a psychic after-effect of the decision to mate. This is the sexuality of homicide–propagation, of killing in order to give birth. As such, family life begins in the unconscious with a primitive homicide and a question is, 'can the couple survive what it has done?' In the weeks and months following the marriage there will be many crossroads. Where to live? In what type of house or flat? Furnished with what sorts of furniture? Decorated in what manner? Bathroom habits in what manner? Breakfasting in what way? Communicating during the day over what in what style? Arranging the meal and dining in what idiom? And sexual life and the erotic in what differing elaborations? And the children that are coming: what names, what schools, what ideals, what visions, what . . .? These are only a few of the many crossings of the new oedipal couple on the road to Thebes.

Each such unconscious negotiation remembers the murder of the families of origin. And yet they are memories of that time, memories laid down as unconscious structures. So how do these structures deal with one another? Can there be a reintroduction of the families of origin, an after-copulation intercourse in which the two sets of fourth objects negotiate their new structures?

Husband: I like coffee first thing in the morning.
Wife: I like tea.
Husband: Well . . . it's a bit much to make both at the same time . . . we are too busy.
Wife: I agree. Why don't you try tea for a while.
Husband: Okay, no big deal.

In a year the husband has not only made the transition to tea, but now he prefers tea. In the years to come, when he is having breakfast with his sons and daughters, they will all be drinking tea.

This is no big deal, fortunately. Hardly the sort of thing to work its way into Sophocles or Shakespeare.

Yet at this crossroads the husband's and wife's fourth objects have met and one element in one set is killed off. The husband, whose father and mother and brothers and sisters always had coffee in the morning, abandons this practice. The wife, in turn – in unknowing turn – agrees to his request that the toothbrushes be put in a glass next to the basin, brushes facing up. The wife has always had her toothbrush in a fitted slot in a rectangular container, she thinks of this as no big deal and soon she is no longer thinking consciously about this so when the children come along, she buys them a mug for their toothbrushes.

In countless acts of unconscious murder, each partner allows elements of his or her fourth object to be killed. Such sacrificial murder allows the self to *lose the familiar*. In time, the family of origin becomes a *holy family*, a set of memories of the way things were. The holy family – presided over by the holy ghost – is the original fourth object now simply a principle presiding over memories. What is now just memory *was* actually a deep unconscious structure, but the murderous work of marriage has resulted in a de-structuring of some aspects of the original fourth object and its restructuring through the many years of its rebuilding. Of course, we know that nothing is lost on the system unconscious and the original fourth object is not abandoned as a thing-in-itself. But its status has been removed. From the only fourth object, from the primary fourth object, it has been displaced. It has been sent to a holy place in the mind. After its murder, which is associated with sacrificial necessity, it goes to mental heaven where the self feels that it shall forgive the self its murderousness.

Of course, the transition any two people face who make the momentous decision to marry is hazardous in the extreme. It is the most dangerous decision of a lifetime. For years and years both partners will be killing off each other's inner psychic structures in an act of rebuilding constituted out of sexual lust and love. For it shall be this primitive love between the two that becomes its own law, originally a narcissistic law, eventually transfiguring into a different type of law. Sex-love will metamorphose to love-law as the couple survive their mutual destructions and find that self-sacrifice is a part of human intimacy, from which a higher principle derives and serves the couple as they proceed to bring forth children who shall be more primitive even than the sex-couple were and who will need 'guidance' from the parents, love guidance. The parents will convey the law of the family: that the love of family, or the family as love, must preside over any individual claimant's private rights to vengeance, or over any child's horror over the arrival of a newborn child.

If the parents have successfully formed their own new fourth objects, a matrix composed in the dialectic of difference, then they will have a psychic structure in place that can be communicated to the children. This object, which we may now term 'the family', is of course separately held in each person. Marital therapy alone illuminates how this object differs as a psychic structure within each partner – this object recognises that – indeed, the fourth object is a psychic space that opens out to the illusion that it is a shared internal object, one always open to dialectics of difference, one operating according to an essential ruthlessness that nonetheless is not destructive of the rights of the other. The other is killed but the self accepts its own killing in that kind of essential ruthlessness of which Winnicott (1969) writes in his seminal essay 'The Use of an Object'. The fourth object is a principle of ruthless creativity in which the self seeks the unconscious communications of all the others in the group who are unconsciously negotiating in this field.

A family of five people chatting just before dinner:

Father: So . . . ah . . . John (15) are you playing football tomorrow?
John: Yeh, can you come?

Father: Ah . . . I . . .

Mary (8):   Mom, I thought we were all going to the sea?

Mother: . . . well . . . John . . . what time is the match?

Peter (2):   What's a match?

John: It's football, Peter, remember . . . I think it's at 1 or 2 or something.

Peter: Play? play football?

Father: That would split the day in two.

Mother: Well . . . what's the weather like tomorrow?

Mary: I think it's fine . . . I don't know . . . can Sue-Ellen come to the sea too?

Peter: Ellen, Ellen, Ellen, Ellen . . . yeah!

Father: What should we do (thinking out loud).

Mother: How about the sea on Sunday?

John: That would be good for me.

Mary: Oh no, Mom, I told Sue-Ellen Saturday!

Mom: You told her already?

Mary: Well . . . I thought you said . . .

Father: Well . . . let's call her mother and ask if she can come on Sunday and if she can't then . . . what's up for next weekend?

[and so it goes].

The family is engaged in trying to solve a simple spatial–temporal problem. All the members are taking part although with differing points of view and with unspoken conscious ideas not to mention countless unconscious 'disseminates'[1] evoked by this moment in time. The family does not break down into malignant discord because each member is now functioning not simply as a member of the group, although that is true, but each is involved in object relations structured by the fourth object.

Yet if Peter is clearly clueless about this object and Mary and John are still involved in their individual formations of it, how could we say that the family is functioning according to this psychic structure?

For a very long time, in the evolution at first of the new couple, and then for a long time during the psychic formations of the growing children, this object exists in primitive form as a law: the love-law. Because we love each other, this law goes, we get along. It does not mandate that we must get along. That would be the law of the group, but not the law of the family. The family law asserts 'blood' or its psychic equivalent, to form a more

---

1 To coin a word, a 'disseminate' is a single particle of a dissemination. It would be a 'loose thread' from a former fabric, now constituting part of the self's disseminations of all prior psychic intensities that form an infinite 'meshwork' (cf. Freud) in the system unconscious. A disseminate is any particle out of the dissemination of mental contents that is evoked by any new psychic event and attaches itself to it.

primitive assertion: as blood has brought us together, so we love each other, and this love asserts its law over all of us. It is the law that derives out of the oedipal conflict, out of a set of murders that leaves each participant with blood on their hands, and blood-connected by intercourse.

It is an extremely primitive form of transitional order. But it often works.

In the domestic scene portrayed above, the family members know in differing ways that this law prevails. Even if one of the children had run off in tears to a room and refused to go along with the family's decision, it would not have destroyed the fourth object, a principle that governs forms of unconscious communication between the members.

We can see it in the above, although only in a glimpse: the fourth object is that psychic structure that receives and transmits at the level of unconscious communication the differing unconscious interests of members of the family group. It is governed by a primitive law of love that serves to stave off primitive forms of hate in the children, long enough usually for the children to mature and then cultivate this inner structure that operates less primitively. In time the children will feel the inner benefit of such openness. They will derive inner nourishment from this object that has survived personal distress within the group – especially moments of intense hate towards one or another of the other members of the group – and come to consciously appreciate the unconscious benefit of 'knowing' how to be open to the dialectics of difference in the group.

Of course, in the modern world we know that many families have other qualifying elements that further complicate matters. Second and third marriages often bring ready-made families or sets of previous families into a 'new family'; much depends on the previous marriages and the status of the fourth object formation in the children. If they have fourth object structures forming within them, then they have lived according to a law – not according to an affect – that suggests to them that love should prevail and this edict – the law of the family and the family as law – helps new members of prior families to 'mesh' together. Murder has always been a feature of marriage. The fact that former spouses may be active targets of hostility on the part of one or both members of the new family does not help, but equally it is not alien to the overall act of murder that constitutes family life.

Implicit in the fourth object is its own eventual structural destruction. This knowledge also curiously informs its character as one knows that, however essential it is to one's self, eventually it will be displaced and the self will go on either to new fourth-object relations – if we refer now to the adolescent looking to his future – or the self will know that its own status as fourth-object progenitor will be eradicated by the new generation's homicide and of course, and most tellingly, by death itself.

Indeed families know this, don't they? They meet at a generational intersection. The parents are walking down the hill toward their graves and the children are walking up the hill to the future crests of their life. They pass each other again and again on this hill, and repetition of this family hike increasingly informs the fourth object in each that something generationally prescient exists within and between them and in turn within and between themselves and all the other families who have lived in the hundreds of generations that preceded them. The *Epic of Gilgamesh* and *The Old Testament* give ordinary humans incredibly long lives, so that one generation seems to live many generations, reaching far into the future, rather capturing ironically enough, the simple place of the single family, passing along a common route on the journey of man and woman kind.

So what makes up the number 4? We have played with the idea of a psychic numeracy available for psychoanalysts to count as they add things up when considering their patients or try to account for where they are. We have argued that $1 + 1 = 3$, but that an additional integer is needed to create 4. We have been intentionally illogical and maintained that the additional integer is supplied by the number when it arrives. We may now argue that the additional integer is 'love-law'. Only when the group of 3, the after-effects of sexuality, have added a primitive element, is the fourth object now to be counted.

I have discussed in another essay the number 5 (Bollas 1999), which I use for the group.

It may seem odd that it is a 'higher' number, especially as I have already said that 3 is a group. I shall have to qualify this. Three is only ever the after-effects of intercourse. Three people may be present, but in fact they are lost in their collectivity until and/or unless they become a family. But members of every family will find that, even after they have counted to 4, the addition of a new psychic number destroys the promise of the number 4 as a psychically efficacious container. For the additional integer I believe stands for the self inside the social group which obeys the laws of psychosis, not the love-law, and it is here that the self's attachment to the family is destroyed.

But let us remind ourselves of what we mean by destruction in psychoanalysis. All of the integers remain in the unconscious, even if further additions destroy them. 1, 2, 3, 4, and 5 survive any combinations that would seem to add up to more. When the child goes off to school for the first time and discovers that he is inside a group that is not his family, that does not know the ways of his family, he is psychically shattered. As Bion teaches us, this group life follows basic laws operating along a psychotic axis, one certainly not processed by any self through his family. But the fecund life of any self's imaginary is *also* more than the fourth object can bear. As the child discovers he has a mind, as he invents many mothers and fathers, he is no longer held within the comforting illusion that he is being looked after by his family of origin. Fortunately, however, we are not referring to figures, but to their functions. By the time the child is four or five he or she will have begun the structure that is the fourth object, that will communicate and receive communications made for family life. The fifth object will break the hegemony of this structure as a promise of all future mixtures of people: the illusion of family as the only assembly will be dispelled. But the structure and its elements will remain and it shall be available for the self in the years to come as it processes the generational act of family life.

The fifth object – that is specifically life in the group – is 4 + 1, 4 plus that which is outside the family, the group within which one takes part. This is a very harrowing experience for all people and it is common enough for individuals to begin a secret subtraction when they count to 5. They may pair up and form themselves up with another to complete a young couple: hence 5 − 3 = 2, ridding the self even of the third object, to resume life in the more comforting arms of the dyad. They may even retreat into 1, seeking refuge in daydreaming or the like. Fortunately most keep on counting and though each new psychic integer destroys the former higher addition, and eradicates the seeming sanctity of its former structure(s), new structures, new numbers, also cure the self of the very damage inflicted. 6 is the self's addition of his or her place in a 'universal order' when the self can find in universal assumptions and laws of civilisation a new unconscious set that indeed helps the self to survive difficulties in all the prior combinations, but especially when dealing with the madness of the group. During the Holocaust, when many lost their belief in man, others drew strength from the sixth object, from memory of and relation to the aims and aspirations of the human order – or man's humanity to man. At any one moment in time, the group (5), may lose grasp of 6. The Nazis lost an integer. But in such moments our memory of 6 – perhaps useless as an unconscious factor in the life of society – is crucial to our own psychic survival.

REFERENCES

Bion, W. R. (1962) *Learning from Experience*, New York: Basic Books.

Bollas, C. (1999) *The Mystery of Things*, Routledge: London.

Ellis, B. E. (1985) *Less than Zero*, New York: Simon & Schuster.

Freud, S. (1919) 'The Uncanny', *S.E.*, 17: 217–256, London: Hogarth Press, 1964.

Rickman, John (1950) 'The Factors of Numbers in Individual and Group Dynamics', in *Selected Contributions to Psycho-Analysis*, London: Hogarth Press, 1957.

Winnicott, D. W. (1965) *The Maturational Processes and the Facilitating Environment*, New York: International Universities Press.

Winnicott, D. W. (1969) 'The Use of an Object', *International Journal of Psycho-Analysis*, 50: 711–716.

Chapter 14

Dynamic mathematics in mental experience. I: Complex numbers represent psychic object relations

David E. Scharff and Hope Cooper

Derek, a shy 17-year-old, reported that for several months he had been almost unable to function. Everyday events such as an airplane flying overhead, a fire engine's siren or his mother picking him up two minutes late, brought panic. Derek's father, an accountant, had died a year earlier from a heart attack. Derek had few school friends. His social contact consisted of playing Dungeons and Dragons weekly with older men. He said he was neither sad nor depressed and yet he presented with strikingly flat affect and an odd way of thinking that was creative yet mechanical. In his second year of treatment, Derek reported a dream:

> I was taking a Latin exam but it wasn't on Latin – it was on Dungeons and Dragons. There were 8 questions and we had to answer 3 of them. The first question was numbered 23 and the second 28. The third one didn't have a number, and after I'd finished it I realized I'd done the wrong question and didn't have time to go back and do the correct 3rd question. At one point I looked at my watch and it was 12:41. As I was doing the test I looked at the time at 12:52, 12:54, and 12:58. I woke up depressed because I had done the test wrong and it was something that I knew – I could have gotten it right.

Derek associated mainly to the numbers. An 8 made him think of the sign for infinity (∞), which is a sideways 8. He said that he'd always found 3 to be a difficult number, something incomplete. The numbers 23 and 28 were important in a video game he played – they had to be divided by half in the game. He noticed that the 3 and the 8 were this time coupled with 2s. Derek said that the numbers sequencing 41/52/54/58 reminded him of a math problem that he often played in his head: somehow it ends up with 8, 4, 2, 1, 4, 2, 1 (4, 2, 1, repeat). This math problem has something to do with proving that a particular formula always works. Derek was testing it to see if he could find an integer that wouldn't work.

Derek said, 'I felt depressed because the problem was something I knew. How could I get it wrong? I don't want to mess up. I should be good at math like my dad. He could do complicated math in his head, and he would try to teach me to do that. In physics I sometimes discover that I've done a problem wrong when I really know the answer. In physics class we're working on the principles of tension. Dealing with tension messes me up. I *know* I know the right answers. My father loved math and used to tell me he looked forward to helping me with physics, too, because he was good at it in college . . . I don't want to be not doing physics right.'

Derek's dream provides a vivid example of the significance of numbers in the inner world and how they convey multiple meanings. It shows him using numbers to try to contain his own anxiety through mathematical skills that maintain the link to his lost father. The numbers help manage his inner tension and chaos that follow the loss of his idealized father. Perhaps the splintering of experience into chaos is signified by the sideways 8 of infinity, a state that he feels inside as the threat of infinite confusion. He tries to bring the infinite quality of his loss and worry down to a more bearable, a more thinkable 3, but even 3 presents problems, as it feels to him so incomplete – and therefore linked to the infinity of his worries. He tries pairing 3s and 8s with 2 to make 23 and 28, but in the dream he gets everything wrong. None of his manipulations of numbers solve his inner problem. So he begins the math problem by checking the time, something he often did during sessions, saying he does this to 'organize myself when things feel chaotic'. Numbers function to contain Derek. They become transitional objects that link him to a less threatening state of mind and to a reassuring identification with his mathematical father. His dream illustrates how numbers, particularly for some mathematically minded people, are an extraordinarily symbolic creation and a connection to reassuring relationships.

A NEW USE OF MATHEMATICS

Numbers and geometry can be used to represent mental and relational situations. In this chapter we want to see if we can make a range of complex psychological matters more susceptible to certain kinds of theoretical manipulation and understanding. We are following a tradition undertaken by Bion (1965, 1970) and Matte-Blanco (1975, 1988) to see how mental phenomena are organized like certain aspects of mathematics. Although psychoanalysis, family and group therapy, use the numbers 1, 2, and 3, most psychological experience takes place beyond the simplified parameters of 1, 2, 3. Theory has yet to make much use of mathematics or geometry to represent, illuminate or explore complex ideas and dynamic relationships. Because numbers and mathematics contain an essence of experience that can be manipulated and juxtaposed with other symbols, they can be used to describe aspects of states of mind, reflective function, and projective identification. Numbers are currently part of psychodynamic language as we attempt to represent the patterns of internal object relations abstracted from the specific characteristics of a particular person or introject. Closely allied with the numbers 1, 2, and 3, the concepts of 'self', 'couple' and 'oedipal triangle' are abstracted to discuss aspects of personal function and interaction. However, larger numbers rarely show up. An exception is the recent interest Bollas (see Chapter 13 in this volume) has shown in an expanded numerical dimensionality. We believe our discussion carries abstraction further to allow easier manipulation of the patterns of individuals and group, both in external interaction and in internal psychic pattern.

While Freud did not deal directly with numbers, he did make important comments on the mathematics and dimensions of time and space. For instance:

> We approach the id with analogies: we call it chaos . . . It is filled with energy reaching it from the instincts, but it has no organization, produces no collective will . . . There is nothing in the id that could be compared with negation; and we perceive with surprise an exception to the philosophical theorem that space and time are necessary forms of our mental acts.

> (Freud 1923: 74)

Bion was preoccupied with the idea that mathematics could be of use in representing developmental and psychoanalytic ideas scientifically in order to present a more rigorous set of principles that could be followed and tested. He wrote, 'Mathematical formulation is not yet available to the psycho-analyst though there are suggestive possibilities' (Bion 1962: 51). After proposing the beginnings of such a system, he added, 'The scientific deductive system may be further abstracted to yield the equivalent of an algebraic calculus which would represent it' (1962: 71).

As a first step in moving closer to these problems, we propose using complex numbers to represent internal object relations that contain the images of people in primary relationships that are internalized and split in relationship to parts of the self. Our use of numbers only begins to deal with the complexity of this situation and of one person relating to others. Fairbairn's (1963) formulation of six basic parts of the self in dynamic flux also calls on us to invoke geometry to try to describe the complex dynamic interaction of parts of self and object in constant dynamic internal interaction. Ultimately, and far beyond the scope of this chapter, we could ask about mathematical representation of brain circuitry, and could wonder at what future point the complex algorithms of the mind might intersect with those of the brain. In the geometric arena psychoanalysis currently uses only simple metaphors like 'space in the mind', 'space for thinking', potential or transitional space, distance and closeness, and the oedipal triangle in relationships.

A more dynamic use of geometry corresponds to the non-Euclidean geometry of fractals and fascinating patterns – called strange attractors – that emerge out of a dynamic system with apparent disorganization. Chaos theory, or theories of dynamical systems, helps understand numbers as part of systems in motion rather than as static representations (Gleick 1987; see also Scharff and Scharff, Chapter 16 in this volume). Chaos theory studies alternations between pattern and disorder in dynamic systems characterized by continuous feedback and sensitivity to small differences in initial conditions. These are both characteristics of biological and psychological systems. Applying chaos theory lets us see that the small numbers and relatively simple geometric patterns we use in psychoanalysis to denote individuals in dyads and triads are limited 'fractals' of much larger systems – that is they are small, easily recognizable patterns embedded within the much larger and infinitely complex patterns of human interaction. This new field of fractal geometry enables us to see the importance of pattern similarity across different levels of magnitude in complex systems – for instance, the way an overly careful pattern in a minute of a patient's session is similar to the obsessional quality of his whole personality. A fractal is a representation of pattern on one order of scale (the moment of interaction in the session) that bears similarity of pattern to other levels (the patient's personality).

To deal with these multiple dimensions, we will use what mathematicians term 'complex numbers' that exist on more than one axis. Small complex numbers stand for internal object constellations inside the mind in order to represent the multiplicity inside the individual and the way the individual is represented inside the many. We will deal first with the complexities of the multiple parts of the self that are usually studied by object relations, and with the complexity of object relations involved in the simplified terms dyad and triad.

First a brief introduction to complex numbers. In mathematics, simple numbers fill the east–west axis from –infinity to +infinity. Complex numbers qualify the simple numbers by providing another dimension on the north–south axis that also runs from –infinity to +infinity. A complex number is mathematically written $3 + 2i$, where 'i' originally stood mathematically for 'imaginary number'. Mathematicians no longer consider the complex number to be imaginary, so the use of 'i' is now only convention. From this perspective, simple numbers (e.g. 1 or 4) are a special case that really means $1 + 0i$, or $4 + 0i$. We have chosen to write our complex numbers differently, as 1^{+2} or 1^{-2}, and sometimes 1_{-2}, because it better fits with the idea that the complexity is inside or completely attached to the original number, representing internal object relations. *We do not mean to signify the mathematical action of squaring or multiplying the original number*. We think of this notation as the equivalent of drawing a cartoon 'bubble' for speech or thoughts above a cartoon character. In our use, the superscript number represents an internal number carried in the mind as an organizing inner structure that has mental linkage to the person's representation of self. When we are representing the inner number of a group of 2, 3 or more persons, we want the superscript number (e.g. 2^{-1}, or 3^{-2}) to represent the group's shared unconscious treatment of one or more inner objects in their shared mentality.

SOME FUNDAMENTALS OF NUMBERS AS STATES OF MIND

Derek's dreams show how numbers represent states of mind and the ways in which numbers can be symbols or less developed concrete representations for mental operations and organization, for anxieties and defenses. Numbers convey bare bones of interior experience, part of the state of mind of a person or of each participant in an interaction. More than one number would be needed to do justice to the complexity of a person's state of mind, of their potential mental states, or of two or more minds relating to each other. Here we are saying that the large number denotes the size of the group (one person, two, a group of three); the superscript denotes the mental attitude of the person or group to another single person or grouping in his or her or the group's unconsciously shared mind. (Although the notion of a group mind is a controversial idea in some quarters, Bion (1961) and Foulkes (1965) suggest that elements of unconscious life permeate all intimately interacting groups, especially family groups. See, for instance, Hopper (2003a).)

The mathematical equations we construct have an arbitrary quality and could just as easily be written in several other forms or with other numbers because people are continually moving between differing internal equations all the time in a flux that could only be represented by a dynamic mathematics like calculus. Here are some examples: We propose that a 1^{+1} can be used to denote a positive libidinal attachment to a single other; a 1^{-1} an aggressive link. The same applies to the inner orientation to groups of 2 or 3: a 1^{-2} denotes a person armed against the idea of an internal couple, while a 2^{-1} represents a couple that excludes a person. A 2^{-3} is a couple unconsciously armed against the idea of a group of three (for instance a couple unconsciously armed against an oedipal group), and 3^{-1} is a triad that aggressively attacks one of its members or has trouble keeping that member in mind. In the current state of our usage, the whole configuration would then represent simply an internal number: 1^{3-1} represents a person who has an internal triad that attacks one member. This gray area – whether the large number is an external group or the group inside an individual – stems from the fact that a group can have a shared attitude that is in many respects like the mentality of a single individual, so that the notation can be used for either situation.

These notations give better *representation* of the internal links that Bion (1970) and others have discussed (Volkan 1981). By using these complex numbers more of the live dynamics of object relationships and the shifting states of mind in the inner world can be seen. For example, the self begins not just with the number 1, but also within the number 2 that stands for the dyad, the mother–baby couple; the individual selves of mother and baby contain the number 1 for each of them that must combine to produce a 2. Until the baby has internalized an inner '2', that is, experienced itself as separate from mother but linked to her, it cannot move into the experience of 3, even though the number 3 is implicitly there, all around the infant from the beginning. (See Chapter 11 in this volume for Poulton's detailed discussion of the complexity of the numbers 1 and 2.)

Because complex numbers have a dimensional quality, they allow us to look inside internal objects to see how numbers are carried and internalized. Thus, the mother's mind in the mother–baby dyad can be represented by parent + a child = 1^{+1} and also by 1^{-1} when the child is not only absent from her mind but the link to the child is through hatred – –H in Bion's (1970) system. Likewise with the triad: we could represent the couple with a child as 2^{+1} because the couple thinks of themselves as a dyad with the child in mind, but in another state of mind they could be represented as 3^{-1}, representing an interacting triad that, as a group, cannot keep the child in mind. In that moment, the parents have 'forgotten' or hate the child, and the child experiences herself as forgotten by them. However, the difference between hating and forgetting is a major issue, and for that reason we have considered the use of the number zero.

Even before 1, 2, or 3 is zero (0), a state of mind that the baby encounters – or at least risks encountering – because it is dependent on the mother to have a mind of its own. Although 0 is theoretically not completely achievable, nevertheless it is the state that the self dreads from the beginning. Before birth there is a primitive encounter with zero – a relational one between mother and fetus, as the baby communicates with the mother through its movement and both may approach zero when the baby isn't moving. 'The most direct threat to the unborn child's physical survival is the danger of miscarriage' (Maiello 2001: 108).

The zero state of mind is something like psychic annihilation. Infant observation has shown the many ways that babies hold themselves together so that they don't reach 0. This is also to say that the baby is doing relational mathematics – it knows the psychic difference between being held in the mother's mind (1^{+1}) or being hated even temporarily (1^{-1}). If the mother is suffering from depression and is unable to hold the baby in mind, the baby feels pushed towards a nothing state of mind (1^{0}). This experience is absorbed in numeric form into the baby's inner object world. The oscillation between these states of mind can be represented by an equation:

$$1^{+1} \leftrightarrow 1^{-1} \leftrightarrow 1^0.$$

This equation shows the mental transformations that occur in the movement between the infant's experience of feeling himself in an external relationship with mother who thinks about him, then is hatefully rejecting (carries the mental representation as -1) and then does not have him in mind and so he internalizes the experience of feeling forgotten by the mother (1^0). The incorporation of a mother who is failing to contain by hating the baby – that is the mother who contains the 1^{-1} experience – may be a transient state, or may be a way station in a move by the infant to the point of experiencing himself as a 0.

SIGNS AND OPERATIONS

Numbers themselves carry primary and rudimentary meaning. Modifying complex numbers by the sign (+ or –) characterizes the libidinal attitude towards the internal object; a (+) sign is one of loving tie or affiliation – the move towards the object; a (–) sign is one of hate or aggression – the move away from the object. *Other* mathematical operations can be used to indicate different mental operations. Division (/) is the factor that splits the wholeness of the object or its relatedness, and may tend towards splintering, fragmentation and aggregation (Hopper 2003b). The process of fragmentation can also be symbolized as $1/\infty = 1/a + 1/b + 1/c \ldots 1/\infty$, producing a sense of self that is so splintered that the person feels herself in bits, each of them equal to or less than 1, with the most severe case being that of fragmentation into infinitely small bits – the effects of psychosis, trauma, multiplicity and of falling into pieces. 0 is a number denoting absence in the mind, but it is also a sign. In a simple way, multiplicity is an aggregate of the fragments produced by division. Multiplication (×) is the force that pushes towards merger, or an aggrandizement of self or object in slightly varying forms. For instance, the operation of multiplication that produces an aggrandized sense of the self leads to a self that seems to be everywhere, swamping the object world. The state of grandiose multiplication of the sense of self can begin to be captured by $1 \times \infty = 1^\infty$ where the ∞ stands for the infinitization of experience (Matte-Blanco 1988). When we think of 0 as a sign (rather than as a number), it also has the effect of introducing an infinite quality of trauma or merger into the relationship between numbers or into the mental state. What should be clear by now is that mental operations can transform the meaning of an internal object and its number. The change in sign from + to – can occur instantly, changing love to hate.

The change from + to 0 instantly changes from love to an experience of the void. Paradoxically, the change from – to 0 also signifies the move to the void that happens at the moment a person feels forgotten by a person to whom they have a hateful link, but one that is nevertheless organizing to their sense of self. The interactions of relationships externally or unconsciously through projective identification and containment – particularly its active element, reflective functioning – can all be thought of as ways we perform mathematical operations and change signs in the process.

Transformation of numbers overlaps with Bion's (1970) idea of the way that mutual projective identification results in containment – how the mother is able to receive from the baby its unbearable states of mind (–1 or 0) and digest them – transform them into something bearable for the infant through a projective identification of +1. If the baby has cried for the mother and in the mother's absence the baby has moved into a –1 or 0 state of mind, the baby relies on the mother's mind to unconsciously transform –1 or 0 into +1. Then the baby also introjects the mother's capacity to transform numbers, which we can represent mathematically as giving the baby a state of mind that moves from $1^{-1} \leftrightarrow 1^{+1}$ or $1^0 \leftrightarrow 1^{+1}$. When the baby introjects the container itself, we can represent this as $1^{-1} \rightarrow 1^{+1} \rightarrow 1^{(1+1)} = 2^{(+2)}$. An example describes this mental function in operation.

A small boy is in his mother's lap being read a bedtime story. His experience is of being held in his mother's mind. But then he feels angry with his mother because she tells him he must go to bed and leave Mommy and Daddy together. He tries to tear the book and then throws it. Mother yells at him, and carries him off to the bedroom. The child is now crying and feeling sad. The mother is able to process the angry experience they had with each other and is then more able to offer the child comfort, so that the child can go to sleep.

The child began in his mother's lap with the (+) state of mind (+1, +2, and perhaps 3^{+1}), but this suddenly turned to (–) when he felt mother wanted to get rid of him (go to bed) or attacked him (go away to bed). Love changed to rejection or even hate. This was a difficult state of mind for the child to bear, because he loves and needs his loving mother, so he projects this angry, attacking, state of mind into his mother, who enacts it by yelling at him and putting him to bed. The child is left feeling sad and abandoned $(1^{-1}, 2^{-1}, 3^{-1})$, approaching (0) if he fears his mother will forget him, but the mother is able to transform this back into + so that the child does not fragment (functions of [/] that would splinter the self) and can fall asleep. Both the child's capacity to project and the mother's capacity for containment through projective identification (to receive and digest the projections through reflective understanding of the child's fears) are part of how signs change, and change again as they move back and forth between mother and child, and as they move dynamically inside both the mother's mind and the child's mind.

THE NUMBER ZERO AND NOTHING STATES OF MIND

Zero is not only a sign, but also is a number that denotes a state of mind without a sign. It signifies the idea of an emotional black hole – a number void of a sign, which makes it all the more powerful. Zero is symbolic of a state of mind that might signify psychic death, an experience of being dropped, or a retreat from the pain of relating – a state that pulls all the other numerical possibilities into its own bottomless mental pit. The nothing state of mind is the feeling and fear that one no longer exists (Mitchell 2000). Prolonged periods of 0 can lead to a massive withdrawal, as in psychosis or autism, but we all have at least momentary experiences with 0 throughout our lives.

An observer watched 12-week-old Mary retreat into a nothing state of mind in reaction to her mother's inability to identify with her and maintain emotional contact with two children. The mother was giving the baby a bottle. Older brother Tom approached and began sticking a pacifier in the baby's mouth. [A (-1) state of mind in each of the children.] The mother told him to stop. Tom pushed harder until the nipple of the bottle was forced out of Mary's mouth. The mother took out the pacifier and put the bottle back in Mary's mouth. Tom then hit the bottle. The mother told him to stop. He hit the baby's arm. Mother told him to go away. Milk dribbled out of Mary's mouth (a 0 state of mind for the baby, a 1^{-1} for Tom.) Mother tried again to feed but milk continued to dribble out. Mother sat Mary on her lap, with Mary's back to mother's stomach. Mary's eyes were glassy and she stared straight ahead, not looking at anything in particular. The she begin to rock, back and forth, against mother's stomach, still staring straight ahead. This is not an autistic baby, but in that particular moment she felt unprotected and dropped from the mother's mind – so one might say she protectively moved into an autistic or nothing state of mind, seen in the staring at nothing and rocking movement that kept her away from the pain of having been 'forgotten'. The autistic rocking reaffirms her body as a somatic defense against feeling the pull towards 0. Ultimately, the mother was able to 'retrieve' baby Mary (Alvarez 1992) and they could once again be in contact, so that this state of mind did not get frozen in time – although scenes like this were repeated and probably did reinforce a 0 state of mind as one position for Mary.

FAMILY NUMBERS

We now turn to a consideration of how numbers can help us think about the family. Most of us do not grow up as an only child, the only family situation for which the number 3 might be adequate. (In the next chapter we will consider the problem of numbers greater than 3. See also Bollas, Chapter 13 in this volume.) We need a way to think about how the child's state of mind shifts in relation to the numbers in the family. For example, the birth of a sibling confronts the child with the dreaded possibility of being pushed aside or forgotten – that is to say, towards the 0 state of mind. A sibling changes all the relational mathematics in the family. In the child's mind 3 + 1 does not only equal 4; it also equals a complex variant of 3. The 3 might be the family as it was before the birth of the second child, signifying that the child's aggression has killed off the new baby; or it could be the parents and the new baby – the new baby taking the place of the older child and pushing him out of the mother's mind. The new baby may confront this problem right from the beginning, being –1 or 0 in the parent's or parental couple's mind. Multiplication and division may also feature in each child's attempt to find a place in the complex interactions of the family if the child feels fragmented in the interaction with family members or infused with a multiplying grandiosity of self or object.

Let us go back to the earlier observation material: Mary was born into a family in which her $2\frac{1}{2}$-year-old brother, Tom, never ceded her a place. The observer (HC) who visited the family weekly could see that Mary had to fight for space next to mother and in mother's mind. When Mary failed to attract mother's attention, she slid toward a nothing (0) state of mind, as a degradation product from the hatred of 1^{-1}, or 2^{-1}, or 3^{-1}; or it could be $1^{(0\leftrightarrow-1)}$ – meaning there is an oscillation between a sense of 0 and of –1 in her mind – depending on whether our focus is on her as an individual, a member of the dyad with mother or with her brother, or a member of a triad of all three of them, and depending on whether the experience is being excluded from mind through hate (–) or through absence of mind (0). When we consider the addition of father, or an observer or therapist, to this family group, the math has to hold another level of complexity. From the point of view of the observer trying to hold the whole situation in her mind, the situation might alternate between two or more representations as mother and Tom oscillate between excluding and admitting Mary to their emotional group:

$$3 \leftrightarrow 3^{-1} \leftrightarrow 2^{-1} \leftrightarrow 2^{+1}$$

Another situation we can now represent is the way an internal object is itself complex. For instance, baby Mary introjects her mother's mind, which itself has complex numbers that signify its state. We might think that Mary's $^{-1}$ also contains mother's history, so that the $^{-1}$ should contain the complexities of mother's split internal objects. We might say Mary introjects her mother to produce a number like:

$$1^{1(-2)}$$

This signifies that Mary now contains her mother's mind or mental state that itself also contains an attack on pairing or on the possibility of forming a couple. Numbers can be used to represent Mary internalizing mother's mind as it attacks the possibility that they can be an emotional couple, the baby's processing of that attack, and the group of three participating in this phenomenon. The entire area written in superscript is an introjection of a complex experience within this family subgroup, since the father did not participate in the observation. The observation would have been even more complex if he had been there, or even if we could represent the action of his representation in the mental states of the three who were there.

It is also possible that our notation could be done with letters with more clarity than numbers, a more algebraic form of notation. In this way each letter stands for an individual. Person A has person B in mind represented by a small b as an internal object. A^b represents A's positive libidinal view of B. A^{-b} is the negative, aggressive internalization. AB^{-c} would mean the dyad of A and B attacks the link to C. If we want to signify that Mary contains her mother's mind or mental state that itself also contains an attack on pairing or on the possibility of forming a couple, we might represent this with algebraic notation where B is Mary and a is her mother's mind, b is the internal object for Mary's self. This would give the notation:

$$B^{a(-ab)}$$

This represents the way Mary has internalized her mother's hatred of the two of them as a couple. ABC^{-c} is the family triad that unconsciously attacks the idea that its member C should play a role in the minds of the three as a group.

THE CONTRIBUTION OF MATHEMATICAL REPRESENTATIONS

It becomes obvious that the complexity even of simple situations exceeds our capacity for representation. What, then, can a system of mathematical representations contribute to our potential for understanding states of mind and internal dynamics, since the first thing we note is that using mathematical notation tells us less about an interaction than a verbal description? The answer lies in the way that all research notation or classification simplifies complex phenomena in order to isolate the field of observation and increase understanding of small parts of complex systems. We believe that mathematical representation of mental states denotes a configuration of internal objects in relation to the self, an internal form of structure in mental space that has a life of its own apart from the specific qualities of particular internal objects at a specific moment. Numbers or algebraic representation show something beyond the verbal description of experience in signifying a relational configuration that itself organizes the mind and that can move from one internal object participating in this configuration to another that is recruited to take part in an internal structure. These numbers have dimension like the north–south dimension of mathematical complex numbers, except that here it is an internal dimension. Sometimes these configurations come and go, representing momentary positions of mind. But when they are traumatically introjected, they form what Bollas (1999: 113) has called 'interjects', encapsulated enduring configurations that represent more or less permanent anti-relational numbers that disrupt normal mental flow. In marking certain mental space as no-go areas, they are akin to the way a space-occupying lesion in the body is impenetrable to healthy physiological processes.

CONCLUSION

We began this chapter with Derek, whose dream used numbers to try to find a formula that would order the chaos of his loss of a mathematical father. He sought a reassuring mental pattern that could come out right when so much had gone wrong for him with his father's death.

A week later, Derek reported another dream. 'I was watching what seemed to be a real scene but it was a fight calculated by numbers – the way you play Dungeons and Dragons. The numbers were appearing around the people and the people moved according to the numbers. The two people fighting were Andre and John from my volleyball team. They each had a sword. I woke up before the fight ended.'

Derek began to give associations. About the people in the dream, he said, 'Andre is the captain of the volleyball team. He's the best player but he can explode. He really gets angry. John just joined the team. He's quiet and nervous. He substitutes for Andre's position.'

Then, without being asked, he talked about the numbers. 'It's like the numbers are a third person in the fight. Maybe numbers represent logic because with numbers you always get the right answer. They will always be right. I've always liked adding and multiplying better than subtracting and dividing. Adding and multiplying – you get normal answers. But with subtracting and dividing you get strange things – remainders and negative numbers. It's not neat. Plato says there are three parts of the mind – spirit, desire, and logic. Logic keeps the other two in check. Numbers are like logic because they make things consistent.'

Derek's dream centers on a two-person contest that is presumably about two parts of him in conflict – the part that threatens to explode angrily and the quiet, nervous part. They are circled by numbers that represent a containing third person abstracted into the force of logic that might be able to keep the conflict from doing damage to one or the other part of his internal. Here the numbers, which we have been discussing as representing internal states of mind concerning relationships, become characters of the dream, showing dynamically how Derek sees them as operating to keep his inner conflicts between warring parts of his personality in check. When he talks about liking the regularity of addition and multiplication he is speaking of the positive libidinal quality of his relationship to his objects. He dislikes the 'strange things' that result from the negative forces of subtraction and division, the strangeness of the phenomena of loss of his father and the fragmentation of his family. We can speculate also that his numbers and the mathematical operations are representations of his relationship with the therapist to whom he entrusts this task. For Derek, the numbers are friendly, reliable inner characters that are more than abstractions. They are inner signposts to an ordering of his troubled mind.

Derek's propensity for bringing numbers to life has helped us to think about the role of mathematics in the organization of the psyche and of unconscious interaction. While he is unusual in this way, we believe he is able to tell us something about aspects of ordinary numerical organization of mind and interaction that are usually concealed by verbal logic and dream imagery. Patients with idiosyncratic styles of thinking can offer lessons in universal components of the human mind. For some mathematics is a passion: numbers speak to them and they speak best in numbers. For others, numbers and geometry seem to be from another world. We hope that we have demonstrated that numbers are of us and in us. Often hidden, they are nevertheless fundamental parts of our organization and functioning. Learning how this is so can increase our overall understanding of the human condition.

REFERENCES

Alvarez, A. (1992) *Live Company: Psychoanalytic Psychotherapy with Autistic, Borderline, Deprived and Abused Children*, London: Routledge.

Bion, W. R. (1961) *Experiences in Groups and Other Papers*, London: Tavistock.

Bion, W. R. (1962) *Learning from Experience*, London: Heinemann.

Bion, W. R. (1965) *Transformations: Change from Learning to Growth*, London: Heinemann.

Bion, W. R. (1970) *Attention and Interpretation*, London: Tavistock.

Bollas, C. (1999) *The Mystery of Things*, London: Routledge.

Fairbairn, W. R. D. (1963) 'Synopsis of an Object Relations Theory of the Personality', *International Journal of Psycho-Analysis*, 44: 224–225.

Foulkes, S. H. (1965) *Therapeutic Group Analysis*, New York: International Universities Press.

Freud. S. (1933) 'The Dissection of the Psychical Personality, Lecture XXI', *Standard Edition*, 22: 57–80, London: Hogarth Press, 1964.

Gleick, J. (1987) *Chaos*, New York: Viking Penguin.

Hopper, E. (2003a) *The Social Unconscious*, London: Jessica Kingsley.

Hopper, E. (2003b) *Traumatic Experience in the Unconscious Life of Groups*, London: Jessica Kingsley.

Maiello, S. (2001) 'Prenatal Trauma and Autism', *Journal of Child Psychotherapy*, 27(2): 107–124.

Matte-Blanco, I. (1975) *The Unconscious as Infinite Sets: An Essay in Bi-Logic*, London: Duckworth.

Matte-Blanco, I. (1988) *Thinking, Feeling, and Being*, London: Routledge.

Mitchell, S. A. (2000) *Relationality: From Attachment to Intersubjectivity*, Hillsdale, NJ: The Analytic Press.

Volkan, V. D. (1981) *Linking Objects and Linking Phenomena: A Study of the Forms, Symptoms, Metapsychology and Therapy of Complicated Mourning*, New York: International Universities Press.

Chapter 15

Dynamic mathematics in mental experience. II: Numbers in motion, a dynamic geography of time and space

David E. Scharff and Hope Cooper

In our first chapter (Chapter 14 in this volume) on numbers in psycho-analysis, we developed the supposition that numbers could be used in new ways to symbolize configurations of internal objects, links to objects, attacks on links and reparative efforts in the mind. We illustrated this through the case of an adolescent and his dreams, and through the example of the shared mentality of a small family group with two children.

In this chapter we explore an expanded use of mathematical notation by moving into the domain of non-Euclidean geometry, Matte-Blanco's exploration of the unconscious as infinite mathematical sets, and chaos theory, also called dynamical systems theory. We believe that such exami-nation can provide a particularly rich conceptualization of certain highly complex family systems.

SYMMETRIZATION AND THE PROBLEM OF HOLDING LARGE NUMBERS IN MIND

We want to deal with the fact that psychoanalytic theory has not yet found a way to consider numbers greater than 3. (An exception to this is a recent essay on numbers by Bollas (1999). See also his Chapter 13 in this volume.) Since life is mostly lived in the complexity of a world characterized by large numbers, it is striking that we have no math or geometry for families with more than one child, or for other dynamic groups. To consider the family with several children, the dynamics of life among siblings, the extended family, the social group, society, and existence in the larger world, we need a capacity to consider large numbers. Freud (1923: 333) theorized the notion of a 'family complex', implying the idea of dynamic phenomena of sibling displacement, jealousy and rivalry in family groups, and the effect on the child of such group events. We have come to think that the human mind is not well-equipped to consider large numbers psychologically. Perhaps 6 or 7 is the largest group size for which we can 'hold in mind' the individuals who make up the group. If this is true, what happens at this psychological limit? How do we consider the mathematics and geometry of ourselves as part of a larger world or of the vast universe?

While parents certainly consider the family as a group, they have difficulty holding 3 or 4 or 5 children in mind as individuals. In our earlier chapter we explored the way the internal object relationships and unconscious group relationships of each family member are better represented as a set of changeable complex numbers. This allows us to represent the ways that links to others are carried as unconscious structure, often as a fixed, single integer, like, for example, the stereotypic '3' which refers to a triangular or the oedipal situation. The problem becomes even more difficult when we turn from small numbers to family numbers greater than 4 or 5.

We propose that understanding the dynamics of large numbers relies on different methods of mental processing than for relatively small numbers. Large numbers are understood on different orders of scale. When numbers get to a certain size – say 6 or 7 – our minds have difficulty wrapping around them or keeping them in focus. Instead, we begin to see them as a group, no longer keeping the discrete qualities of each individual (or integer) in mind, because our minds become dominated by an experience of the group. We perform a particular kind of mental operation which elides thinking of each discrete person: we use small numbers to stand for the whole group. This is similar to Bion's (1961) concept that one person in a small group stands for a quality of the whole group, for instance, the group's aggression or dependency. This idea – that the idea of the group overtakes representation of the individual – has a good deal in common with Matte-Blanco's (1975, 1988) theory of bi-logic thought (the simultaneous existence of two dominant modes of human thought), which posits contrasting symmetric and asymmetric patterns in unconscious and conscious thought (Rayner 1995). In this system, the unconscious works principally by considering classes of things or experience, by finding sameness or symmetrization, instead of the differences or asymmetries that are predominantly the province of conscious and verbal thought. Affects, especially strong affects, tend to merge experience symmetrically. Matte-Blanco's idea of symmetrization of thought – that all members of a class are thought of by qualities they have in common rather than as individuals with discrete qualities – helps understand the mental representation of a group by one of its members. It is virtually impossible to describe a group experience while being faithful to that of its individuals. The best one can do is to alternate between descriptions of the atmosphere (symmetrization) that organizes such a group, and the focus on individuals who embody certain aspects of the group experience. Focusing on one or two individuals might be a matter of asymmetric thought that discriminates difference, but it may function to condense symmetric thought into the idea of the one person inside or outside the group who embodies it. This operation is accomplished by the right mind, by unconscious process, but the thinking is then often returned to the left mind where it is experienced as though thoroughly logical. Stereotyping of members of an entire group is another frequent result of symmetrization carried out by people outside that group.

Another feature in Matte-Blanco's description of symmetric thought is infinitization of experience, extending it as if forever – a common feature of unconscious thinking. Infinitization is also a feature of unconscious or psychotic thought in which a thought or event is treated as if it is always or completely true (see also Stadter's discussion of time-far experience, Chapter 2 in this volume). In the process, a part is treated as equivalent to the whole. Strong affects tend to infinitize. For example, a minor setback or failure makes someone feel the whole world is bleak and will be so forever. Experiences in large groups have a tendency to infinitize. Anger in the group may be felt by a person that everyone hates her and that the affect stretches on forever as total, permanent and unalterable.

SYMMETRIZATION, GROUPS AND PROJECTIVE IDENTIFICATION

The idea of symmetrizing aspects of group experience is also embodied in Bion's (1961) description of unconscious group leadership where one person speaks for dependency or aggression in the group, or two people pair to speak for the capacity of the group for libidinal combination. The small numbers, individuals, pairs, triads, come to embody the larger group. We think of groups, even relatively small family groups, in a similar way: one or two individuals stand for the common qualities that characterize the group, and this symmetrization of family experience is lived out psychologically by projective identification that unconsciously actualizes the shared mental activity of housing a group trait in one member. For example, in a family characterized by pessimism, a parent may feel a son's poor grades doom him to failure in life forever. The tendency to think in and of groups in this way becomes even more marked when we try to comprehend very large groups of hundreds or thousands. Here, we use a different mental processes, thinking of the group as a conglomerate characterized by its common qualities; or we may enter what is essentially a confusional state that we then organize by the dynamics of chaos that defensively employ limited patterns of understanding and small number situations to simplify complex large number, multidimensional situations.

A large family by its very numbers will have to confront the difficulty of holding the numbers 3, 4, 5 and 6 in mind, and by having varying sub-groups present large combinations of numbers in interaction with each other. Often, one child will contain the anxiety about individual recognition given the overall size of the family. The following example shows how a family of six engaged in this process:

An $8\frac{1}{2}$-year-old girl, Kelly, came with her family who had discovered she had written notes suggesting that she and a neighborhood boy repeat some genital activity. The girl was attempting to compensate for her loneliness and sense of being left out in the family that had been accentuated by the birth of a fourth daughter in the family eight months earlier. Because the older sisters were close and Kelly felt alone, Kelly was 'given' the baby who now slept in her room. Initially pleased, Kelly soon realized that a live baby interfered with her life. There was a history of loss in the family because of two moves that left everyone feeling bereft, and there had been many months in which the father had been away on extended business assignment. When Kelly was 5, her mother had to be rushed from the house in the middle of the night with a life-threatening ruptured ovarian cyst. In the family interview Kelly said tearfully, 'Mommy didn't say good-bye to me.' She was voicing a deficit in mothering felt by each member of the family (including the mother) that constituted a symmetrized group level experience.

In the notational terms we described in our earlier chapter (Chapter 14), this experience could be represented as an experience for the mother as 1^{-1} or 1^0 and in the maternal internal object that all 6 members shared as 6^{-1}. A -1 symbolizes an individual experience of being attacked or neglected, and the '0' notation represents a pull to being nothing, to the void or black hole. However, on this occasion, the whole group was experiencing symmetrization of the $(-1 \leftrightarrow 0)$ mentality, that is $6^{-1\leftrightarrow 0}$, an unconsciously shared group affect and mentality. This notation signifies that the family group of six shared the attack which can either be seen as beginning as an attack on the mother and on her role, or as beginning as a group experience that then condenses onto the mother. Further, this shared experience had been treated by group projective identification, and through this process, put also into Kelly as a $1^{-1} \leftrightarrow 1^0$ experience on behalf of the whole group. This represents oscillation between a mentality of being hated or neglected – moving towards annihilation. Kelly and her mother take turns expressing this individually and, through symmetrization, on behalf of the group. Then, again on behalf of the group, Kelly tries in a symptomatic way to effect a transformation by manufacturing a solution through premature sexual intimacy, living out the internalized number (2^{+1}) in a fantasy image of the parents giving each other a sense of mothering through their sexual relationship. In trying to solve her own internal problem, she is also trying to help the family group through the return projective identification of a repaired group symmetrization.

This little girl's anguish communicated her anxiety in relation to the mind's capacity to hold numbers greater than 4 or 5, an unconscious awareness of the numbers and their impact in the psyche. This example also illustrates how there is a great deal more than the classical oedipal triangle's number 3 at play, both in larger families and in individual internal worlds. Developmentally, perhaps the main thing about moving from home to school is the emergence into a world that is numerically chaotic, needing to be recorded and processed by a different mental capacity than the smaller numbers of the home. In developmental regression, we condense our understanding to the home's small numbers (and the mind's greater capacity to think asymmetrically with small numbers) in order to make experience affectively comprehensible. The frequent failure to comprehend these larger numbers may trigger a confusional state, one that can lead to a regression to the small number state of mind. The struggle each person undergoes to wrap the mind around large numbers has the potential to lead to an enlarged capacity to hold new dimensions in mind, but it can also lead to regression to symmetric logic that distorts the group relational experience.

NUMBERS IN MOTION AND CHAOS THEORY

Building on our earlier studies of chaos theory and our previous chapter (Chapter 14) on complex numbers, we now propose that internal numbers are constantly on the move. Everyone is constantly moving psychically between differing internal equations in a flux that could only begin to be represented by a dynamic mathematics like calculus. A number is not a fixed thing in the mind, but a state of the moment, something that is here-and-gone. Therefore, (1) self, (2) the couple dyad, and (3) the oedipal triangle are more like constellations to be used for internal orientation than they are fixed internal numbers. A number is not so much a thing in itself as it is an address of a mental phenomenon or organization, but only for a given moment in patterns that change constantly with time. Each person is a dynamic system whose internal numbers are in flux. Numerical or algebraic notation for the flux show different frozen frames during the flux. The number is an address for a point in the flux, as is a single frame in a movie that shows individual moments of the larger pattern that ordinarily pass by too quickly for individual recognition. States of mind and the numbers and equations that represent them are on the move. The mind's capacity to organize and re-organize new object numbers is essential for adaptation and development. How open is the internal world? Is it able to take in new experiences and 're-group', as it were, to hold new sets of numbers in different relation to one another? Because numbers are in motion, they are part of a system that safeguards the capacity for adaptation that is inherent in chaos (Gleick 1987).

When discussing numbers in motion, we can only describe them at certain points at which we catch them, points on the excursion of dynamic systems that form complex arcs that never precisely repeat but that produce patterns we can learn to recognize. But as soon as we recognize a pattern, things change again and we see something different at another moment. Numbers seen in this way present essential paradox: they are not so much things-in-themselves, as they are themselves patterns that organize experience for the moment. Experience – a state of mind in movement – is captured as it materializes momentarily in a number, but the number itself is in flux. That flux to another numerical constellation signifies the change in the state of mind of the kind that characterizes transformations, and change of a kind that is stopped by trauma. It is only severely, even pathologically, limited individual and relational systems that closely repeat. In health, individuals and relational groups have chaotic patterns that confer adaptive capacity to life's changing situations. People have to bear chaos, even as infants, to negotiate the vitality of relating. Part of development involves enlarging this capacity. Neither math nor language is fully adapted to the challenge of describing numbers, equations, and geometric patterns that are in movement, of taking into account the dynamic variability of living psychological systems.

This description has important implications for analytic thinking that emphasizes repetitions and re-enactments. We consider the ordinary repetitions of life – as shown in the recognizable pattern of character or the patterns of daily life – as *self-similar* repetition (characterized by the chaos theory term 'strange attractors'). These show recognizable pattern, but do not have the deadly or self-destructive *self-sameness* of those unchangeable elements we call the repetition compulsion or repeated enactments of neurotic behavior. (These are characterized by the chaos theory term 'limit cycle attractors'.) The *self-same* repetitions are repeated effects of mental organization of fixed internal numbers that do not have the adaptive flux of ordinary, adaptive mental life (Scharff and Scharff 1998).

Another intriguing feature of numbers is that they are essentially zero-dimensional points. They are a point, not even a line that makes full use of one dimension, lacking the two dimensions of drawings. On the other hand, the phenomena we are thinking about are so complex that four dimensions are not enough to represent them. But mathematics can represent this problem (Matte-Blanco 1975). When a multidimensional situation has to be represented in only two or three dimensions, one must use duplication to show parts of the situation multiple times. We can illustrate this through the exercise of showing triangle 'abc' – a two-dimensional object – in one dimension.

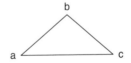

To do so, we draw a line that represents the unfolded triangle, but we then have to repeat one of the points that represent the angles. Notice that point 'a' has to be shown twice to represent the unfolded triangle.

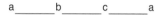

The same idea of duplication applies to representing a three-dimensional object like a cube in two dimensions, showing some lines more than once in the process. To represent the three-dimensional cube in two dimensions, each square side will be unfolded and be represented once, but some lines will appear more times, and each point is duplicated even more often (Matte-Blanco 1975). When it comes to representing four or more dimensions, these principles of duplication apply: a process or form in a higher dimension can be represented in fewer (say the two or three dimensions of a dream) by using processes of duplication to represent the added complexity of the higher dimensions.

Now we move to a discussion of numbers in motion. Here we have to use geometry more than calculation, something that can show the motion of a point in many dimensions and over time. There are at least four dimensions of mental space as soon as time is invoked as the dimension through which three-dimensional things move. Therefore, representation will involve multiple duplication of the kind dreams employ to show different aspects of the self over time.

Holograms can represent the idea that space and time are continuously folded into each other and that each point in space and time holds the representation of the entire universe. Negroponte (1995) described a hologram as containing all potential views of a scene which collects them into a single plane in patterns of light modulation. Constant movement is intrinsic to its pattern. Holograms give three-dimensional spatial form to non-linear equations of dynamic systems that have the quality of similarity across orders of scale. Each part of the pattern contains the seeds of the whole pattern. Sutherland thought the hologram was an apt metaphor for representation of the self, an overarching, emergent organization in which any one part contains the potential of the whole (J. S. Scharff 1994; Scharff and Scharff, Chapter 16 in this volume; Gleick 1987). When we capture a fixed mental number or configuration, it contains the seeds of the rest of mental structure because it is in motion and therefore relates to other points in the extremely complex pattern that is the whole of mental structure. Holograms can also be used to show structures that change over time, with alternating configurations that move and are in tension with each other; they evolve with time even while retaining pattern that contains earlier states of mind, in the way that evolving development contains condensed traces and patterns of earlier time.

TRANSFORMATION OF NUMBERS IN SPACE AND TIME

The two major organizers of thought into primary and secondary process thinking – the right- and left-brain, or right- and left-mind – process experience differently (Schore 2003a, 2003b). From Freud (1933) on, it has been understood that the quality of time is different in secondary process thought than in primary process – dream thought, creative condensation or psychosis. As we have seen, the geometry representing in three dimensions the complexity of dimensions greater than three involves multiple representations of the same thing in the visual space, and this capacity is part of the way the right mind represents experience.

Freud wrote that there is no time in the unconscious and '. . . where it is possible, the dream work changes temporal relations into spatial ones and represents them as such' (1933: 26). We prefer to say that time is represented in the unconscious, but in the complex way that shows its role as a fourth dimension. When time is processed in the affective right brain, events from different times are juxtaposed and overlap without *apparent* regard for the experience from which they are drawn having been at different periods in the person's life. The thought processes involve matching of qualities of experience, finding likenesses that span time, for instance through affect-matching. In another way, we might say that this process tells us a great deal about both the limits and the functions of time, about the likenesses the unconscious identifies that causes it to leap over time as a dimension that separates things. To put it another way, *time does exist as a crucial part of the thinking of the right mind, in the sense that it is addressed and illustrated in the limited experiential dimension available during dreaming*. Time exists, but it exists as dimension differently from the way it does in left-mind's logical thought: it exists to join things across dimension, not merely to sequence them in secondary-process linear fashion. Time folds back on itself, creating the kind of fractal representation as in a hologram that has infinite internal dimension and that repeats on itself in order to create meaning. (As discussed in Chapter 16 in this volume, fractals are patterns found in dynamic systems that are similar across different levels of scale. Fractal geometry is the study of such non-regular patterns produced by non-linear equations. See also Gleick (1987) and Scharff and Scharff (1998).) Time is an active factor and the possibility of superimposing time is precisely the point. That is to say, time is not disregarded, but seen as a multidimensional phenomenon requiring superimposition in order to be fully represented.

In the unconscious, following Freud and Matte-Blanco, the multiple dimensions of the unconscious exist simultaneously because that is the point of right-mind thought. All number representations exist simultaneously. Dream thinking superimposes these dimensions on each other. An event, a thing or a person shows up at several places in a dream to represent the multiple dimensions of experience of that event, thing or person in different situations and with differing affects in order to represent the multiple dimensions of experience. In this way, events of differing linear time are 'purposely' superimposed in non-linear space in order to propose new arrangements and meanings.

EXAMPLES OF TRANSFORMATIONS IN SPACE AND TIME

> I (DES) dreamt of seeing my father passing at the foot of my bed silently while I was in a room where my brother slept in another bed. He was a young man, of perhaps 35. At the time of the dream, I was 38 or 39, older than the 35-year-old father I saw in the dream. In the associations, I realized that during the time of difficulty between us, he was younger than I was at the time of the dream. I had children who were older by then than I was in the dream. The configuration of the beds was like that of the beds in my parents' room, recalling an incident when I was 5 and had wandered into their room and stolen his cigarette lighter, which I used with my brother to start a fire while he slept, resulting in calling the fire department.

In this example, dream thought transposed at least three times in my individual life and the life of my family – my childhood at age 5, my father five years later (close to the time of my parents' separation and my difficulty with him) and myself in the present as dreamer. It also transposed space – my parents' bedroom and my childhood bedroom that I shared with my brother, along with the bed in which I dreamt as an adult and the analytic couch on which I would certainly report the dream. In juxtaposing these elements of time and space, it became a 'dream that turns over a page' (Quinodoz 2002), because it permitted transformations in space and time. I could suddenly see that as a child I had attacked my father and my parents as a pair, and that the anger I felt coming from him was, at least in part, projective identification born out of my own youthful immaturity. The point here is that the unconscious dream thoughts use time and space transposed in a moving hologram, using fractal geometry to create meaning, even though understanding that meaning also requires left-brain decoding.

All transformations of number occur in time and space. Numbers represent object relations patterns that move through mental space or do not have space to move or expand. The numbers acquire new patterns by repeating over time, by juxtaposing processes of right- and left-mind, and by moving through different mental spaces. Numbers that have been constrained acquire, over time, new flexibility and the ability to exist in more than one form.

In the dream reported above, the numbers change as the images are folded, superimposed in differing time and space. The -2 of my relationship to my father, the $+2$ of my relationship to my mother, or the 3^{-1} of my vision of an oedipal struggle, is superimposed on a new $+2$ of the internal object relationship with him, and that reconfigures the 3 with my mother, and many aspects of myself, from a 1^{-2} that had elements of intolerance for an internal couple to a 1^{+2} that is a more settled self-image. And there is also the pairing with my younger brother as a substitute $+2$, a factor that has been folded into the moving equation. The point here is that the transformation of numbers occurs by the folding of multiple dimensions of space and time in ways that make them interchangeable in order to create meaning.

Here is another example showing the action of time in psychotherapy. Alternating states of mind reflect the work of transformation, as can be seen moment-to-moment in a therapy session. In this example, time marks a slow transformation in the transference and the quality of object relations available to the patient. Time figures both in the details of sessions and in the larger-scale passage of time.

> A chronically depressed mother brought her 9-year-old daughter, Jenny, to therapy with me (HC). Mother said that her daughter follows her around like a shadow and cannot sleep unless she is in mother's bed. For the first year of therapy, Jenny carefully watches the clock and tells the therapist, usually with a deep, sad sigh, how much time is left in session. It never feels like enough. She looks at the calendar and counts how many days (the numbers taking on meaning) until her next session. After nearly two years of treatment, Jenny introduced something new near the end of sessions: she said that her stuffed animal would be calling one of the therapist's stuffed animals in the week between sessions. They will stay connected. But when there are only five minutes left Jenny becomes despondent and quiet; she asks whether there is another patient after her.

Jenny rarely experienced herself as being a $+1$ in her mother's mind. She needed to stay physically close to mother to ensure that her mother did not forget her, so that she did not drop into the bottomless pit of her mother's depression. She feared becoming -1 or even '0' in her mother's psychological mathematics. Over time she began to feel held, a $+1$ in the therapist's mind: this transformation of numbers is expressed in the play of the stuffed animals in the space of the therapist's office, able to keep each other in mind (in mental space) as live numbers across time. The experience of '0', or -1 becoming $+1$, is also seen in how Jenny values her time in session, how she wants more, and wants to know when she'll have it again. The separation at the end of the session shows how fragile this was for her, as the idea of another child who might push her out of the therapist's mind, brought her back to anxiety about −1 and 0. The numbers here are charged with meaning and affect and they are in a constant state of movement in the session and between sessions. Time and space are dimensions in the anxiety, in the change of mental state about number, and in the process of movement and transformation between −1, 0 and +1. Jenny felt there was too little time for being held in mind or for transformation. As time passed with a steady place in the therapist's space and mind, she could experience the move from +1 to −1 with each week's separation, then form a conjunction of $1 + 1 = 2$, let that go, reconfigure it so that an internal space moved from $1^{-1 \rightarrow 0}$ to 1^{+1}, from 2^{-1} as an isolate without enough time, to 1^{+2} state of mind in interaction: $1^{+1} + 1^{+1} = 2^{+2}$. Now all of these numbers could co-exist to overcome the separation of time.

ENCAPSULATED AND SATURATED NUMBERS

Numbers have versatility of form and meaning. Like all mental experience, they can be made to hold a range of qualities. In this section we briefly explore how numbers are useful in thinking about the nature of traumatic encapsulation and saturation. The unconscious juxtaposes numbers and experience across time so that numbers can move into new configurations, form new complex numbers by being combined or put into new sets. An encapsulation is simply a constellation of numbers that cannot be in movement or in interaction with other numbers and therefore cannot be transformed or given meaning. It assumes the quality of a fixed mental object, and therefore becomes a limit-cycle attractor or even a fixed attractor – a focus of deadness and immobility in the mind (see Chapter 16 on chaos theory). Thus the number 1 as a fixed object does not allow new combinations into 2 or 3, or into a larger grouping, and even could shun becoming a complex, moving 1. There are other impediments to the spontaneous capacity for recombination of numbers, but trauma may be the most severe.

A middle-aged man sought therapy after the failure of his third marriage. In each case he precipitated divorce by having an affair. The man reported boyhood memories of hearing his parents argue late at night when they thought he was asleep. His father's affairs sent his mother into deep depressions. His inability to be in a couple (without enlisting a third) suggested that he may have encapsulated the number −2 to represent the warring, attacking parental couple. The encapsulation of this number was an organizing factor in his internal world and led to the pathological repetition – in this case, his parents' trauma and his traumatic experience of it.

This man kept trying to find a +2 experience, but has also carried other limit-cycle numbers: $2 \leftrightarrow -2$ with his wives. He also has persistent use of 3^{-2} that attacks the possibility of +2. This number does not get transformed. It just gets repeated.

Bion's (1970) notion of saturated experience relates to the idea of encapsulation. A saturated experience ceases to have authentic meaning because it gets repeated and held on to in a way that drains its vitality. When this happens with a numbered situation, the number may have the kind of magnetic, repeated pull (or in chaos theory terms, it functions as a basin of attraction) that this man's internal situation had – the repeated searching for a +2 situation that was saturated with –2, forming the fixed, self-same cycle that repetitively pulled his relationships towards self-destruction. When mourning occurs, the internal situation can once again become unsaturated and ready for a newly vital experience.

> A 4-year-old boy would initially only allow me (HC) to communicate with him via puppets: two on my hands and one on his. Lamb and Bear were to talk with Dog and could say anything they liked, but if they tried to address the boy directly he became violent and would attack the puppets. We might say that he only had room for three in his mind, the three puppets. After nine months of treatment, he began to allow there to be four or five of us into the room – the three puppets, the boy, and me. Dog would feed Lamb, Bear, and me a breakfast of pancakes and then the boy would talk with the four of us about the breakfast. The therapeutic space had the effect of creating more space in his mind for more complex numbers, and of course for people in new combinations of relationships.

In this example, we see the initial collapse of a capacity to number into an encapsulation. The therapy allows expansion of mental capacity so that there is room for more numbers. It also promotes the fluid flow of numbers back and forth so that they can transform into one another given therapeutic opportunity and the dimension of the passage of time. Doing so also involves enlarging the inner space in which transformation occurs.

Movement of internal numbers creates the fractal internal geometry of mental space and the invisible transitional geometry of interpersonal relations that is necessary for transformation and growth, and for the maintenance of normal vitality. In therapy, this occurs in the movement of the patient's or the family's static internal numbers that is brought about through the repeated passages through the mind of the therapist – that is through the matrix of transference and countertransference. The mind of the therapist has a multiplicity of number and geometry that is charac-terized by adaptive chaotic pattern, the ability to tolerate the projective identification of saturated and encapsulated numbers into a more mobile space, as the therapist lets herself disorganize into creative confusion and chaos, and through tolerance of numerical rigidity alternating with con-fusion, to reorganize the geometry of the separate and shared internal worlds. Chaos – numbers, shapes and spaces without tangible order – alternates with order and pattern as new possibilities for number and geometric pattern emerge. The possibility of such creative transformation of numbers is the goal of our work.

CONCLUSION

Patterns of numbers and shapes express mental configurations. In the process of forming these patterns, the unconscious establishes similarity of emotional experience of object relations in numbered representations and geometric relationship and puts them next to each other in dreams or in the dream-like action of art and fantasy. The right-mind is built to make patterns in this way – to use symmetrization to create meaning. Numbers produce geometric shapes that are both a combination of points on the plot of pattern and notations of pattern themselves, contributing to larger patterns that eventually become recognizable. These patterns do not dis-regard time or space. A dreamer has, in the background, a sense of the simultaneous presentation of two or more time frames, and of items from different spaces brought together to form a multidimensional juxtaposition. The right-mind does not so much disregard time to make new meaning as it juxtaposes events from different times in order to construct new multi-dimensional meaning about the passage and non-passage of time in which events are similar but not exactly the same. It uses space in a similar multidimensional way, playing with space and spatial relationships to create new meaning.

Now we have a picture of moving numbers, points that make up the alternating holographs that are being constantly manufactured by the juxtaposition of right- and left-minds, of logic and affect in continual interaction, each making its own pattern. Then the dominant pattern comes from the combination of the two, which, however, soon breaks down because it is inherently unstable, and therefore chaotic. Bion (1962) has likened this to the use of two eyes to create three-dimensional vision. Mathematically, the left, logical, linear brain does something like Euclidean geometry and simple math – squares, circles and triangle shapes, simple numbers and equations, straight-line reasoning and simple Freudian pat-terns. That simplification of pattern has great advantages in helping us to navigate the physical world, and to impose understandable pattern on the emotional world where complexity exceeds our grasp. But the patterns of the right-mind are formed by non-Euclidean shapes and geometry, by complex numbers, by non-linear equations that begin with the entrainment of mother and infant's right brains in a vital pattern (Schore 2003a, 2003b) and produce the alternating confusion and pattern we see in modern psychoanalysis. With simple math and geometric thinking, we make the world more available for understanding and manipulation, but we also rob it of its much-needed chaotic capacity for adaptation, and of much of the way its beauty reverberates across many dimensions. Having simplified it, we can put things into operation, but they have to be re-transformed into the more complex pattern in order to be given richer meaning, and this alternation between the two universes of organization goes on oscillating between the alternating holographs of discrimination and synthesis, reason and dream. To understand both modes of thinking we need both simple and complex mathematics to plot the oscillation between order and chaos that generates meaning in our lives.

REFERENCES

Bion, W. R. (1961) *Experiences in Groups and Other Papers*, London: Tavistock.

Bion, W. R. (1962) *Learning from Experience*, London: Heinemann.

Bion, W. R. (1970) *Attention and Interpretation*, London: Tavistock.

Bollas, C. (1999) *The Mystery of Things*, London: Routledge.

Freud, S. (1923) 'The Development of the Libido and the Sexual Organizations', *Standard Edition*, 16: 320–338, London: Hogarth, 1964.

Freud, S. (1933) 'Revision of the Theory of Dreams, Lecture XXIX', *Standard Edition*, 22: 7–30, London, Hogarth, 1964.

Gleick, J. (1987) *Chaos*, New York: Viking Penguin.

Matte-Blanco, I. (1975) *The Unconscious as Infinite Sets: An Essay in Bi-Logic*, London: Duckworth.

Matte-Blanco, I. (1988) *Thinking, Feeling, and Being*, London: Routledge.

Negroponte, N. (1995) *Being Digital*, New York: Random House.

Quinodoz, J.-M. (2002) *Dreams That Turn Over a Page: Paradoxical Dreams in Psychoanalysis*, New York: Brunner/Routledge.

Rayner, E. (1995) *Unconscious Logic: An Introduction to Matte Blanco's Bi-logic and its Uses*, London: Routledge.

Scharff, J. S. (1994) *The Autonomous Self: The Work of John D. Sutherland*, Northvale, NJ: Jason Aronson.

Scharff, J. S. and Scharff, D. E. (1998) *Object Relations Individual Therapy*, Northvale, NJ: Jason Aronson.

Schore, A. (2003a) *Affect Dysregulation and Disorders of the Self*, New York: Norton.

Schore, A. (2003b) *Affect Regulation and Repair of the Self*, New York: Norton.

Part IV

State of mind

The fourth dimension: state of mind

David E. Scharff and Michael Stadter

As editors, we experienced an ambivalent state of mind in the process of making the decision to include a part on 'states of mind' in this volume. This is familiar territory. All analytic writing is about one or another aspect of state of mind, so why here? On the other hand, the culmination of thinking represented throughout this book is the application of the basic elements of psychotherapy to the questions posed in this Part IV. Can an examination of number, space and time as basic dimensions lead to an increase in our understanding of them as elements of and metaphors for development and pathology? Similarly, can we examine how states of mind organize and integrate the basic dimensions of number, time and space? The state of mind of each participant in individual, group or family therapy influences the total interactional field, and, in turn, the total field influences each involved person. The complexity of such dynamic involvement is beyond calculation, drawing as it does on the multiple aspects of personality within each individual, and the essentially unpredictable influence of the sum of their conjoined and interacting personalities.

The four chapters in this part demonstrate this organization and integration in different ways. The first by Jill Scharff and myself (DES) is grounded in mathematics and physics. It also bridges Chapter 15 on numbers in motion as a model of mind that ended the last section. Chapter 16 in this part explores the use of chaos theory to explain processes of alternation between non-integration and integration that characterize normal development, that show how we can understand alternation of states of mind in a patient, and that provide the ordinary oscillation between periods of knowing and not knowing in psychotherapy. In that way, this chapter forms the bridge between the aspect of this book based in the more literal aspects of time, space and number, and their use as something crossing the ambiguous area between literal model for mental and interpersonal processes and their use as metaphor. Jill Scharff and I see chaos theory as offering a fundamentally new psychoanalytic paradigm, grounded in information processing and complexity, in juxtaposition to the original ephemeral clarities of psychoanalysis based on the physics of the nineteenth century. We propose that mental states in development and in therapy move in and out of recognizable pattern, and that there are long periods of time in all modalities of therapy when it is not possible or advisable to try to know too much.

The chapter by Sheila Hill deals with psychological space and the mental organizations that characterize traumatically sequestered space. She traces the history of thinking about the boundaries of inner and outer space of the mind, the way that intense early injury drives individuals to construct walls and boundaries that are designed to limit their continuing vulnerability to the outer transactional world, and the ways in which these second skin or psychic retreat constructions limit access in treatment. Through her case vignettes, she gives ample illustration of the kind of mental organization that takes over in pathologically limited situations, inhibiting the normal processes that are more chaotically in flux in the service of the continual adaptation and variety that characterize psychological health.

The third chapter explores two states of self: a state of complete fulfillment unbounded by time or space and a state of self-experience and development that comes from interaction with and awareness of limits and loss. Charles Ashbach uses the paradigm of Being and Becoming. He begins by noting the philosophical roots of these ideas. He then connects Being and Becoming with Bion's work, especially the concept of 'O' (origins) and extends it. Offering a clinical example, he illustrates transference/countertransference issues that arise. Ashbach ends his chapter with a discussion of the implications for therapists as they face their own narcissistic issues and he cites Bion's advice to avoid promoting a 'cozy' therapeutic relationship which obscures the fundamental aloneness of both therapist and patient.

In the final chapter of the book, Theodore Jacobs provides both a retrospective and an update of his own innovative work on countertransference, extending his thinking into the way mental states play out in the body and in the analyst's mental processing of the surface trappings of the patient's clothes and behaviors. This line of attention culminates in Jacobs' attention to enactments – those inevitable, valuable and often embarrassing interactional constructions that can show the therapist deep and abiding patterns that patients are unable to show verbally. This level of analytic understanding most illustrates the transformation of the elements of time, space and number into deep and strong patterns of co-constructed behavior that influence and are influenced by abiding mental states. These sweep therapist and patient alike into living things out that, only in this way, become accessible to new understanding. Here paradoxical elements of the everyday come to life in new ways that deepen our understanding of unconscious life.

Chapter 16

Chaos theory and object relations: a new paradigm for psychoanalysis

David E. Scharff and Jill Savege Scharff

After two years in analysis, Celia King began a session by saying, 'I can't believe what's happening to me. I think of myself as someone who doesn't mess up, but suddenly I feel like I'm turning into Calamity Jane. I scratched my car on a post in the garage, and I pulled something out of the icebox and spilled grease on myself. I have a headache. I can't do anything right. Before analysis, I was unhappy but I knew who I was. I don't know who I am or what I'm supposed to do.'

Many patients find that the more they discover about themselves, the more at a loss they feel. They begin by organizing treatment in patterns similar to the way they organize their lives, only to find that unexpected happenings of treatment throw them into turmoil. They become more confused. The inner turbulence is unwelcome, yet offers new possibilities.

In this chapter, we attempt to show that deterministic chaos theory – grouped with other theories called complexity theory, dynamic systems theory, and the theory of self-organizing systems – offers a new paradigm for thinking about the way the inner turmoil that emerges within the treatment process offers such new possibilities. To this end, we will introduce elements of chaos theory and apply them to concepts in object relations theory and practice: Fairbairn's theory of the self as a dynamic system of subsidiary ego, inner object relations developed by splitting and repression; Melanie Klein's (Klein 1946; Segal 1963; J. Scharff 1992) ideas on positions and on projective and introjective identification; Winnicott's (1963) concepts of the environment mother and the object mother, of transitional space; Ogden's (1994) analytic third; the clinical application of transference and countertransference in the light of Bion's (1970) application of projective identification to the container/contained, and his proposal that the analyst should eschew memory and desire; the role of interpretation; Sutherland's (J. Scharff 1994) conception of the self as a self-organizing system; and Fairbairn's (1958) axiom that the action of psychoanalytic treatment rests fundamentally on the nature of the therapeutic relationship. Chaos theory explains similarities of pattern at different levels of magnitude in personality, therapeutic process and social systems, offering a scientific rationale for the postmodern proposition that interpretations of psychic meaning are never absolute because they always depend on the vantage point of the interpreter.

Chaos theory derives from the study of non-linear equations that characterize dynamic, self-organizing systems. The findings that began to accumulate in the 1970s were first popularized in the 1980s (Gleick 1987; Briggs 1992). In the 1990s writers in psychology and psychoanalysis began to explore the value of chaos theory for understanding unconscious process, ego development, and therapeutic interaction (Spruiell 1993; Galatzer-Levy 1995; Ghent 2000; Levenson 1994; Masterpasqua and Perna 1997; Palombo 1999; Piers 2000; Quinodoz 1995; Scharff and Scharff 1998; van Eenwyck 1997). When Sutherland conceived of the self as a complex self-organizing system (J. Scharff 1994), no scientific framework was yet recognized that could be applied to his hypothesis. He had no access to non-random chaos theory, which now makes possible a more sophisticated understanding of individual psychic organization and of personalities in the dyads, groups and institutions.

PRINCIPLES OF CHAOS THEORY

Just as the theory of relativity and Hegelian philosophy offered new vistas for psychoanalysis in the middle of the twentieth century, chaos theory underpins the philosophy of deconstruction and postmodernism that themselves offer new ways of seeing psychologically and psychoanalytically (Birtles 2002). Chaos theory comes from the study of formerly unsolvable non-linear mathematical equations and from the new field of non-Euclidean geometry, also called fractal geometry (Gleick 1987; Briggs 1992). In this section, we will describe selected principles of chaos theory (Table 1). In the following section, we will show their relevance to the psychoanalytic situation.

1. Dynamic systems are characterized by continuous feedback

An iterated equation is the basis for a continual process of feedback in a system. In an *iterated algebraic equation* where 'X' is the unknown, the equation is solved, and then the answer is taken as the next starting point. For instance, $X^2 + 0.0001 = Y$ is solved. Then Y becomes the new X as the equation is solved again: $Y^2 + 0.0001 = Z$. Such an iterated system always begins the next cycle at a place determined by the solution of the previous cycle.

All biological life systems work as iterated systems. Individually, as a community, as an entire human species – we begin each moment by starting

Table 16.1 Selected principles of chaos theory

1. An iterated equation is the mathematical description of a continual process of feedback in a complex system.
2. Because complex non-linear systems demonstrate sensitive dependence on initial conditions, prediction is impossible.
3. Complex dynamic systems are chaotic and unpredictable, but, in non-random chaos, the patterns they create are recognizable.
4. Chaotic systems tend to self-organize.
5. Non-linear dynamic systems show self-similarity when examined at different levels of magnitude, a phenomenon called fractal scaling.
6. Attractors organize the form of a system, although paradoxically, they are also formed by the action of the system they characterize. There are three main types of attractors: *fixed attractors*, *limit-cycle attractors*, and *strange attractors*.
7. Small perturbations may effect major pattern changes when a system is chaotic, but are likely to be dampened near basins of attraction.
8. In biology, non-random chaotic rhythms afford a high degree of adaptability. Relatively fixed rhythms are a sign of pathology or lowered capacity for adaptation.

at the point we have arrived at so far, and then use the same operating equations to take the next step. We begin with a new X that is the sum of everything so far. For instance in each analytic session, the analytic dyad begins with an X that is the sum of experience between patient and analyst in previous sessions.

2. Sensitive dependence on initial conditions

An example of the process of iteration in the psychoanalytic process occurs when the analyst simply repeats a thought of the analysand's, restarting the equation at the point just reached, also inevitably introducing small differences to the next iteration through unnoticed variation in tonal inflection or phrasing. Edward Lorenz discovered that in computer simulation of complex weather systems, small differences in starting conditions produce unpredictable results. Theoretically, the flap of a butterfly's wings in Brazil could produce a small current that unpredictably amplified could become a hurricane in Texas, hence the name 'butterfly principle' (Gleick 1987). In complex systems, it is not possible to know in advance what difference even unnoticeable differences will make.

Humans have lifelong sensitivity to initial conditions. Small differences in neurobiological events and constitution, parent–infant factors, school, chance conversations, and trauma have effects beyond expectation. In psychotherapy, small differences in therapists' listening, or the way therapists' vocal inflection necessarily changes over time make distinct differences in the following iterations. Over time, small incremental differences have a large impact.

3. Unpredictability

Periodically, psychoanalysis has been criticized for being unable to predict the outcome of development or treatment. Chaos theory helps explain how we can know much and yet be helpless to predict. One hundred years ago, the mathematician Poincaré found that he could almost determine mathematically the effect of two celestial bodies on each other, but when a third body was introduced, it was no longer possible to predict results (Gleick 1987). Similarly, we cannot predict multivariate systems such as personality development or family interaction in families, but we can often understand them in retrospect because of our capacity to recognize complex patterns.

4. Chaotic systems tend to self-organize

Chaos theory has shown that self-organizing systems seem to organize out of apparently random chaotic patterns (Briggs 1992). When complex equations are iterated millions of times, and the solutions plotted in *phase space* – the mathematical space in which the system's activity is charted, the solutions may follow a definable curve at first. Then the curve splits at a place called a *saddle point*: two groups of solutions form a double or saddle curve. As iterations continue, each curve doubles at another saddle point, until a *cascade of period doubling* breaks pattern into apparently random chaos. The successive solutions become unpredictable. But if one keeps iterating and plotting, out of the edge of chaos, a pattern suddenly emerges that resembles the original one. An alternation between chaos and form develops.

In psychotherapy, we see corollaries of period doubling and cascades into and out of chaos. When a patient's mood determines whether a situation is seen as satisfactory or frustrating, there are two interpretations (or solutions) to the same situation. Which solution or interpretation is dominant depends on the affective tone accompanying the situation. As these alternate, the patient may become confused (breaking into chaos) as to the meaning of such events, only to emerge from the confusion by reverting to the old familiar alternation of positively and negatively toned interpretations.

> Mrs King had come to analysis with an idealized view of life. She was highly competent and served others unselfishly. Her life was enviable. That picture served to cover an inner emptiness and frustration of which she was hardly aware: that everyone else came before her. Her compliance to others' needs masked a resentment without words. In terms of chaos theory, she had two solutions to her life's equations: the sunny, idealized compliant one on the surface, which alternated with the empty, wordless, deeply buried frustration and resentment. In

analysis, as the iterations of her story joined with the analyst's feedback, she slowly saw the repressed 'solution' to her daily equations. The perturbation caused by this disturbing new awareness caused, at first, an oscillation between these two ways of understanding her daily experience, and then periodic cascade into confusion and emotional chaos. She no longer knew who she was. Periodically, she would solve the problem of feeling lost in chaos by returning to the familiar patterns. She preferred reinstating the idealized view of her life, but when someone frustrated her, resentment and anger also appeared, now more on the surface.

5. Non-linear dynamic systems show self-similarity at different levels of magnitude, a phenomenon called 'fractal scaling'

When iterated non-linear equations are plotted by computer, they show *self similarity at different scales of magnification*, a feature Bernard Mandelbrot has called 'fractal scaling' (Gleick 1987). A fractal is similar pattern at varying levels of scale – the 'footprint' of a dynamic system. The mathematics of chaos is easier to visualize in natural geometric images of fractals than in formulas. Fractals are found everywhere in nature and art (Briggs 1992). A leaf pattern of branching veins at varying levels of magnification is similar to its overall shape, again to patterns of leaves on twigs, twigs on larger branches, and trees in the forest. Branching neural dendrites and the pattern of veins and arteries into smaller units demonstrate fractal scaling. In art, self-similar fractal patterns at differing orders of scale – as for instance in the detail of exterior decorations of the Paris Opera matching its overall architectural structure – produce the most aesthetically satisfying images. In analysis, Galatzer-Levy (1995) has shown fractal similarity between patients' speech patterns, the structure of a session, and personality structure, and also similarity between the process in any session and the overall shape of treatment.

6. 'Attractors' represent the form of a system as plotted in phase space

A 'fixed attractor' is a *point*, the kind of pattern to which a pendulum powered by gravity tends. As the pendulum runs down, its arc acts as though drawn by the point at which it will eventually stop.

A 'limit-cycle attractor' is a *fixed pattern* that holds all the points in phase space through which movement occurs. The arc of a pendulum powered by electricity is a simple limit-cycle attractor. Clinically, frozen, encapsulated time-stopping phenomena of trauma act as limit-cycle attractors.

A 'strange attractor' is a pattern of random, non-repeating points, seen, for instance, in the movement of celestial bodies or biological rhythms. Although there is a pattern to the equations or movement of objects, the exact location of movement in phase space does not repeat. Paradoxically, strange attractors have a predictable overall form, but that form is made up of unpredictable details (Briggs 1992). The pattern of a whirlpool offers a good visual image of a strange attractor, with the small eddies found nearby and within the larger pattern as fractals of the overall pattern.

A strange attractor appears to organize its system, but the attractor is actually produced by the system of which it is a part. Both these qualities of strange attractors are useful in understanding human development. For instance, the brain of an infant is organized by repeated interaction with parents (Schore 1997). The attractors that organize the infant–mother interaction are formed by it, and also act on it. Although exact sequences do not repeat, the patterns are recognized by both mother and infant, and can be measured by researchers. The concept of strange attractors is also useful in the conceptualization of psychotherapeutic process, as we will demonstrate in the clinical example below.

7. Perturbations more easily effect major pattern change when the system is chaotic, but are likely to be dampened near 'basins of attraction'

Strange attractor patterns resemble those in systems of turbulent flow, such as a waterfall or the patterned chaos of leaping flames, where certain patterns repeat, then give way to randomness, then suddenly emerge out of the chaos to form an ordered pattern, and then revert to chaos again. For instance, turbulent water near a whirlpool seems to be sucked into the pattern of the whirl. Near the attractor, the system seems to be swept into the current in an area called a 'basin of attraction'. It seems that matter in the 'basin of attraction' of an attractor is pulled into it, although it paradoxically also produces the continuing pattern by its behavior in being near the attractor. Near the basin of a strange attractor, the system is less susceptible to influence by small perturbations or intrusions that disturb the system. In disorganized areas of chaotic regions, perturbations may have relatively large effects. By analogy, the force it takes to get a ball rolling is relatively slight at the top of a hill (like a chaotic region) while it takes a much larger force to get the same effect in a valley (like a basin of attraction) (Piers 2000).

The concept of 'basin of attraction' and its implications for change in a system have been applied to psychoanalysis by Palombo (1999), who labeled as 'infantile attractors' those unconscious models that influence current behavior to follow infantile patterns. Analytic material close to the infantile attractor's basin is held more fixedly in the old pattern, while material further from the basin is more easily susceptible to influence from the analytic process. The 'tuning variable' – the strength of perturbation that it takes to destabilize orderly flow in a system or change chaotic, turbulent flow into a pattern – depends on many conditions, an important one of which is the proximity to a more organized pattern or basin of attraction. Quinodoz (1995) has suggested that the strength or weakness of object relationships form a tuning variable for anxiety and psychic integration, both during infantile development and in the transference to the therapist.

8. In biology, chaotic rhythms afford a high degree of adaptability. Relatively fixed rhythms are a sign of pathology and lowered adaptability

Self-similar patterns – those characterized by strange attractors – are the norm in dynamic systems. *Self-same* patterns, more like those characterized by a limit-cycle attractor, are often signs of pathology. A marcher's pace, so-called regular heart rate, normal EEG rhythms are all healthy biological rhythms that show chaotic irregularity. The frequencies are ever-changing and when plotted mathematically reveal patterns of strange attractors. Only in disease do these biological rhythms become essentially regular. Chaotic irregularity confers a much higher degree of adaptability than lock-step regularity. Current neurobiological research has begun to demonstrate that the brain is also organized by the principles of non-random chaos theory as seen for instance in the way the mother–infant exchanges that are similar over time but never exactly the same, form strange attractor affect patterns that determine the growth of the infant's right orbitofrontal lobe in the first 18 months (Schore 1997). It is not that complete randomness is healthy. It is the slight chaotic irregularity within an overall pattern of stability that produces healthy capacity for adaptation to unpredictable needs.

APPLYING PRINCIPLES OF CHAOS THEORY TO THE CLINICAL SITUATION

We view psychological experience as a matrix of fractals that shows self-similarity across scale. Aspects of healthy experience are organized by movement between varying strange attractor patterns. In such a matrix, linear elements of progression and regression – such as psychosexual stages, repetition compulsion, or the concept that developmental fixation and regression are the foundation of psychopathology – can be seen as limit-cycle attractors. These linear models do not sufficiently address the facts of life within a complex matrix of experience made up of conflicting meanings and relationships, and multiple truths. Bion (1970) and Winnicott (1971) described the task of living in the fundamentally paradoxical situation in which conflicting and irresolvable elements have to be experienced without choosing one over the other. In this synchronic mode, conflicting meanings coexisting. Psychological experience is organized by varying patterns that have a complex relationship to each other. This complexity more accurately describes psychological experience, but Freud's limit-cycle attractors have a continuing validity as clinically helpful approximations that frequently describe pathological breakdown patterns because limit-cycle attractors often simplify overall pattern at the expense of the adaptability of chaotic flexibility. This provides a scientific way of understanding why psycho-analysis has always been better at explaining psychopathology in retrospect than at predicting or even describing health, since health consists of more complex combinations of patterns of behavior.

CLINICAL CHAOS

Celia King, a 35-year-old, highly functioning divorced mother and successful entrepreneur, came to analysis with me (DES) with an inner sense of emptiness that led, over the first two years of work, to a sense that she did not really know who she was. Married at 19, she immediately had a son, then a daughter, and divorced at 23. Her children, now young adolescents, did well academically, socially and in sports, but they complained and whined at her a good deal. She had chest pain found to be neither cardiac nor esophageal in origin that had disappeared on treatment with a small dose of SSRI antidepressant. In analysis Mrs King regularly presented her family and colleagues as offering her mainly persecuting and rejecting experiences: her live-in boyfriend was unreliable, her children refused to help, and her employees lacked initia-tive. She handled irritation by becoming obsequious, doing favors, failing to set limits, and other 'too good' excited object behavior, thereby keeping her painful internal objects split off from central, satisfying experience.

Superficially, Mrs King's pattern appeared to be a flexible adaptive strange attractor. Underneath, it resembled a limit-cycle attractor designed to allow no conscious connection with painful affects, a stricture producing inner meaninglessness. Mrs King's limit-cycle attractor pattern of self-organization was less adaptive than a more chaotic strange attractor pattern. It offered predictability and control at the expense of spontaneity and access to feelings. It led to somat-ization of her 'heartache' into chest pain. In analysis, she regained contact with experience split-off by repressed anti-libidinal, limit-cycle attractors.

Analysis introduced destabilizing perturbations. Taking her complaints seriously, I began to challenge her affective disconnection by linking adult patterns and somatic pain to current and childhood disappointment. I came to realize that Mrs King's idealizing transference and compliance produced a complementary countertransference of me as a good analyst who, however, was superfluous and empty of real function. In chaos terms, iterations of our interaction produced an excited countertransference pattern that also contained her emptiness. With minor exceptions, she agreed with what I said. Her trust was too-good-to-be-true, an excited-object projective identification designed to keep me from becoming a persecuting object. Using my counter-transference sense that her unquestioning trust made me less useful, I began to show her the transference pattern in which she used projective identification to keep me feeling good but untested to avoid friction between us. This friction introduced a tuning variable between us, a destabilizing force that could throw things into or out of chaos and confusion.

As I interpreted the limit-cycle nature of her pattern, Mrs King began to voice small annoyances towards me. These gentle criticisms represented the first excursions away from the basin of attraction of her character defenses. Introducing small perturbations into the initial conditions of the iterations of our interactions had produced unpredictable changes in subsequent interaction because of sensitive dependence on these initial conditions. Slowly we moved away from the basin of attraction in which both of us felt empty, and the analytic relationship and discourse began to oscillate across a wider and less comfortably predictable range.

Mrs King now experienced a slowly increasing inner chaos she had foreclosed because of threat of disintegration in her family growing up. She complained about her parents and her current family, voiced resentment, but soon denied it. I pointed out her retreat from awareness of resentment to avoid the threat of being pulled back into the chaos of the family. She was avoiding the infantile basin of attraction where family dysfunction was pooled. Successive iterations of descriptions of her childhood, her current family experience and my interpretations slowly produced new patterns. Where pain had been avoided by cutting off affect, there was now room. Just my saying to her that she was disappointed in people or that she resented them, created a perturbation in her fixed reactions, a new turbulence that moved her toward tolerating the chaos of ambivalence and futility, the pull of split-off and repressed gravitational bodies – inner painful objects she had kept out of her conscious universe. Having lived with rigid predictability, she was disconcerted to be less predictable to herself.

As the pull of the compliant, excited object relations basin of attraction loosened, the resentment, rejection, and longing appeared. With more awareness of her resentment came her realization that she feared being like her parents, irresponsible, abandoning and damaging to children and partners. She had taken care of her sisters, and then of her children, boyfriend and employees to avoid being like her parents. Her denied unconscious identification with bad internal objects based on deprivation and impingement, led to her relentless need to repair old objects. Each of these isolated patterns had become limit-cycle attractors constrained from becoming adaptively chaotic. As I commented on the contrast between the way she presented herself and the way her unthinkable anxieties reached me through iterations of projective and introjective identification, the whole range of my input into our shared interaction produced small repeated perturbations in her psyche. Mrs King faced more affect than she had previously allowed, providing the inner tuning variable that moved her from one attractor to another.

Dynamically, the situation worked like this: each incident that might trigger resentment could either evoke a rejecting object constellation, or could quickly lead to an idealizing compliance. In terms of chaos theory, these were saddle points at which the equation split into two opposing solutions determined by contrasting affects. Before analysis, the resentful anti-libidinal attractor had been largely unconscious, subject to intense repression by the idealized excited object attractor. As analysis proceeded, Mrs King was transported across one saddle point after another – branch points in her identifications. The tuning variables that propelled her into chaotic, anxiety-ridden experience came from previously repressed affects. The rapid unconscious crossing of the saddle points (choice points of how to be organized) she now experienced in anxious situations became a destabilizing cascade of 'period doubling' or of emotional solutions for her internal operating formulas, until chaos ensued in the form of confusion about her sense of herself. Now Mrs King could no longer maintain an identity as 'the good-natured fixer'. She no longer knew who she was.

Influenced by the overarching new attractor pattern formed within the analytic matrix, analyst and analysand form a new shared pattern of unconscious strange attractors identified by Ogden (1994) as the analytic third, by which both participants were influenced. Mrs King interacted consciously and unconsciously with me as an external object with both environmental and object-related elements that were gradually internalized (Winnicott 1963). We interacted through continuous cycles of projective and introjective identification, forming the container/contained (Bion 1967, 1970). In this process, the analyst's mind becomes a new region of phase space through which the analysand's anxieties travel repeatedly in each iteration, and this is also represented in the potential or phase space between them, in the atmosphere of the analysis that itself forms new strange attractors that pull the patient away from old ones and old basins of attraction.

Analysis is an iterated experience. Through the repetition compulsion – which constitutes reliance on limit-cycle attractors, patients repeatedly use formulas. Each repetition is a fractal of the patient's personality and of her relationship to others. The repetitive transferential patterns are self-*same* rather than self-*similar*. Mrs King used an outer shell of exaggerated depressive position functioning to maintain the repression of frightening aspects of paranoid/schizoid object relations (Klein 1935, 1946). The result was blocked movement between the positions, rather than the chaotic fluctuation between psychic positions characteristic of psychic health (Bion 1962, 1963; Ogden 1989). She was in a static position or psychic retreat (Steiner 1993), a limit-cycle attractor that protected her from a collapsing sense of self. Change was like pushing a ball uphill out of a deep basin of attraction. But each therapeutic repetition becomes subtly different because of sensitive dependence on initial conditions – because extremely small differences can potentially make disproportionate differences in fixed patterns. Slowly Mrs King became able to move out of these basins to experience the chaos of the unknown, and move slowly through the analysis of transference toward a more integrated experience. As she did so, the foreclosed analytic space began to open into a more functional transitional phase space. This space was characterized by some states of more adaptive chaotic irregularity in which new attractor patterns could develop.

Two dreams

Two dreams from Mrs King demonstrate Fairbairn's (1944, 1954) proposition that dreams represent 'shorts' of a patient's endopsychic situation. We now see them as fractals of personality, and as iterations of dynamic endopsychic structure combining cognitive and affective organization. Dreams also represent an analysand's relationships including the transference relationship (D. Scharff 1994), and illustrate new psychic strange attractors evolving in the transference–countertransference encounter.

Mrs King said, 'I had two dreams last night. In the first I was a teenager hiding from a strange boyfriend who was going to beat and rape me. I went into the library where you were reading. You didn't look up, so I went into the ladies' toilet. I felt trapped because the dangerous boyfriend was still outside. A woman said, "We'll help." Some women gave me a military uniform and snuck me out a window. I joined a military parade and marched away to some barracks and felt safe.

'The second dream upset me more. I was living in a one-level ranch house with a low roof. My real boyfriend was there and said, "The cats are out tonight." There were tigers and panthers. He said he was going to look for our dog. I didn't want him to. He's in the jeep with the roof off. He drives into the carport without putting on the brakes and crashes. Then he comes into the house carrying my son's head. It's obvious it was the cats that got him. I dial 911. The person answers, "Once the cats target you, there's no hope!" I go on the roof and shoot 11 of the cats, but I know there are always 12. I decide the 12th cat is in the house, and I don't know if it's going to go after my son, my boyfriend, or me.'

Mrs King's boyfriend had a jeep, but she said the dream car also represented my cars usually parked in the carport in front of my office, a low-roofed one-story building. This led her to an image of the car crashing into my office, driven now by me. In the first dream I sat reading, although she was in danger, and she had to hide in a toilet associated with the one off my waiting room. This reminds her of the time she and her mother hid in the bathroom when her father threatened to shoot them. The military women could defend her against armed men related to her father with the gun. The lions and tigers of the second dream reminded her of the color of bees buzzing in my garden she can see from the couch. In the last few days she has felt afraid of them. As Mrs King gave these associations, I felt sadness at the threat she was feeling in our relationship, a loss of transference idealization. At the same time, because I knew the idealization had limited our work, I felt an inner quickening in response to her bringing the previously excluded danger into the room.

These dreams show the cracking of the projective identification of an excessively too-good-to-be-true holding pattern (a limit-cycle attractor pattern) that had protected us from knowing the ways in which Mrs King feels unsafe, a dawning awareness of an unconscious lack of safety, of the invasive, rapacious and even murderous persecuting objects previously excluded from our relationship. They are fractals of Mrs King's unconscious internal object relations, her developmental history, and the transference–countertransference interaction. The sense of danger that characterized her childhood has returned. She does not feel I will look up from my books to protect her. I appear as myself ignoring her and as the dangerous boyfriend. She uses the toilet to hide from danger emerging in the transference. The military woman refers to her mother in that situation and also to my wife, whose office is across the waiting room, who she has often fantasized could help her. Only her militant women friends will defend against the marauding men.

The second dream iterates the same problem with her boyfriend in a more helpful role. She has previously been unable to speak of unconscious fears, unsupported because of my lack of awareness of her inner fright.

Through projective and introjective identification, I have been participating in a pattern in which we both exploited an attitude of exaggerated trust to keep the cats at bay; therefore her fear that they would never rest until they got her could not be acknowledged. I am the 12th cat that is still out to get her.

The dream fractals of Mrs King's internal situation and of the transference–countertransference exchange locate the cats as the ever-present sense of threat. I fail to defend her, and then pounce on her with interpretations. The dream communications to herself and to me are fractals of her overall psychic organization, self-similar to larger patterns in which she is on guard because no one understands. They are also fractals of her relationship to her primary objects, and of the aspect of the analytic relationship in which she feels I do not understand, and that only a longed-for but unknown woman could arm her against the night.

The analysis with Mrs King has seemed on the surface to be conducted in the depressive position, but these dreams indicate that it has been a limit-cycle, relatively fixed version of the depressive position. As the dreams surface her paranoid/schizoid themes, I can loosen the protective, rigid pseudo-depressive pattern – a basin of attraction that has gripped much of our interaction. As I feel her fear, I see the splitting and repression of her encapsulated psychic retreat (Steiner 1993). Sitting in my chair behind her, looking past her to the magnolia tree in my garden, I silently think about how she watched protectively lest its buds be frozen before they could bloom as happened in the previous year. I imagine a cat on a branch, stalking a bird in the tree. I feel the danger lurking everywhere for Mrs King. There has been a perturbation in this session, in this iteration, a move away from the basin of attraction that has held therapeutic action at bay. Now she is able to convey fear in such a way that I have been able to take it in. And it connects, too, to the blossoms we can both see outside. The terror and the beauty are closer together. They do not have to be as limited as before, not so rigidly held apart.

THE ANALYST'S SURRENDER TO CHAOS

Balint urged therapists to allow a 'harmonious interpenetrating mix-up' (1968: 136) in order to promote a therapeutic regression cathected by the therapist's primary love in order to offer a 'new beginning' for an analys-and's emerging self. Bion (1970) proposed that analysts eschew memory and desire, giving themselves over in each moment to learning in the immediate experience of the session. In a related vein, Winnicott (1971) urged parents and analysts to allow babies and analysands to live with irresolvable paradox. *Each urges us to tolerate chaos!* When we truly surrender to the moment, we give up what we already know in favor of what is not yet known, to the chaos inherent in complex self-organizing systems that frees us from old limited attractors, and opens to the excursions of new strange attractors. One can almost feel the pattern oscillate between analyst and patient, feel unnamable influence, let it seep in and change the inner patterns with which it resonates, and then feel the force of a strange attractor as the atmosphere of the session changes, as the analysand takes in our words, tone or facial expression in a slightly altered way. New shapes gradually form out of the 'analytic third', the new strange attractor co-created by analyst and analysand.

Beyond the surrender to chaos, what difference can chaos theory make clinically? In most ways, it is too soon to know. Practice changes more slowly than theory. We are still learning from the discoveries of Klein, Fairbairn, Winnicott, Balint and Bion. Clinical practice is changing in multiple directions. The new openness to mutuality in the therapeutic relationship removes much of the imposed certainty of Freud's linear theories. Many of Freud's propositions are limiting attractors. Newtonian physics is still extremely useful as a working approximation to mechanical problems. Like Newtonian physics, Freud's propositions are based on a limited point of view that offers valuable approximations to operational truths. But it is time to open ourselves to the uncertainties that allow new understanding to form from experience. In complex systems, limited attractors can form part of the pattern, just as Euclidean geometry forms a guide to building a house. More complete understanding of dynamic systems calls for strange attractors.

We find it helpful to think of strange attractors and basins of attraction as we experience the iterations of the therapeutic experience, as we surrender to the unpredictable swings of clinical hours. The metaphors of fixed, limit-cycle and strange attractors, the movement from self-same patterns of psychic retreats and encapsulations to the self-similar fractal patterns of health allow us to see variance in repetitive behavior. Self-similar patterns demonstrated in a patient's speech, behavior, dreams and transference (Galatzer-Levy 1995) offer the analyst opportunities to intervene at any level, knowing that a perturbation on a small scale may eventually produce profound effects at larger scale.

The many uncertainties of working in an intersubjective field, and anxiety about the durability of knowledge in the postmodern era, raise questions that are easier to parse with help from chaos theory. Analysis has struggled for a long time with the charge that our interpretations stem from pathological certainty, bias, and medical omnipotence without scientific foundation. But in the postmodern philosophical context, all knowledge and all interpretation of experience are seen as relative, all constructed from the vantage point of the culture, the current intellectual framework, and the experience of the interpreter. There is no absolute truth. Using chaos theory and the ramifications of the Heisenberg principle – that all observation changes the phenomena observed – we can see that pattern recognition in complex systems is always open to multiple interpretation, and that analysis is not unique in having to live with ambiguity.

Fairbairn's model of personality (1944) introduced the concept of dynamic flux of complex factors into psychoanalytic theory. The clinical concepts of the fluctuation between Klein's psychic positions mediated by mutual processes of projective and introjective identification as the organizer both of the mind-in-development and of the therapeutic process, the concepts of the holding relationship and of container/contained, dreams as fractals of personality and of the transference/countertransference exchange, the role of interpretation in inducing change, concepts of psychic and interpersonal splitting as pattern doubling at saddle points, and Bion's dictum that analysts should work without memory or desire, are theoretically explained by chaos theory. More than a metaphor, chaos theory offers to ground psychoanalysis in a modern paradigm that fits current trends in psychoanalytic thinking. A theory of complex self-organizing systems that tend towards higher levels of organization, it provides a fitting new model for the psychoanalytic process. We are, after all, biological organisms governed by the principles of the physical universe in which we live. The universe and all who inhabit it are governed not just by the known principles of gravity and relativity, but by the complex theories of non-random chaos, which, with the aid of slowly advancing knowledge, we begin to perceive dimly. Within the limits of what we know so far, it is not possible to predict how far the strange attractor of chaos theory will take us from its use as metaphor coloring our thought, to paradigm shift galvanizing new understanding.

REFERENCES

Balint, M. (1968) *The Basic Fault: Therapeutic Aspects of Regression*, London: Tavistock.

Bion, W. R. (1962) *Learning from Experience*, New York: Basic Books.

Bion, W. R. (1963) *Elements of Psycho-Analysis*, London: Heinemann.

Bion, W. R. (1967) *Second Thoughts*, London: Heinemann.

Bion, W. R. (1970) *Attention and Interpretation*, London: Tavistock.

Birtles, E. F. (2002) 'Why is Fairbairn Relevant Today: A Modernist/Postmodernist View', in F. Pereira and D. E. Scharff (eds.), *Fairbairn and Relational Theory Today*, London: Karnac, pp. 36–52.

Briggs, J. (1992) *Fractals: The Patterns of Chaos*, New York: Touchstone.

Fairbairn, W. R. D. (1944) 'Endopsychic Structure Considered in Terms of Object-Relationships', in *Psycho-Analytic Studies of the Personality* (1952), London: Tavistock with Routledge, Kegan Paul, pp. 82–136.

Fairbairn, W. R. D. (1954) 'The Nature of Hysterical States', in D. E. Scharff and

E. F. Birtles (eds.) (1994), *From Instinct to Self: Selected Papers of W. R. D. Fairbairn*, vol. 1, Northvale, NJ: Jason Aronson, pp. 13–40.

Fairbairn, W. R. D. (1958) 'On the Nature and Aims of Psychoanalytic Treatment', in D. E. Scharff and E. F. Birtles (eds.) (1994), *From Instinct to Self: Selected Papers of W. R. D. Fairbairn*, vol. 1, Northvale, NJ: Jason Aronson, pp. 74–92.

Galatzer-Levy, R. (1995) 'Psychoanalysis and Chaos Theory', *Journal of the American Psychoanalytic Association*, 43: 1095–1113.

Ghent, E. (2000) 'Motivation in the Light of Dynamic Systems Theory', paper presented at the American Academy of Psychoanalysis, New York, January 2000.

Gleick, J. (1987) *Chaos*, New York: Viking Penguin.

Klein, M. (1935) 'A Contribution to the Genesis of Manic-depressive States', in *Love, Guilt and Reparation and Other Works: 1921–1945* (1975), London: Hogarth Press, pp. 370–419.

Klein, M. (1946) 'Notes on Some Schizoid Mechanisms', in *Envy and Gratitude and Other Works: 1946–1963* (1975), London: Hogarth Press, pp. 1–24.

Levenson, E. A. (1994) 'The Uses of Disorder: Chaos Theory and Psychoanalysis', *Contemporary Psychoanalysis*, 30(1): 5–24.

Masterpasqua, F. and Perna, P. A. (eds.) (1997) *The Psychological Meaning of Chaos*, Washington, DC: American Psychological Association.

Ogden, T. (1989) *The Primitive Edge of Experience*, Northvale, NJ: Jason Aronson.

Ogden, T. (1994) *Subjects of Analysis*, Northvale, NJ: Jason Aronson.

Palombo, S. R. (1999) *The Emergent Ego: Complexity and Coevolution in the Psychoanalytic Process*, Madison, CT: International Universities Press.

Piers, C. (2000) 'Character as Self-organizing Complexity', paper presented at the winter meeting of the American Academy of Psychoanalysis, New York, January 2000.

Quinodoz, J.-M. (1995) 'Transitions in Psychic Structures in the Light of Deterministic Chaos Theory', *International Journal of Psycho-Analysis*, 78: 699–718.

Scharff, D. (1994) *Refinding the Object and Reclaiming the Self*, Northvale, NJ: Jason Aronson.

Scharff, J. S. (1992) *Projective and Introjective Identification and the Use of the Therapist's Self*, Northvale, NJ: Jason Aronson.

Scharff, J. S. (1994) *The Autonomous Self: The Work of John D. Sutherland*, Northvale, NJ: Jason Aronson.

Scharff, J. S. and Scharff, D. E. (1998) *Object Relations Individual Therapy*, Northvale, NJ: Jason Aronson.

Schore, A. N. (1997) 'Early Organization of the Nonlinear Right Brain and Development of a Predisposition to Psychiatric Disorders', *Development and Psychopathology*, 9: 595–631.

Segal, H. (1963) *Introduction to the Work of Melanie Klein*, London: Hogarth Press and the Institute of Psycho-Analysis.

Spruiell, V. (1993) 'Deterministic Chaos and the Sciences of Complexity: Psychoanalysis in the Midst of a General Scientific Revolution', *Journal of the American Psychoanalytic Association*, 41: 3–44.

Steiner, J. (1993) *Psychic Retreats: Pathological Organizations in Psychotic, Neurotic and Borderline Patients*, London: Routledge.

van Eenwyck, J. R. (1997) *Archetypes and Strange Attractors: The Chaotic World of Symbols*, Toronto: Inner City Books.

Winnicott, D. W. (1963) 'The Development of the Capacity for Concern', in *The Maturational Processes and the Facilitating Environment* (1965), London: Hogarth Press, pp. 73–82.

Winnicott, D. W. (1971) *Playing and Reality*, London: Tavistock.

Chapter 17

Hideouts and holdouts

Sheila Hill

> How good to be safe in tombs,
> Where nature's temper cannot reach
> Nor vengeance ever comes
>   Emily Dickinson, *XVI Refuge* (2000: 207)

Some patients, born into the world, cannot abide here. They are so afraid of development that they have created a hiding place or hiding places, which provide protection against an incapacitating terror. They construct a defensive carapace from whatever comes to hand or to mind in what for some is an endless variety of enclosures, which enable them to holdout and hold back genuine contact with others and the world. These patients are a clinical challenge since they usually work in treatment in what appears to be an ordinary way until the therapist realizes that no progress has been made or, when genuine emotional contact is made with a hidden aspect of their personality, they respond with withdrawal at best or fear and loathing.

Donald Winnicott (1945), Esther Bick (1968, 1986), Wilfred Bion (1970), Donald Meltzer (1992) and John Steiner (1993) have all described the various ways in which people construct defenses against the experience of primitive anxieties: of having no one to hold onto and no one holding on. Winnicott, Bick and Bion describe the most primitive anxieties or states of mind and the defenses or mental spaces in which to hold those states of mind. Meltzer and Steiner include in their work the defenses against emerging from the defensive carapace which both argue is a defensive organization made up of a variety of states of mind expressed in what for some is an endless variety of hideouts from the posture of being a holdout from life.

I shall first describe the situation in which many of these patients find themselves, the defenses they employ, some techniques for working with them, and then discuss the need to remain alert to the levels and cycles of primitive anxieties that often manifest in a session especially when patient and therapist are working well with one another.

The conceptualization of mental states within a mental space proceeds from Melanie Klein's assertion that human beings move not only from one psychosexual stage to another but also from one state of mind to another. She asserted that those states of mind are accompanied by particular anxieties, defenses, and qualities of relationships. She further asserted that in normal early development, later in life in the absence of development, or under stress, these states of mind are 'ejected' from the mind by a process she called projective identification. The consequent notion is that from birth one projects into something and someone (Klein 1946). Then the self maintains a relationship with the object projected into in which it recognizes the projected states of mind as its own (Etchegoyen 1991).

Wilfred Bion in 'Attacks on Linking' (1959), advanced the notion that projective identification is not only a process of evacuation but also a process of communication to a recipient/container capable of modifying the projected contents into a form which can be taken back and made use of for the development of thoughts that can be thought about and feelings that can be held. The recipient/container in this formulation is the mother and the projected is the state of mind contained within the baby. Bion's concept is usually called the 'container/contained'.

The need for a mother as a holding space in which thoughts and feelings are held, processed, and then returned describes a model of relationship and relating that takes Melanie Klein's formulation forward in development. It is often mentioned that Klein's 1946 paper, in which she introduced the thesis of projective identification, made use of the work of Fairbairn on schizoid states, what he called the *basic position*, and the active splitting process he described as a schizoid mechanism. It is often overlooked that Klein was also very familiar with Winnicott's work of the same period on *states of primary unintegration*. This is a primal state that precedes the development of mental structure (Winnicott 1945, 1948, 1949; Likierman 2001).

Ester Bick focused on that phase of early development in which a baby begins to construct the notion of the structure of a containing space from its skin to skin contact with the mother. Her thesis was that 'in its most primitive form the parts of the personality are felt to have no binding force among themselves and must therefore be held together in a way that is experienced by them passively, by the skin acting as a boundary' (Bick 1968). She likens the process to the development of a psychic skin as a container for psychic contents. The psychic skin covers the personality and holds the parts of the personality together within a bounded place creating in so doing, an inside and an outside. Thus anxieties are contained in a way conducive to growth (Emanuel 2001).

Bick's thesis is that until a containing object exists and is taken inside by the infant the attainment of the phantasy of internal and external space is impaired both in the infant's psyche and also in its experience of the other.

Projective identification of the evacuatory kind continues unabated in such a situation. Introjection of a containing space and of a mind capable of processing experience does not occur. There is not, in the absence of the development of a mental experience of inside/outside, the development of the dimensions of life: no length, no breadth, no thickness, no time, no holding in, no holding on, no someone else.

Bick, in her paper, 'The Experience of the Skin in Early Object Relations' (1968), described what she called 'second skin' defenses developed as replacements for a containing presence. These 'second skin' defenses involve sticking onto the surfaces of objects in an *adhesive identification* because there has not been a taking into the mind of another. These kinds of defenses include hyperactivity, muscularity, and mindless business. They are a way of living inside one's second skin as a compensation for not having taken in a psychic skin. Surviving outside, sticking to, an object on which one could not depend for mental refuge is a precarious state. Often patients with this kind of early experience present with a compulsive need to exercise, to sew or knit, and to engage in mindless activities, which provide a feeling of being held together, of movement with little sense of aliveness and no pleasure. Living outside the 'second skin' is unthinkable, however, as life outside presents the possibility of there being no limiting boundary.

Separation for these patients becomes an experience of being torn away from the object to which they are clinging or to which they have adhered (Bick) or a tearing away of the object and the experience of rupture (Tustin 1986; Meltzer 1992). The 'second skin defenses' defend against the fear of falling to pieces, disintegrating, liquefying, life spilling out (Bick 1968). There is, as Holden Caulfield describes in J. D. Salinger's 1951 novel, a need for a 'catcher in the rye' or all the children go mad and then over the cliff.

It was Donald Winnicott's (1948, 1949) thesis that when introjection of a containing space does not occur that states of unintegration become states of disintegration and the child is left open to taking in the state of self-preoccupation that is the caretaker's state of mind. In a series of papers about the varieties and degree of maternal absence and presence, the states of mind in between and most importantly the journey from one to another, Winnicott developed the idea that one can either traverse the experience of the absence of maternal presence in an alive way or one can deaden the experience by keeping alive internally what has died. No transition takes place. One holds onto something as opposed to thinking about it.

Both Winnicott and Bick describe patients who hold the therapist outside their emotional experiences relating not to the person of the therapist or to the therapeutic process but rather to the furniture or art in the office, the odor in the room, the presence or absence of certain objects, or the therapist's clothing. They emphasize their own activities and belongings as things to hold onto not as expressions of interests or personality with meaning. The material objects and the sensual and physical experiences are 'second skin' hiding places. From inside the 'second skin' these patients can simulate a participation in life without any genuine contact. They have a variety of ways of filling a session with both non-verbal and verbal information in which the style of the communication is more important than the contact. For these patients, however, Bick argues that, when the setting has been extremely constant and the technique firm, the very early anxieties will become available in the transference, often presenting as terror and a heightened state of paranoia.

Helen, an attorney in her late thirties, had been born and raised in the Middle East. She came to see me eight weeks after the September 11, 2001, attack on the World Trade Center. She presented as a screaming, terrified woman sent to therapy by her married lover of ten years because he could no longer help her with her fears. Helen talked to me in a manner in which her words and their delivery reminded me of a machine-gun strafing the space between us. She spoke in staccato fusillades of angry accusations designed it seemed to both hold me at a distance and to communicate her fear. There were 'second skin' defenses in the rough timbre of her voice, rigid body posture, and clenched fists. She reminded me of the 'boxer' baby in Bick's 1968 paper, fighting the air and struggling for self-containment. When I said that she feared that she had no one to hold onto and that no one was holding onto her she softened her body and her voice, relaxed, and began to cry.

As we have worked together in three-times-a-week psychotherapy she has related her history of serious and early feeding problems and her experience of being 'tossed aside' at the birth of her younger brother. At the time of her birth her mother had been depressed over the death of the mother's brother in an automobile accident. Helen says she was told that she was a good baby because she was willing to accept a rag 'titty' of scented cotton to suck on and with which to preoccupy her when her mother was unavailable. Perhaps, Helen said, that explained her need to hold the neckline of whatever she was wearing to her nose to smell whenever she felt anxious. Her need to hold onto herself while she worked meant that she preferred to work in private and behind a closed door.

She has commented on the scent in my office and has noticed any change. After two years of treatment she noticed and commented on a painting on the wall she faces as she enters the office. She observed that she felt safe enough to look around, to notice, and to comment on the restful scene she thought the painting depicted. She had taken it in. I think she had not yet taken me in.

Recently a clearer description of the seriousness of her early feeding difficulties has come to light in her pursuing family conversations about the feeding problems of her infant niece. She learned that her parents feared that she would die from her mother's inability to breastfeed her. Only when she became dangerously thin did her parents decide to bottlefeed her. Then she often refused the bottle. In the transference she complained about the horrors of her weekends, presenting herself as friendless in the first session of the week with no acceptable companionship. She also complained about her inability to get herself into my life, and the too-long gaps between sessions. Her reactions fit Bion's description of my absence as a non-existence, which becomes 'immensely hostile and filled with murderous envy'. Space becomes 'terrifying or terror itself' (Bion 1970: 20).

The first session of the week on Monday is often very tense and difficult, the second an oasis, and the third a mixture of work and recrimination about the rough time to come. When faced with terror over a lonely weekend, Helen first holds onto her work. She takes refuge in legal research working for long hours at her computer and surrounding herself with books. She sits reading and writing while holding onto and smelling her clothing. When she has calmed herself, she withdraws from the books, papers, and clothing onto which she has been holding and looks for another and more personal object in whom to take refuge.

Often she calls her lover who lives in a distant city. She seeks out one of her many acquaintances for long discussions about the world political situation. Then she brings her preoccupation with the current political situation to the next therapy session usually telling me of her many e-mail conversations with friends. The atmosphere in the session is one of pre-occupation with important matters taken up with others with whom she is in contact over the weekend.

When I say that she sees me as frustrating and unavailable because she does not have my e-mail address so that she could reach me and stay in touch over the weekend, she often sighs and begins to tell me of the frustration of not being able to 'drop in' on people to visit. When I say, again, that she wishes she could have access to me as she wished, to drop in, instead of being on a schedule, she sighs again and reminds me that as an infant she wasn't even on a schedule, so her therapy is an improvement. It is not, however, the reversal of her earlier experiences which she longs for. Recently she commented that at least she less often holds her cotton sleeve to her face to calm herself in the way she held the 'cotton titty' when she was a baby, is smoking less, and is on a schedule of regular eating and sleeping during the week.

When the passive experience of an object outside the self has been apprehended and a limiting boundary has been set, accepted, and used, there is a psychic skin in place. The infant's next task is for an object to introject. The object needed is the nipple in the mouth.

Over time my repeatedly setting time, place, and role limitations has established a boundary for Helen. There are psychic events, which happen inside her mind, then in mine, and within the session. There are events both psychic and material outside the session. Establishing and maintaining that boundary has enabled Helen to take in the existence of a limiting boundary and an awareness of internal contents to speak about and think about with feeling and meaning. She resorts less to smelling, smoking, eating, and explosive arguments as a way of reassuring herself that she is alive and sane. She speaks more directly about what she thinks instead of speaking to me as a critic of a *New York Times* article, which she presumes I have read, 'because you are the kind of American who reads the *New York Times*.'

The achievement of the taking in is dependent on the mother's assistance. It is an 'active experience of acquisition' (Briggs 2002). Recently I came across an episode on TV in which a new mother helps her infant son find the nipple on her breast so he can nurse. Both baby and mother are at first frustrated by their failure and then elated and satisfied by their success. The encounter is portrayed as the mother's work on behalf of her son along with his cooperation. The depiction was of a mutual concordance. The baby had access to a mother willing and able with humor, perseverance, and genuine concern to help him take hold, suck, and eat. When the nipple is in the mouth, the container is closed. When the experience of closure is sustained over time, the infant can take in the functioning container/ contained system described by Bion. Projective identification can then proceed for the basis of communication.

As the setting became secure by becoming dependable and predictable and as I became an understanding and humane person by interpreting Helen's reactions to my limit-setting as both frustrating and reassuring, without becoming either explosively angry or coolly dismissive, she began to communicate more of her feelings in words and less in action, innuendo, or tone of voice. She began remembering and relating with feeling repeated experiences of being an outsider, desperate acts of clinging to anyone willing to tolerate her presence such as a woman high-school teacher who befriended her and became a lover, and an insistence on being taken in by people in whom she developed an interest, such as her married lover. Helen told me of her mother's inability to think about Helen's needs as well as her mother's preference for mindless activities, which filled the hours and kept at bay anxieties about the family's safety in a politically dangerous situation, which was never discussed.

When the process of communication goes awry because there is not a mutual concordance between infant and mother, the infant is exposed to intolerable anxieties. While some infants can only manage an adhesive clinging and physical second skin defenses, some can actively construct a *mental* protective armor or hiding-place in which to avoid the intolerable anxiety. Others do both. They can cling and get inside as Helen longed to with me and then both despair of and fear leaving their hiding place, as she feared to end her relationship with her married lover.

Donald Meltzer has described such a hiding place as a claustrum and John Steiner as a psychic retreat. Klein's delineation of a system of human development described projective identification as a mechanism used to put parts of the self into another, first to rid the self of psychic and physical pain and then as a vehicle for the development of the structure of the personality (Meltzer 1992: 8).

John Steiner's 1993 book, *Psychic Retreats*, gathered together the work of the London post-Kleinians on the cryptic communications of patients in hiding and offered a diagnostic schema, and an interpretive technique that allows the therapist to communicate with them where they are hiding – either in a 'second skin' defense of physicality or the mental armor of what he calls a pathological organization.

Paul told me in one of his early psychotherapy sessions that I would be working with a man living in an igloo under the polar ice cap. It appeared to me that he wanted his treatment to be a warm refuge in which he could maintain his status as a person of superior qualities who was misunderstood and under-appreciated both at home and at work with less pain from the cold of his isolated existence. Some years later he said that he was emerging from his icy retreat inch by inch, like the progress of a glacier moving and melting. Indeed Steiner has observed that one can watch patients emerge from a retreat 'with great caution like a snail coming out of its shell and retreat once more if contact leads to pain and anxiety' (Steiner 1993: 1).

Paul's description of living in and under was his description of the mental organization he had crafted as a refuge from the pain of not being a hero to everyone in his life. He often described the firm at which he worked as a mafia-style organization at which one was obliged to cooperate with madmen and thieves in order to survive. He had devised many strategies which he considered clever and which he could not revise despite their obvious failure to either free him from the firm or promote his success. Joseph (1983) has depicted patients like Paul as interested in using their therapy as a refuge both from the pain of their failure to get inside and control their objects as well as the pain of letting go and mourning their inability to succeed.

Steiner, developing his own ideas and working from Henri Rey's (1979) work on the spatial quality of the mind structured once the ability to use projective identification is established, emphasizes that patients unable to accept a painful reality can evade, distort, and misrepresent that reality by organizing a mental retreat, the contents of which they can control. Their interest is in imposing the retreat on the treatment and inviting the therapist to share it. Thence both patient and therapist hide together and the treatment enables the patient to be a holdout from the realities of life. The organization of the retreat can be multifaceted in that all its members or all its parts are interchangeable and that the patient can change his position at will or, as Paul often explained, 'in a nanosecond'.

Psychic retreats are mental structures as opposed to the sensuous and physical structures of second skin defenses. They are usually elaborate verbal descriptions and catalogs of intimate spaces like those described by Bachelard in *The Poetics of Space* (1958). In each instance the organization or space is a variant of an immense or miniature maternal space in which the patient is either trapped or from which the patient has been prematurely ejected: a house, garret, cellar, drawer, chest, nest, shell, corner, etc.

Steiner proposes that patients retreated into such a world first want to be understood. They need evidence that their projections as messages have been received and comprehended. In that the patient is unconcerned and uninterested in either understanding himself or the other, the retreat is a form of narcissistic organization. To the degree that the retreat is a more or less permanent state of mind and not a temporary, transient respite, it is pathological. Any attempt to assist the patient in understanding his role in his dilemma is experienced by the patient as an expression of the therapist's attempts to foist the therapist's problems onto the patient since the patient, in a state of projective identification, assumes that all his problems are the therapist's problems.

What needs to be understood from the patient's point of view is that he is afraid, if not terrified, of the next step in development. He is hiding from the past failures to negotiate the next step and holding out against another attempt. And, as far as the patient is concerned, it is the people into whom he has projected in the past who were responsible for the failure then and the therapist into whom he has projected in the here and now who will be responsible for the failure if it occurs yet again.

Paul wanted me to understand that his hard work for his family, firm, and me was unrecognized and unappreciated. He could, after all break down completely and refuse to function as his mother, father, wife and boss had at one time or another. If I failed to understand the heroic efforts he made to continue to work and think despite the failures of others, then I also would fail him in the task I had accepted. When confronted with criticism of any kind or anyone, he retreated to a mental world in which he was a hard-working hero and did not want, at this point, to understand the ways in which he contributed to his difficulties. Only after my repeatedly interpreting my understanding of his point of view was Paul after some years able to tolerate understanding the contributions he made to his difficulties.

Steiner points out that patients unable to tolerate a painful reality of any degree can retreat transiently, intermittently, or permanently to a mental hiding place. Communicating with them requires the use of what he calls 'analyst-centered' interpretations. These interpretations often require the therapist to accept the role of the failed or failing other in the transference. The interpretations often take a form in which the therapist observes and describes the patient's experience; the therapist observes that the patient has an experience of the therapist as dangerous, helpful, neglecting, stupid, crazy, incompetent, etc. While one might prefer to present a balance of interpretations which convey both being understood and understanding, a therapy can proceed for a long time with a preponderance of analyst-centered interpretations.

When Helen, the patient with the early feeding difficulties, feels understood, she can elaborate her present experiences and early memories. She moved from screaming her terror about the present political state of the world to the past politics of her earliest relationship with her mother and father and can tolerate, now, interpretations of the politics not only between us but also between herself and others.

When I fail to understand the ways in which I fail to protect her from her fears, she often retreats, particularly on Monday, the first session of the week, first into detailed reports of an article in the *New York Times*. From inside the article she tells me of her superior understanding of the world. I then become the uninformed and stupid author of the article. If and when I understand that, she moves briefly out of the retreat either to share with me some progress in her being able to be in the world and feel safe, for instance, participating in a meeting with people 'who can talk and really listen to one another', or to a memory from which she had been hiding in the article.

In all her sessions she changes positions like the nested structure of Russian doll toys. Only when I understand that she is hiding, and from what, do we become 'people who can talk and really listen to one another'. When we can remain in contact for most of a session, she can leave the retreat, look back on herself, and observe, as she did recently for instance, that she has been 'very angry for forever' and often grits her teeth and refuses to accept help even when it arrives.

Both Steiner and Meltzer describe the resistance to change in patients entrenched in a *psychic retreat* or *claustrum*. Steiner, in particular, develops the ways in which grievances about failed containment can become so important an organizing force in a personality that it becomes impossible to develop out of all the retreats created to survive life's catastrophes and disappointments. Paul remained a holdout from contact with many of the realities of his life for very long. He said he enjoyed the romance of being a 'lone wolf, a desperado'. He terminated treatment having made many changes, including the negotiation of an excellent severance package from his firm and establishing himself at another. Nevertheless he refused to responsibly manage payment of the taxes and fees of car and house ownership and was frequently at odds with the 'state as parent' from which he expected special treatment in redress of his difficult childhood. He said he reserved the right to continue to withdraw from the 'cold facts of life' to the mental excitement of being successful at being above the ordinary rules and that if I could not understand that there was no point in continuing.

Some people cannot abide the world as they find it. For some it is both terrible and a terror. For others it is rejecting and excluding. Some find no cover in another and create a covering for themselves out of whatever they find. Others, once inside a cover, cannot bear to be uncovered and seek refuge in a world of phantasies from which they look out on life. These patients come to treatment needing to have their situations understood if they are ever to gain any understanding of where and why they have hidden themselves from life.

REFERENCES

Bachelard, G. (1958) *The Poetics of Space*, Boston: Beacon Press.
Bick, E. (1968) 'The Experience of the Skin in Early Object Relations', in A. Briggs (2002), *Surviving Space: Papers on Infant Observation*, London: Karnac, pp. 55–59.
Bick, E. (1986) 'Further Considerations on the Function of the Skin in Early Object Relations', in A. Briggs (2002), *Surviving Space: Papers on Infant Observation*, London: Karnac, pp. 60–71.
Bion, W. R. (1959) 'Attacks on Linking', in *Second Thoughts: Selected Papers on Psychoanalysis* (1967), London: Heinemann, pp. 93–109.
Bion, W. R. (1970) *Attention and Interpretation*, London: Heinemann.
Briggs, A. (2002) 'Reflections on the Function of the Skin in Psychosocial Space', in A. Briggs (2002), *Surviving Space: Papers on Infant Observation*, London: Karnac, pp. 188–207.
Dickinson, E. (2000) *The Selected Poems of Emily Dickinson*, New York: The Modern Library.
Emanuel, R. (2001) 'A-Void – An Exploration of Defenses against Sensing Nothingness', *International Journal of Psycho-Analysis*, 82: 1069–1084.
Etchegoyen, R. H. (1991) *The Fundamentals of Psychoanalytic Technique*, London: Karnac.
Fairbairn, W. R. D. (1944) 'Endopsychic Structure Considered in Terms of Object Relationships', in *Psychoanalytic Studies of the Personality*, London: Routledge, pp. 82–136.
Joseph, B. (1989) *Psychic Equilibrium and Psychic Change*, London: Routledge.
Klein, M. (1946) 'Notes on Some Schizoid Mechanisms', in *Envy and Gratitude and Other Works, The Writings of Melanie Klein*, vol. 3 (1975), London: Hogarth Press, pp. 1–24.
Likierman, M. (2001) *Melanie Klein: Her Work in Context*, London: Continuum.
Meltzer, D. (1992) *The Claustrum: An Investigation of Claustrophobic Phenomena*, Worcester: The Clunie Press.
Rey, J. H. (1979) 'Schizoid Mode of Being and the Space-Time Continuum (before Metaphor)', in J. Magagna (ed.) (1994), *Universals of Psychoanalytic Experience*, London: Free Association Books, pp. 8–30.
Salinger, J. D. (1951) *The Catcher in the Rye*, Boston: Little, Brown.
Steiner, J. (1993) *Psychic Retreats*, London: Routledge.
Tustin, F. (1986) *Autistic Barriers in Neurotic Patients*, London: Karnac.
Winnicott, D. W. (1945) 'Primitive Emotional Development', in *Collected Papers:*

Through Pediatrics to Psycho-Analysis (1958), New York: Basic Books, pp. 145–56.

Winnicott, D. W. (1948) 'Reparation in Respect to Mother's Organized Defense Against Depression', in *Collected Papers: Through Pediatrics to Psycho-Analysis* (1958), New York: Basic Books, pp. 91–96.

Winnicott, D. W. (1949) 'Mind and Its Relation to the Psyche-Soma', in *Collected Papers: Through Pediatrics to Psycho-Analysis* (1958), New York: Basic Books, pp. 243–254.

Chapter 18

Being and becoming

Charles Ashbach

INTRODUCTION

Psychology, as a study of the basic elements of human personality, evolved out of philosophy. For two thousand years, before the advent of psycho-analysis in the late nineteenth century, humanity's attempt to understand the human mind and imagination was centered totally within philosophical systems, specifically, within metaphysics as that branch of philosophy focusing on the ultimate nature of reality. In the East, Buddhism emerged in India about 500 BC, and spread to China and Japan. In the West, the work of Greek philosophers, primarily Plato, led to the development of systems of thought which attempted to understand the basic nature and structures of existence. Two central concepts which emerged through these philosophic reflections were those of *being* and *becoming*. From the work of Plato (Buchanan 1948), through Kant (Copleston 1994) and Schopenhauer (1969) and forward to the modern era with the work of Sartre (1974), these concepts have been developed as conceptual tools through which to contact and ponder the ultimate points of human existence.

The philosophic perspective which best embodies these concepts is that of Idealism (Routledge 2000). Idealism is that school of philosophy which holds that mind is the most basic reality and that the physical world is only an appearance or expression of mind. Further, it maintains that there is a more basic, hidden reality behind mental and physical experience, e.g., Kant's 'things in themselves' (Copleston 1994: 213). In Plato, for example, the ultimate reality and source of value are 'forms', or 'ideas', which are the fundamental points of existence (Kraut 1992: 7). The object relations approach to the mind and personality can be seen as a manifestation of the Idealist view. Within object relations theory the ultimate points of psychic experience are the internal objects which are the core and basis of the personality and through which the person derives the significance and meaning of their lives (Meltzer 1967). Like the shadows in Plato's metaphor of the cave (Kraut 1992), interpersonal experience is lived within the shadows cast by primary psychic objects and our experience of them.

Being (Routledge 2000) describes various aspects of human existence. First, it is the state of existence; second, one's fundamental or essential nature; and third, the fulfillment of possibilities or essential completeness. It is also defined as nature, constitution and substance. These definitions reveal a broad and somewhat shifting definition of Being over the millennia. In this chapter we will be focusing on the third definition, i.e., Being as essential completeness, as a way to approach the concept of narcissism from a fresh perspective.

Becoming, on the other hand, is defined as the fact of coming into existence; a coming to be, or a passing into a state (Neufeldt 1997). Essentially, it is a concept that describes the change and transformation of the manifestations of Being, through qualities, characteristics or forms.

We can think about Being and Becoming as operating in a figure–ground relationship. Being is the 'ground' of reality and Becoming is the 'figure' which is contained or realized within Being's realm. The psychological correlates of these terms can be found to exist in psychoanalysis. Freud's topographical model clearly establishes a paradigm where there is a dimension of human experience which is timeless and unchanging. This dimension he calls the unconscious and ascribes the dynamic characteristics of primary process to it. Through language this dimension is connected and transformed into the conscious part of the mind which operates through secondary process, i.e., logic and rational modalities. Freud directly addresses the way in which the unconscious 'becomes' conscious, i.e., the symbolic function of the mind which represents the 'thing presentations' which exist as the primary manifestations of the depth unconscious. The 'becoming' of the unconscious, the collision and integration of ego with unconscious phantasy, is the stuff of the conscious mind. Freud never uses the terms Being or Becoming in the philosophical sense. In the work of Bion (1970), there is a direct reference to Being through his concept of 'O', i.e., the 'origin' of the mind's activity. To Bion, Being is the dimension beyond, i.e., transcendent, unconsciousness. He further goes on to state (1970: 36) that transformations in Being, through 'at-one-ment' with the patient, are the central pathways for all therapeutic change

From a clinical point of view I am hypothesizing that the ego's experience of Being is experienced within the person as the subjective sense of the self's completion and fullness, i.e., a state of narcissistic fulfillment. The ego's experience of Becoming, on the other hand, is felt as a gradual process associated with learning, change and development. The experiential aspects of these two processes are fundamentally different. With states of narcissistic experience there is a coenesthetic sense of fullness and completion. That is, this experience registers from the inside of the body-self and radiates out and 'up' to the mind. It is basic, direct and intuitive and operates outside of time. With states of Becoming there is a sense of time and therefore of struggle and limitation (see also Johnson, Chapter 3, and Stadter, Chapter

2, in this volume). Growth and development always occur as a result of absence and the frustration of needs. The organism is driven, as in Freud's drives, to alter its relationship to reality, both internal and external. The ego is the mechanism which guides the growth process but its efforts always occur within the 'gravitational influence' of the depth phantasies and structures of the unconscious. If we use Melanie Klein's (1946) formulations of her two basic positions, the paranoid–schizoid and the depressive, we would say that narcissistic distortions associated with the encounter of Being generally occur in the paranoid–schizoid position, whereas encounters with Becoming and development occur within the depressive position.

The thesis of this chapter is that, since encounters with Being produce such radical narcissistic experiences, both negative and positive, they are easily distorted by the ego/self's defensive processes. The fullness of the self, during transitory states of blissful expansion, can form the basis for the self's perverse and addicted attempts to control experience in order to stay fused with the wellspring of such euphoria. Pathological states of narcissism can then be said to be linked to the ego's attempt to control or possess the experience of the encounter with Being. States of false-self or perverse functioning would be a sign of the utilization of narcissism as a regressive and greedy attempt to avoid the pains of separation, limitation and vulnerability through a delusional fusion with the sensual manifestations of Being (Green 2001). The encounter with Being is also associated with the sense of ego fragmentation or 'ego death' (Grof 1985: 46). Feelings of loss, sadness, dread or narcissistic injury can all occur when the ego encounters the vastness of Being as it surfaces through experience. Likewise, the ego is threatened by non-being which constantly stands alongside or behind the experience of Being. May states that anxiety, at its core, is the self's experience of the threat of 'imminent non-being' (May *et al.* 1958: 50).

In this investigation I will use the work of Wilfred Bion to establish a way to help us map the ego's encounter with Being. True encounter will produce states of authenticity and growth, i.e., development and transformation. False encounter will produce pathological states of inauthenticity, delusion, possessiveness, addiction and coercion resulting in extreme distortions in object relations and interpersonal functioning. Finally, I will attempt to describe the implications for treatment as these conditions affect both the transference and the countertransference.

BEING AND NARCISSISM: THE PROBLEM OF PERFECTION

We have already employed Freud's distinctions between primary and secondary process to make the connection between Being and Becoming. Primary process is an area of mind without the awareness of time, space or causality. It is ruled by desire and wish and utilizes objects in a plastic and fantastic fashion, as a medium for the accomplishment of its creative need to form its world. Secondary process is ruled by time, space and limitation. It is ruled by the reality principle. These two modes of 'reality', in conjunction with the forces of the Life and Death instincts, were used by Freud to account for the vicissitudes of internal and external reality.

We must reflect on the dire consequences associated with the collision between primary and secondary process. Within primary process is a cluster of experiences which depict a world without limit or frustration, replete with satisfaction and gratification, filled with beauty and omnipotent power. This realm, I believe, is the ego's representation of its encounter with Being. Grunberger (1971) relates this bedrock condition of fundamental narcissism to the child's actual experience and unconscious memory of the 'garden of Eden' which was the pre-natal realm of amniotic perfection. Whatever the source of the experience, there is, undeniably, a stratum within the core of the self that radiates a signal which beckons the human mind, calling it back to a place of perfection and total gratification. We use terms such as 'heaven', 'nirvana', 'Shangri-la' to represent this experience to the conscious mind. Terms such as 'fixation' and 'regression' have been used to refer to this sector of mind. Clinically, we know that states of drug and alcohol intoxication are ways to chemically induce such euphoric conditions which seem to mimic the fullness and merger of states of perfection.

The ego's encounter with reality, limitation, ignorance and suffering are all refutations of this experience/wish of total gratification or pure Being. The pain of growth, the vulnerability associated with learning, and the disappointments characteristic of separate existence all become assaults on the self's sense of its own integrity and of the omnipotent underpinning which form the core of the human identity. Being itself cannot be known directly, but our experience of Being is known directly and passionately through emotional and intuitive pathways. It is this expanded sense of existence which is associated with narcissistic states of omnipotence and grandiosity.

Becoming is known through the limited tools of the conscious mind – reality testing, induction, hypothesis testing – and ultimately through the admission of error and limit. The friction associated with Becoming makes it easy to identify. Being, on the other hand, is so difficult to encounter because it works through a double invisibility. The first invisibility is that of the narcissistic factor which silently attaches itself to the needs of the self and the pressures of the instincts so as to maintain the expansion and wellbeing of the self. This is seen in the way that sexuality is used by narcissism to maintain self-esteem, as opposed to reproduction. The second form of invisibility is the way in which Being attaches itself to the narcissistic factor. Being is the state-of-existence which stands silently behind the self's yearnings for fulfillment and realization. To consciously encounter Being thus requires a special act of attention and imagination.

I want to expand Bion's (1970) ideas on Being and 'O' since his work is fundamental in thinking about Being in the clinical encounter. While accepting the work of Klein, he suggested that the unconscious was structured as an instrument to encounter and transform the very foundation of the human mind which he named 'O', as in 'origin'. Here's what he says about O:

> I shall use the sign O to denote that which is the ultimate reality represented by terms such as ultimate reality, absolute truth, the godhead, the infinite, the thing-in-itself. O does not fall in the domain of knowledge or learning save incidentally; it can be 'become', but it cannot be 'known'. It is darkness and formlessness but it enters the domain of K [knowledge] when it has evolved to a point where it can be known, through knowledge gained by experience, and formulated in terms derived from sensuous experience; its existence is conjectured phenomenologically.
>
> (Bion 1970: 26)

He went on to say that the analyst must focus his attention on O, the unknown and unknowable, and further stated that the psychoanalytic vertex is O. This recommendation of Bion's is a call for the therapist to stop seeking 'knowledge' as a way of controlling experience and to enter into an empathic contact with the Being of the patient through an encounter with one's own Being as revealed and represented in the experience of the countertransference. He recommends renouncing 'memory and desire' (Bion 1970: 33) in order to make contact with O. The therapist must strive toward a state in which the desire to possess mental and emotional experience is renounced in favor of the openness of the self to the uncertainty and evanescence of the therapy process. Our therapeutic Becoming, once grounded in the immediacy of the moment, enables us to encounter the shadow of Being as it is cast upon our person. It should be noted that for Freud and Bion the dream is the most direct access humans have to the shadow of Being as it is cast across psychic experience. This explains why the dream has such a pre-eminent place in psychic work.

If we follow Bion's theory of mental development as represented in his grid (Grindberg et al. 1993: 55) we might understand the following trajectory:

Being (unknown and unknowable) →
unconsciousness → representations/realizations →
pre-consciousness → consciousness.

A clinical example may help to illuminate my paradigm. Mr X, a successful architect, continually acted to undo the impact of the therapy process on his self-idealization. He would eagerly 'accept' interpretations and then subsequently reject them by acting-out his hostility and resentment through attacks on his wife. The essence of his attack was a scornful and condescending judgment and criticism of her using a variety of petty observations, always couched in his multisyllabic and arcane way of speaking. The patient was in three-times-a-week therapy with me and my feelings of frustration, anger, impotence and confusion were the countertransference signals that a perverse form of relationship had developed within the therapy. In spite of what looked like a cooperative and productive partnership, I too began to feel like his wife: mocked, useless and humiliated. My narcissism had been inflated through the projective identification of his own grandiose self-experience onto the surface of our work and through the evocation of my own narcissistic strivings. This experience was realized in a pseudo-intimate mode re-enacting the false self experience with his mother: if he would pretend to be the perfect son she would pretend to love him. The feeling of working hard and seeming to achieve important insights appealed to my sense of self-esteem.

The feelings of impotence and falseness within my countertransference experience showed me that I had experienced a concordant identification (Racker 1968) with the patient. By means of his projective identifications he was able to evoke within me the representation of his striving, adaptive child self and he became identified with the haughty, grandiose and unapproachable mother. He and his brother attended four of the most prestigious universities in the country. The mother always communicated her feeling of being trapped in middle-class surroundings with middle-class intellects. She had a dictionary, on a pedestal, right by the dining room table and would stop dinner any time a word of interest emerged in the evening conversation. She would not only look up the 'precise' meaning but would also expound on the etymology of the word. She essentially made words a fetish: objects to be used to give the impression of power and authority but actually lacking their true symbolic function. My patient had an incredible amount of information but woefully inadequate wisdom about the nature of his situation.

The work has focused on revealing the nature and impact of his grandiose sense of self-idealization. His self-esteem is traumatized when he meets up with the falseness and artifice of his social self. I believe this experience is the clinical manifestation of meeting up with his Being. As it is encountered it collides with false images of himself stored within his ego-ideal and the clash produces shame, and the impulse to counter-attack. When the impulse toward truth is in the ascendancy he also responds with a sense of guilt and a movement toward integration which brings forth a sense of grief and mourning. The mourning concerns the giving up of lost ideal images of himself which were deployed as defenses against the gaping sense of inadequacy and insignificance. The working through process is an on-going oscillation of resistance against and surrender to the truth of himself, which is to say, to his Being.

Let me offer a metaphor to further develop my thesis. Assume you are walking along a beach and you see a paper cup washed up on the shore. It is filled with the waters of the ocean as the tide comes in. Now let's assume further that the cup is a permeable membrane holding the water within it and yet at the same time connecting the cup to the sea. I would say that this cup is the ego-self and the membrane is the gradient unconscious/pre-conscious aspect of mind that links the human psyche to the waters closest to the beach. Perhaps we'll consider this to be the surf that breaks upon the shore. These waters I would call unconsciousness. Beyond the surf is the great ocean of Being. Becoming occurs within the cup and Being is communicated, somehow, through the membrane of the cup.

This membrane also processes signals from the cup itself and monitors its structure and is in touch with the process of the cup's deterioration. Within the meager boundaries of the cup are contained a mere 16 oz. of seawater and yet there is a link and connection to the infinite immensity of the oceans of the world, and to all the life, forces, and dynamics contained within them. This metaphor might then help us to represent the burden of human narcissism. The self is able to experience its connection to the vastness of Being but is continually forced to operate within the limited boundaries of the conscious mind, and the needful, anxious and mortal body which acts as its container.

For my metaphor to work we must assume that the ocean develops, at the tip of the waves which wash upon the shore, a layer of consciousness which enables it to know the land. The land in our metaphor is both the demands of external reality and the material Otherness beyond the scope of the self's omnipotence.

Narcissistically damaged individuals, like Mr X, suffer from traumatic states of separation from the mother. Owing perhaps to the mother's depression or her own narcissistic depletion, the child has too much or too little maternal fusion or has inconsistent fusion experiences. In Mr X's case, his mother was a very depressed woman who suffered the catastrophe of her first-born child being born with cerebral palsy. The shadow of this event cast itself across the rest of her life as a compulsion to drive her two healthy sons to perform at the highest levels possible. The necessary experience of fusion provides the bedrock for the self's sense of security and faith in reality. Since this 'sense' is lost to narcissistically damaged individuals there is the compulsive attempt to 'hijack' the object, to make it its own and to bypass the dangers of separation and contingency.

The mother, which is to say the concrete experience of her body and its phantasied insides, becomes the matrix of Being to the child. The primary object becomes a psychological lens through which the shadow of Being might be encountered. Mr X found relationship with the mother an unattainable challenge. The only path left was therefore identification with the 'imagined' mother, i.e., the mother who will fulfill his deepest needs, completely. It is this object, projectively created and aggressively transformed into the ideal, that forms the core of the narcissistic personality and stands as the manifestation of (false) Being. But since this object has been 'created' and not discovered, that is, it is a fiction produced by the self, there can be no security and no true peace. The self is forever aware, in its own depth unconscious, that the true object which holds Being and love at its core, is missing. It is this central unconscious knowledge, of absence, that powers the relentless activity and searching of such individuals. These individuals are compulsive, insecure, demanding and resentful. They suffer from envy, generally unconsciously, because they begrudge the goodness of the object in the face of the trauma which has created a 'basic fault' (Balint 1979) in their sense of themselves. They seek to 'conquer' the object and through a displacement and projection they frequently conquer aspects of the world. But tragically they are driven, like Oedipus or Icarus, to overreach their mark. Their life is characterized by the use of obsessional mechanisms, manic defenses and acting out, as well as addictions and perversions of every stripe to protect the self from acknowledging the awful truth of their own sense of weakness, brokenness, separateness, and need.

The other form in which these damaged individuals seek to hijack Being is through a schizoid withdrawal into nothingness. They seek to rid themselves of any and all excitation as a means to merge, in a backwards form, with the source of all Being. They do not conquer the sea, they silently sneak into it.

BECOMING

Now what about the dimensions of Becoming? Becoming, because it occurs within the non-manic ego-self always operates against a backdrop of fear, anxiety and uncertainty. The 'cup' can never know what will wash up on the shore the very next moment. It can never be sure how long its structure will hold together. Belief in an object beyond the self, provides the basis for faith in the face of mortality. Becoming, in the shadow of both the limits of time and the limitlessness of Being, is perhaps the only way in which true transformation can occur. The actuality of the self, opens up to that which is beyond the self and in that paradoxical moment a condition of limited transcendence occurs. It cannot be possessed or controlled.

The self in a mode of authenticity would be operating within Klein's depressive position. The aspirations toward immortality and Being are acknowledged and owned. The object is valued in and for itself, not as a means of false transcendence. The work of Becoming occurs within time and yet the links to Being allow for the emergence of timeless truth, beauty, insight or understanding. The paradoxical nature of Becoming reveals itself through the deepening of the self's reliance on the object for genuine contact and growth. Introjective identification with the external object replaces projective identification of an internal self-object.

Becoming is known through the sweat of encounter with limitation. Such discoveries lead to insight and change but not to the total transcendence sought in the flight into false, narcissistic Being. This moment of true Becoming is manifested most commonly during creative endeavors where time falls away as we struggle with a problem. The self grows through its increased linkages with the unconscious. We use 'our' minds and imaginations but the outcome produced actually occurs as an element from another realm which is not 'ours'. Under such conditions of work and inspiration, narcissistic self-idealization ultimately gives way to creative growth of the self, to whatever measure is possible.

A NOTE ON DREAMS AND BEING

Freud (1900) and Meltzer (1963) each have used dreams to depict a pathway through which the deepest strata of the self become available to the conscious mind. The oceanic realm of Being can only be approached by the shadows it casts across personal unconsciousness and this shadow, according to Bion, is the essence of the dream. For the twenty-five hundred years since the writing of *Oedipus Rex* there seems to have been no appreciable increase in the unconscious's openness to being penetrated by the conscious mind. Dreams today are no less mysterious and symbolic. While we have only recently evolved scientific means to probe the unconscious, through the instrument of psychoanalysis, the protective veil that the self drapes across the unconscious has not become more transparent. This may be the evolutionary evidence which supports the idea that the human being needs unconsciousness in order to be able to stay in touch with the deepest sources of the self which I am proposing is the encounter with Being.

IMPLICATIONS FOR TREATMENT

Racker (1968) observes that the deepest motivation that drives most individuals to become therapists rests upon the internal experience of having damaged primary objects in our childhood. The therapy process is then, for the therapist, a way to repair or resuscitate damaged or dead objects. This vital undertaking for the sense of personal goodness and worth of the therapist is tied up with the feeling of having cared for and improved the lot of the patient. This internal pressure is source of all therapeutic ambition and likely to be the place where narcissistic factors in the therapist begin to affect the clarity and function of the therapeutic relationship. The Becoming of the therapeutic process, a condition filled with uncertainty, doubt and confusion, can so burden the narcissistic sector of the therapist's personality that we strive after positive outcomes rather than allowing the Being of both patient and therapist to emerge in the container of the relationship. As noted earlier, it is here that Bion's admonition against 'memory and desire' comes into focus. If we 'possess' knowledge rather than receive it through the mystery of Being we are in danger of imposing a false experience on the true and actual complexity of Being and Becoming. All such behavior leads to an 'as if' mode of related-ness wherein patients cannot be themselves as we strive to be someone other than the limited and vulnerable people we actually are.

Being, in the depressive position, is discovered through the process of Becoming rather than through the merger with the ideal objects of phantasy which are possessed by the self and which are established as alternatives to actual Being. Being is essentially Other and can only be encountered through introjective identification. That is, as Other it must be imported into the self. The use of projective identification creates a sense of 'false Being' wherein the self has projected its own idealized contents onto the Other and has mistaken the now confused, narcissistic self-object as an actual external Other.

In my dealings with Mr X, I fell prey to some disturbance in my self-esteem. It might have been my hunger for his seeming respect for my mind or my method. It may have been associated with his increase of sessions so that his economic contributions to my wellbeing may have begun to play a part. Whatever the actual circumstances that brought about the sense of blockage or deadness, the end-product became a relationship where deeply aggressive and destructive forces were covered over by a veneer of agree-ment, enthusiasm and respect that pointed to a perverse form of therapeutic relationship. By staying true to my sense of deadness in the sessions we were able to understand how we had begun to re-enact the false relationship between him and his mother where his 'acceptance' of her wisdom and knowledge protected him from the unsettling hatred and rage that he felt about her grandiose estimate of her mind and its accomplishments.

As noted earlier, Bion says the only way to authentically encounter the O of the patient is through a process he terms 'at-one-ment' (Bion 1970: 43). Note it is the hyphenated version of the word atonement. At-one-ment means a connection beneath 'knowing' which leads to O which will subse-quently produce the experience of K, knowledge in a more conscious mode. This deeper mode of encountering self, patient and relationship becomes a paradigm for a fundamental therapeutic connection. He further observes

(1970: 55) that at-one-ment should be the clinical basis for all interpretations as this stance is less likely to produce envy and more likely to lead to an experience of shared learning and development.

Bion advises that we must never promote a therapeutic relationship which obscures the radical aloneness of both therapist and patient. We are required to carry the burden of our separate existence and not to overcome it with the collusive comfort of a 'cozy' relationship. Envy is the essential reaction of the cup that seeks to be equal to the sea. We must be aware of this reaction in both us and the patient. It is predicated upon the sense of personal injury and lack and is fueled by a hopelessness that there can ever be a satisfying connection between the cup and the sea. It is the basis for the negative therapeutic reaction, for therapeutic impasse and ultimately for the sense of depressive dread that is the ultimate experience of false Being.

Bion drolly noted: 'Of all the hateful possibilities, growth and maturation are feared and detested most frequently' (1970: 35). Perhaps by applying the concepts of Being and Becoming as we've examined them the practicing clinician might be aided in understanding the enormous forces associated with growth and development. On the one hand is the beckoning experience of totality, fullness and perfection that is the shadow of Being announced through states of narcissistic plenitude. This is continually frustrated by the burdens of Becoming and the danger of non-being.

On the other hand is the suffering and travail of Becoming with its limited victories and partial understandings always opening the self up to the next challenge and the next encounter with ignorance, fear and the unknown.

Of course, for those who persist in the process of Becoming there is the reward of moments when Being is accessed and there is the experience of radical transformation and genuine, but limited transcendence. These moments provide us with a sense of aliveness, truth and beauty which comes from the arduous efforts of Becoming. Hopefully the framework of Being and Becoming as presented here might help us sustain the rigors of containment without the grasping after a false sense of knowledge or transcendence, for ourselves or our patients.

REFERENCES

Balint, M. (1979) *The Basic Fault*, New York: Brunner/Mazel.

Bion, W. R. (1970) *Attention and Interpretation*, in *Seven Servants* (1977), Northvale, NJ: Jason Aronson.

Buchanan, S. (ed.) (1948) *The Portable Plato*, New York: The Viking Press.

Copleston, F. (1994) *A History of Philosophy*: vol. VI: *Modern Philosophy*, New York: Image Books, pp. 180–392.

Freud, S. (1900) 'The Interpretation of Dreams', *Standard Edition*, 4 and 5, London: Hogarth Press, 1953.

Green, A. (2001) *Life Narcissism – Death Narcissism*, London: Free Association Books.

Grindberg, L., Sor, D. and Tabak de Bianchedi, E. (1993) *New Introduction to the Work of Bion*, Northvale, NJ: Jason Aronson.

Grof, S. (1985) *Beyond the Brain*, Albany, NY: State University of New York.

Grunberger, B. (1971) *Narcissism: Psychoanalytic Essays*, Madison, CT: International Universities Press.

Klein, M. (1946) 'Notes on Some Schizoid Mechanisms', in *The Writings of Melanie Klein*, vol. 4, *Envy and Gratitude* (1975), New York: Delacorte Press.

Kraut, R. (ed.) (1992) *The Cambridge Companion to Plato*, London: Cambridge University Press.

May, R. (1985) *The Discovery of Being*, New York: Norton.

May, R., Angel, E. and Ellenberger, H. (eds.) (1958) *Existence*, New York: Touchstone.

Meltzer, D. (1963) *Dream-Life: A Re-examination of the Psychoanalytic Theory and Technique*, Perthshire, Scotland: The Clunie Press.

Meltzer, D. (1967) *The Psychoanalytic Process*, Perthshire, Scotland: The Clunie Press.

Neufeldt, V. (ed.) (1997) *Webster's New World College Dictionary*, New York: Macmillan.

Racker, H. (1968) *Transference and Countertransference*, New York: International Universities Press.

Routledge (2000) *Concise Routledge Encyclopedia of Philosophy*, London: Routledge.

Sartre, J. P. (1974) *Being and Nothingness*, Secaucus, NJ: The Citadel Press.

Schopenhauer, A. (1969) *The World as Will and Representation*, New York: Dover.

Chapter 19

The use of the self revisited

Theodore J. Jacobs

My aim in this chapter is to update, revise, and expand upon ideas concerning the analyst's use of self that I articulated in my 1991 book, *The Use of the Self: Countertransference and Communication in the Analytic Situation*.

My focus in that book was primarily on the phenomenon of counter-transference and especially on the way in which covert, unrecognized and unacknowledged, communications from the analyst can influence the analytic process. As I tried to demonstrate then, such countertransference reactions most often arose in response to subtle communications from the patient of which the analyst was unaware. Thus much of my book was devoted to elucidating the effect on the analytic process of the manifold unconscious communications between patient and analyst that flow beneath the surface of the analytic dialogue.

The impetus to writing the book came largely from my struggle with my own countertransference feelings. In my training, countertransference was not something one talked about. Following Freud's view of countertrans-ference as an obstacle to be overcome and Annie Reich's papers (1951, 1960, 1966) that reinforced the idea that countertransference constituted an interference in the analyst's ability to understand and to respond effectively to his patient, classical institutes in the nineteen-sixties regarded countertransference as a problem to be dealt with privately by each analyst either in his own analysis or by means of self-analytic efforts. A certain shame hung over the whole notion of countertransference. One was supposed to have as little of it as possible and what one did have, was not to be publicly acknowledged. As a consequence of this attitude, there was little teaching about countertransference. It was almost never mentioned in case conferences and students were wary about revealing it in their supervisory sessions. And when in supervision an intrepid soul did acknowledge a countertransference response, rarely was its relation to the patient's material or its impact on the analytic process explored. Rather, the candidate was told that she should take up this matter with her analyst. Clearly the implication was that countertransference represented the outcropping of an unresolved personal conflict that required more analysis.

The attitude toward countertransference had both historical and contemporary roots. Although Freud recognized the phenomenon of unconscious communication between patient and analyst as an important feature of the analytic process, he did not apply this insight to countertransference experiences. Thus he did not recognize that countertransference could be understood in part as representing projected and displaced communications from the patient that register in the mind of the analyst. Instead, as I have noted, he viewed countertransference as an obstacle to analytic work that needed to be overcome, primarily through one's self-analytic efforts. In fact, in a strongly worded statement, Freud (1910) declared that no analysis could proceed beyond the limitations imposed by the analyst's countertransferences.

Freud's negative view of countertransference, which essentially halted effective exploration and use of countertransference experiences, for some forty years, derived not only from his personal experiences in analyzing – he was well aware of his own tendency to be drawn into the transference – but from his concern that certain colleagues, Ferenczi, Steckel, Jones and others, were acting on their countertransference feelings in ways that were potentially destructive to the young analytic movement. It was necessary, Freud thought, to take a strong stand not only against such acting out, but against the dangers inherent in countertransference itself.

It remained for Heimann (1950) in England, to articulate a different and novel perspective on countertransference. Influenced by Klein's emphasis on the importance in infancy, and throughout life, of the defensive mechanisms of projection and especially of projective identification, she viewed countertransference as a creation of the patient's. The analyst's subjective experiences, in other words, could be understood as emanating via projective identification, from the inner world of the patient. Unable to cope with the affects aroused by the warring internal objects that constituted the essence of her conflict, the patient projected aspects of that inner world onto, or into, the analyst. Thus by focusing on his or her subjective reactions while analyzing, the analyst had a window on, if not a pipeline to, the unconscious of the patient.

This essentially Kleinian view met with strong opposition in the USA. Although arising in part as a consequence of Freudian analysts' rejection of Klein's ideas concerning infant development, and their strong championing of Anna Freud in the historic Freud–Klein debates of the nineteen-fifties, this opposition was also based on substantial clinical experience. Drawing on her many years analyzing candidates, Annie Reich, who was the chief American spokesperson for the Freudian view of countertransference, amply demonstrated the troublesome effects of countertransference in both its acute and chronic forms. So persuasive, in fact, were her arguments that for the next quarter century in the USA it was the Reich–Freud view of countertransference, and quite exclusively that view, that dominated theory and practice.

It was not until the early nineteen-eighties that things began to change. At that time, several classically trained Americans, notably Gill (1982), McLaughlin (1988), Poland (1986), Chused (1987) and Jacobs (1986), began publishing articles that described not only the manifold ways that countertransference could manifest itself in the analytic situation, but its effective use as an important element in technique. Some years before that, Searles (1959) and others in the relational school had demonstrated the power of countertransference not only to impede but to advance the analytic process; but it was not until more traditionally trained analysts began writing and speaking in a similar vein that a revision in thinking about the roles of countertransference and the analyst's subjectivity took hold in the USA.

The change was due to a number of factors. In American institutes, the influence of the European émigré analysts, fiercely loyal to, and defensive of, Freud, was beginning to wane, objectivity and positivism in the allied fields of literature, history and philosophy were under attack and were being replaced by a relativistic point of view, the British object relations perspective had become more widely known and appreciated, and Kohut's (1971, 1977) writings on self-psychology focused attention on the profound effect that failures of empathy – essentially enacted countertransference responses – could have on the patient's sense of self and the ensuing analytic material. In addition, there was greater appreciation of the dyadic aspect of analytic work, a perspective stimulated by the infant research of Stern (1985) and others – research that supported the idea that, from birth on, human experience is profoundly affected by interpersonal as well as intrapsychic influence. All of these factors coming together in the late nineteen-seventies and -eighties contributed to the newer perspectives on countertransference and process, the subjectivity of the analyst that were rapidly developing.

My own work as an analyst was markedly at variance with what I heard at our institute. There, even in advanced clinical seminars, countertransference was very rarely mentioned. The focus, quite exclusively, was on patient's material. And while the understanding of that material frequently seemed accurate and the presenting analyst's interpretation insightful, oftentimes the patient did not progress in the way that one might expect. What seemed to be missing was the effect on the analytic process of the analyst's subjective experiences and the covert communications between patient and analyst that were taking place beneath the surface of the manifest exchanges.

I had found that my countertransference responses, conveyed both verbally and in non-verbal behavior, affected the analytic process, including the emerging material, in ways that were equal to, and often outweighed, the insights gained through interpretation.

In an effort to make sense of what I was experiencing and the impact of my subjective experiences on the analytic process, in the early nineteen-seventies I began to take notes on this dimension of my analytic work. Eventually I published a series of papers (Jacobs 1973, 1980, 1986) on countertransference and related issues which, when collected in a single volume (Jacobs 1991), formed the core of my subsequent book.

This publication was not greeted favorably at my institute. The older, more traditional, analysts regarded the kind of open discussion of counter-transference issues that I described in my book as inappropriate and in violation of an unspoken taboo. Consequently I was viewed as suffering from an exhibitionistic/masochistic problem that required further analysis.

Elsewhere, however, my approach found a receptive audience. A good many colleagues, it seemed, had been waiting for someone to take the lead in opening a discussion of key elements of analyses that heretofore had been kept under a veil of secrecy. Spurred by the writing of the colleagues I have mentioned, as well as my contributions, in the last two decades, there has appeared in America a virtual flood of publications dealing not only with countertransference, but with the closely related issues of enactments, neutrality, abstinence, self-disclosure, co-created experience, and the uncon-sciously shared assumptions between analyst and patient that have been designated the analytic third (Ogden 1994). Stimulated by many of these innovative and creative papers, by the important findings of infant researchers, and by increased clinical experience, I have sought to expand as well as to revise some of the ideas concerning countertransference, non-verbal communications, enactments and the question of self-disclosure that I discussed in my 1991 book.

In what follows I will touch on several of these issues without attempting to include them all. The first issue that I wish to discuss is the question of non-verbal communication in the analytic process.

Although given impetus by the contributions of McLaughlin (1987, 1992), Pally (2001), and other colleagues who have enlarged our under-standing of the significant role that non-verbal communication plays in every analysis, the study of non-verbal behavior and its relation to the verbal exchanges of patient and analyst remains a frontier that has yet to be fully explored. In my own work I have been impressed by the way that close attention to the facial expression and bodily movements of patient both in the waiting room and as they enter and leave my office has opened path-ways to the exploration of centrally important ideas and fantasies that had not been verbalized in sessions, either because they were not conscious or because there was a strong resistance to their verbal expression.

Such was the case with Mr N, a bright and able young man who sought treatment because at age 25 he had not been able to choose a vocation nor develop an intimate relationship. It was clear that he was floundering in life and that he had little purpose or direction. Until he was 17 years old, Mr N was viewed as an exceptional young person. Handsome and talented, he was an outstanding student and an extraordinarily gifted musician. In addition, he was an outgoing, friendly and thoughtful individual who was instantly liked by all who met him. A rising star in his community, Mr N was expected – and expected himself – to achieve great things in life. Then when Mr N was a few months past his seventeenth birthday, his father, a distinguished and accomplished man in his own right, suddenly developed a progressive neurological disease. Within a year, Mr N's father was incapacitated. Placed in a nursing home, this once powerful man was reduced to being a helpless child who was unable to care for himself. He died within two years of contracting this debilitating disease.

The effect on Mr N was dramatic. Crushed by losing the father whom he relied on for support, guidance and encouragement – and with whom, unconsciously, he was in fierce competition – Mr N fell apart. He could not concentrate on his studies, became morose and increasingly isolated, and lost interest in his friends. Increasingly he clung to his mother who soon became his chief companion. Some brief therapy and a trial of medication effected little change. Although he was admitted to a prestigious college, Mr N had little interest in his course work, or really in anything else. He became a desultory student, drank a good deal, took drugs, and eventually left school in his sophomore year.

For the next couple of years, Mr N alternately traveled abroad and spent time at home, but seemed to have no purpose in life. He had only a few old friends, and had no sustained relationship with a woman. On occasion Mr N would begin a relationship with a new person, but within a matter of weeks it would end, and usually because Mr N found some reason to break it off. Clearly he was afraid of intimacy and of being attached to someone who might disappoint him. He found it safer to remain emotionally tied to his mother, a relationship that for her own reasons, she encouraged. Mother and son, then, clung to one another, each using the other as a substitute for the man that both had lost.

Given Mr N's history and current situation, I became convinced that to make progress he required an in-depth approach, one that would uncover the roots of the profound regression into which he had fallen and that would help him work through the loss that precipitated it. Accordingly, I recommended that he begin an analysis, a suggestion that he readily accepted. For a period of almost eighteen months, the treatment went very well. Mr N took easily to analysis, associated quite freely, brought in dreams, and early on developed a positive dependent transference that in essential ways reproduced the relationship that for many years he had with his father.

Then, a year and a half into the analysis, everything changed. Instead of communicating openly in sessions, with his thoughts readily shifting between past and present and ranging freely over a variety of topics, now Mr N focused repeatedly, obsessively, on a single issue: his relationship with C, a new woman in his life. In session after session, Mr N described every facet, every nuance of their relationship. While, initially, I thought this material to be an important expression of Mr N's efforts to master an anxiety-producing situation – C was the first woman with whom he had been able to establish an on-going relationship – in time I realized that his preoccupation with this single matter, important as it was, was also serving a defensive purpose. By focusing so persistently on this one issue, Mr N was screening out other problems, ones that, unconsciously he associated with unmanageable anxiety.

What these other issues might be, however, I had no idea. I strongly suspected that something had happened in our relationship – Mr N now scrupulously avoided any references to me – that had frightened him and had caused him to retreat, but it was not at all clear to me what might have evoked such a response. I decided to wait and to see if I could pick up something in Mr N's associations that would help us both understand the source of what appeared to be a rapidly developing impasse. That understanding came from another, quite unexpected, source.

It so happened that at that time I was seeing Mr N in my home office. Since he had an early morning appointment and I did not want to wake my wife when I got up, I often dressed in semi-darkness. This I could usually do without difficulty, but one morning, being short on time, I dressed hurriedly and went quickly to the office. As I greeted him, Mr N looked at me quizzically, but said nothing. At the end of the hour, as he rose from the couch, he again looked at me in what I thought was a puzzled way. Then, without another word, he departed.

After that session I went into the house for a cup of coffee and, seeing me enter the kitchen, my wife burst into laughter. 'Are you conducting an experiment in subliminal perception this morning?' she inquired. 'If not, I suggest that you change your jacket to one that matches your trousers. Otherwise you are going to have to deal with a bunch of very confused patients.' What happened was this. Dressing in semi-darkness, I took from my closet the trousers belonging to one suit and the jacket from another, similar in color, but differently patterned. Encountering me that morning, Mr N was startled to see me wearing a clearly mismatched outfit, and also that I seemed unaware of the error. This sight terrified Mr N as it evoked memories of his neurologically damaged father and led him to worry as to whether I, too, was showing signs of organic impairment.

Actually this was not a new concern. For several months, Mr N had noted that I seemed to be distracted and forgetful and he had the idea that I was showing signs of deterioration. This idea so frightened him that he avoided mentioning it in sessions for fear of discovering that it was true. In fact, Mr N was not wrong in what he had observed. For a number of months I had been making a series of mistakes. I misplaced some bills, made errors in others, nearly forgot one appointment, and generally was acting in a distracted, if not confused, manner. While I was aware of these mistakes, I rationalized them as being due to overwork, fatigue, and concern about one of my children who had health problems. What I realized only later, when I reflected on my behavior, was that it had developed after my father suddenly suffered a stroke. Ordinarily an exceptionally well-dressed and well-groomed man, after this cerebral accident my father dressed indifferently. Now he often wore mismatched and ill-fitting clothes, with the result that he appeared unkempt and slovenly. Cognitively damaged, he had difficulty reading and remembering what he read. His short-term memory was impaired as was his judgment and thinking.

In an effort to cope with this loss and the complex feelings it evoked in me, unconsciously I identified with my impaired father. Like him, I made numerous errors, became distracted, and forgetful, and, in choosing a mismatched outfit, began to look like him. All of this so frightened Mr N – he imagined that history was repeating itself and that I, like his father, was going to disappear on him – that he became paralyzed. Unable to speak of his fears, all he could do was avoid them.

Following the mismatched suit incident, I waited to see if Mr N would bring up this troubling experience in subsequent sessions. He did not. Instead Mr N avoided the issue and concentrated once more on his relationship with the girlfriend. One day as I approached the waiting room to fetch Mr N, I noticed that he was looking at me in what I thought was an intense, piercing way. It was the same kind of intense look that he had given me when I appeared oddly attired for his session. Now on the couch, Mr N made no reference to the waiting room incident but carried on as before with a description of the latest incident with C, the girlfriend.

When during a moment of silence an opportunity arose, I asked Mr N about the waiting room incident. I described what I had observed and asked Mr N if he was aware of the way that he had looked at me. I asked him, too, if he was aware of any feelings toward me that might have prompted what seemed to be intense curiosity. For a period of a minute or so, Mr N remained silent. Then, finally, he spoke. 'Is there anything wrong with you,' he wanted to know. 'Or do you always buy your clothes at a Salvation Army store?' For several months, Mr N revealed, he had been watching me make one error after another. He had been unable to bring up the matter, but he was pretty sure that something was very wrong with me. He wanted to know if I was sick and, if so, whether I would be ending his treatment.

In response, I confirmed the accuracy of Mr N's observations and told him that a personal matter had been preoccupying me and had caused me to become distracted and to make the kind of mistakes that he had noticed. I also interpreted the connection that he had made between his father's illness and my behavior and explored with him the complex feelings that were aroused by his observing the difficulties that I was having. For the first time, Mr N realized that he felt some satisfaction in seeing me, the doctor, the superior one, have problems of my own. This insight led to others and Mr N came in touch with the rivalrous and resentful feelings that he harbored toward me and his father. And in time he understood and could work through the profound feelings of guilt – and need for punishment – that he experienced for harboring hostile wishes toward both of us.

Thus in this case it took the understanding of enactments – non-verbal behaviors, on the part of both patient and analyst – for an impasse that could have destroyed the treatment to be resolved. This is often the case with enactments which in many instances represent complex interactions between patient and analyst that are conveyed in non-verbal form. And as was true in this situation, the analyst needs to observe not only clues contained in the patient's postures, gestures, movements and facial expressions, but his own bodily responses as well, for it often happens that the key to understanding what is transpiring at a given moment in analysis lies not in the words spoken by patient and analyst, but in their non-verbal behavior.

Sometimes it happens that a communication of great importance is conveyed not in an action taking place in the analytic hour, but by means of the patient's dress and physical appearance. This was true of Ms Y, a young woman who sought analysis through our institute and who was assigned to me as her analyst. A poet and musician, Ms Y placed little emphasis on clothes and regularly appeared for her sessions dressed in a wrinkled blouse and torn jeans. There was, however, some notable exception to this mode of dress. On Thursdays, I noted, my patient either wore a skirt and tailored blouse or an attractive and fashionable dress.

I thought, at first, that this change in her appearance was due to some professional activity of Ms Y's – she gave music lessons and held a part-time job – that required her to look more professional. This, however, turned out not to be the case. The change was due to a quite different, and unexpected source, one that it took us many months to uncover. It was not, in fact, until material concerning Ms Y's applications to the Treatment Center spontaneously arose in the course of an hour that I began to understand her behavior. It turned out that in the course of the interviews that she had in connection with her application for treatment, Ms Y met the director of the clinic. She immediately liked this kindly man who reminded her of her beloved grandfather. The loss of this grandparent when she was 6 years old was a severe blow to the child and for many years, she had unconsciously been seeking his replacement.

During the interview with the director, Dr G, he was suddenly called away by an important phone call. During his absence, Ms Y could not control her desire to know what Dr G thought of her and, yielding to temptation, she glanced at the notes that he had jotted down as they spoke.

What she read in his notebook delighted Ms Y. In his description of her, Dr G had observed that she was an attractive, articulate young woman who appeared for her interview fashionably dressed in a matching skirt and blouse. Ms Y was pleased by this description, just as she had been pleased when, dressed up to meet her grandfather on Sundays, he always complimented her on her outfit.

Ms Y very much wanted Dr G to be her analyst and was keenly disappointed when she learned that his role was limited to being one of her interviewers. Through certain misinformation that she had obtained from a friend who was being treated through the clinic, Ms Y came to believe that Dr G was to be my supervisor. Moreover, she figured out that Thursday was the day that I had supervision and through me she sought to make a good impression on Dr G. Thus, believing that I would be talking to him about her and describing her appearance as well as the content of the hour, Ms Y made every effort to look attractive on Thursdays.

It was on that day, too that Ms Y often brought in dream or fantasy material. And so with my patient's mode of dress, it took some time for me to become aware that the content of the Thursday session was different and more 'analytic' than on other days. Here, too, by giving me interesting material that I would then report to Dr G, Ms Y was trying to impress the grandfather figure who evoked so many fond memories and whom she so sorely missed.

Interestingly, at that time I did have supervision on Thursdays, although not with Dr G. How it happened that Ms Y detected that Thursday was my day for supervision is in itself a most interesting question. No doubt I communicated something to her on that day that was different from other days. Reflecting on this question, I concluded that the quality of my listening in the Thursday session was different from other hours. I recognized that I was more alert, tracked her associations more closely and in preparation for supervision, no doubt jotted down more notes than usual. Although these clues were subtle ones and not easily perceived by a patient lying on the couch, clearly Ms Y had picked them up and had responded to them with changes of her own. And it was through understanding the changes that Ms Y enacted in the Thursday sessions that ultimately we were able to reconstruct an aspect of Ms Y's childhood that had had an enduring influence on her personality development, her fantasy life, and her later object choices.

From the examples that I have cited thus far, it is evident, I believe that non-verbal behavior, and the enactments so closely related to it, regularly occur on both sides of the couch and form a kind of mini-drama within the analysis that often is the vehicle for the playing out of conflicts and fantasies that are of the greatest importance in the patient's psychology.

Since most often there is a mutuality to these enactments, the question arises as to how the analyst should deal with his or her side of the equation.

Should she simply confine herself to observing her own behavior, seek to understand its relation to the patient's material, and attempt to use that understanding to frame an interpretation? Or should she share with the patient some of her subjective experiences? If so, what would be the purpose of such a revelation? What gain would the analyst hope to achieve by employing it?

This is not an easy question to answer. In fact, it is one that currently is the focus of much discussion and debate. And as one might expect, there are no clear answers to this conundrum. Each situation must be dealt with individually, recognizing that self-disclosure of any kind by the analyst has a powerful and often enduring impact on the patient. In what follows I will briefly outline three situations in which I chose to disclose to a patient aspects of my countertransference that were enacted in sessions. I will try to explain why I did so, and what effects these disclosures had on the patient. As will be evident, at times self-disclosure proves useful in opening up closed doors, that is, in overcoming certain tenacious resistances or impasses, thus allowing the treatment to move forward. On other occasions, however, self-disclosure may have an inhibitory effect that is not easily detected. The analyst has to be aware that, although on a manifest level the disclosure may enhance the patient's understanding of an aspect of her psychology, less consciously it may have the unintended effect of increasing the patient's resistances. Understanding and interpretation of this covert reaction is vitally important if the patient is to progress in the analysis.

Some years ago I was working with a young woman with strongly obsessional features who tended to externalize her conflicts and to see her problems as resulting from the fault of others. For many months I interpreted this tenacious defensive structure with only a slight loosening of it becoming evident in sessions. I was relieved, therefore, when in the third year of analysis the patient brought in some new and potentially important material. This had to do with the fact that at age 5 she had been sexually fondled by a beloved male cousin, a boy of 15, who regularly read to her at bedtime. While I did not believe that this experience was, by itself, the key to Ms K's neurosis, clearly it had a significant impact on her and I was eager to learn more about it.

As quickly as it had emerged, however, this material disappeared. It went underground and in its stead the patient returned to the old complaints about friends and family. In response to this reactivated obsessional defense, often I found myself feeling bored and sleepy in sessions. On one occasion, partly to help keep alert, I picked up a notebook reserved for Ms K and began to leaf through the pages. Shortly thereafter I realized that she had heard what I was doing, but had chosen not to speak about it. I interpreted her avoidance, but quickly thereafter sought to explore her associations, to overhearing a man behind her making strange noises. Ms K got the message and quickly began to relate the sounds that she heard in our session to the traumatic childhood experience with her cousin. This consisted of the boy reading to her, turning over pages in the book, and then slowly caressing her legs and genitals. While, clearly, these memories and the related material were of importance and were, in fact, stimulated by the noises that I made, by entering so rapidly into an exploration of this earlier experience, Ms K and I entered into a collusion. Not wanting to focus on my countertransference response, and my inappropriate behavior – I had allowed myself to be distracted and had not been attuned to the patient – I led the patient down a path that while meaningful in its own right, was being used at the moment to avoid dealing with my own countertransference behavior. Ms K went along with me because she was terrified of her own anger and wished to avoid a potentially explosive confrontation. As a result, both of us joined together in the creation of a resistance that on the surface looked like meaningful analytic exploration of an important experience in childhood.

I realized that if I continued on this track the patient would never again trust me as some part of her would know that she had been double-binded. When the time seemed right, therefore, I reviewed with Ms K what had happened between us, told her that her perceptions had been correct, that, in fact, my mind had wandered and that I had become distracted. In turn, Ms K told me that she knew that this was true, but had avoided confronting me with the truth for fear of a clash between us that would lead to the ending of our relationship. Once the air was cleared in this way, we could go on to explore both the factors between us that contributed to my reaction and Ms K's need to keep me at a distance by unconsciously seeking to evoke such a response.

Some colleagues maintain that it is an error to acknowledge a mistake or a piece of countertransference behavior to the patient. This approach, they say, functions to alleviate the analyst's guilt and does nothing to help the patient know themself. It is far better and more useful to investigate the patient's reactions to what they have perceived. In that way, they maintain, one is continually investigating the patient's psychology and avoiding unnecessary distractions. While I understand this thinking, I believe that it overlooks the profound effect on a patient of not acknowledging the truth of her perceptions. This puts the patient in a double-bind, leads to profound mistrust, and in my view, by enacting a deception, undermines the entire treatment. I do not think that a patient will feel safe enough under these conditions to truly reveal the most vulnerable parts of herself.

In another situation, I found myself at times unable to make effective contact with a patient who, when angry, remained silent, withdrawn, and totally unapproachable. When retreating in this way, Mr D lay on the couch huddled over with knees drawn up, looking as though he was folded into himself. In many respects Mr D's withdrawal mimicked his father's behavior. A bitter and angry man who suffered much physical trauma in his youth, the father spent long hours sitting alone in a dark living-room, silent and unapproachable. When as a boy Mr D tried to reach out to his father, he was either ignored or snapped at in a way that terrified the child. When he was angry at me, usually because I had missed a session or otherwise disappointed him, Mr D would retreat into his protective shell. Then nothing I would say or do would bring him out of it. There was, in fact, no interpretation that at one time or another I did not offer. Typically, Mr D would listen, curl into himself and not respond. Only when he was ready to do so, usually several days later, would he begin to emerge from his fortress.

One day I returned from a brief vacation to find Mr D in a sullen, and angry mood. Huddled into himself as usual, he remained stubbornly silent. Totally unmovable in the face of my efforts to reach him. After offering a few interpretations having to do with Mr D's reaction to my absence and receiving no response whatsoever, I found myself withdrawing, struggling with a wish to end the session and get away from this impossibly frustrating man. For some time the two of us sat in silence. The atmosphere in the room was heavy. Then, probably in response to the enormous frustration that I was feeling, I found myself speaking in a way that I had not done before.

'I would like to share with you what I am experiencing at this moment,' I said. 'I am sitting here feeling totally shut out, totally helpless. It is as though a steel door has dropped down between us and there is absolutely no reaching you. And I know that no matter what I say or do, no matter in what way I knock at that door, it will remain shut tight. From what I am experiencing, from what I am feeling in my gut, I believe I know really in a way that I did not know before, how utterly helpless you must have felt as a child, trying to reach that unreachable man sitting in darkness. Because now I am that child and you are that man.'

Mr D was silent for a moment. Then, suddenly, he broke into tears and wept for fully five minutes. When he composed himself he remarked that although the essence of what I said was no different from what I had said many times before, he experienced my words in a totally new way. 'You really do know what it was like for me,' he said. 'I feel that for me that makes all the difference. Before, you were speaking words, ideas. Today you spoke feelings. I don't trust words, but I trust the honesty of raw feelings.'

For a number of years I have pondered over this response and its meaning. It addresses an aspect of psychoanalysis that is not well understood, but that seems of great importance. While clearly related to the communication of empathy, it involves something more. What is transmitted is a sense of authenticity communicated through affects that convey the analyst's identification with the patient's emotional experiences. For many patients this kind of response on the part of the analyst is more meaningful and evokes greater trust than the more usual quiet empathy that is an inherent part of the analytic technique.

My final example is of a different sort. It illustrates a kind of difficulty that one may, at times, encounter in the use of self-disclosure. Mrs R was a woman who suffered early and severe losses that left her an angry, often embittered woman, but also a person who continually sought the approval of others. This conflict – the constant desire to express her pain and fury, on the one hand, and her fear of alienating others on the other, caused Mrs R to be an expert at the indirect, oblique, subtly expressed, put-down. She also became an injustice collector, tallying every possible slight or hurt that came her way and using them as justification for the expression of her long-standing rage.

In our sessions Mrs R was often critical of me but always in an indirect way. Quoting so-called experts, she would sharply criticize psychoanalysis as well as colleagues with whom I worked. She was also indirectly critical of my office, having negative things to say about old-fashioned doctors' offices, furnished in styles similar to mine. Quite remarkable was the fact that, although she would launch these attacks, Mrs R was quite unaware that she was being negative and critical toward me. Although I was accustomed to Mrs R's criticisms, on occasion they got to me. That happened one day when listening to Mrs R's attacks on colleagues, the field of analysis, and related issues, I found myself feeling tense. My body was tight, my guts felt knotted and my face was flushed. Then, spontaneously, as happened with Mr K, I found myself speaking. 'As I listen to what you are saying Mrs R,' I began, 'I am aware that I am feeling tense and ill at ease. My guts feel all roiled up and my whole body feels tight. And I realize that your comments are making me angry because indirectly, in the guise of criticizing others, you are actually attacking me and putting me down. But because your attack is indirect, it is hard to respond to it and this causes me to feel angry and helpless.' There was silence in the room. Mrs R looked surprised, then puzzled. 'Does what I've said make any sense to you?' I inquired. At that point I was feeling rather foolish and unprofessional for having come out so directly with what I was experiencing. I shuddered to think what my former supervisors would say if they heard me speak in this way.

'Actually it does,' Mrs R replied. 'For years my husband has been telling me the same thing, that I'm always criticizing him and getting at him in an indirect, roundabout way. He is so crazy himself, though, I don't listen to him, but if you, someone who I know well and trust are telling me the same thing, I have to take that seriously.'

Although I felt uneasy about my spontaneous self-disclosure, I was pleased by Mrs R's response to it. She was able to reflect on what I had said, take a step back, and examine herself in a way that she had not done before. She was, I thought, on the threshold of obtaining a new and centrally important insight about herself. In fact, partly through my intervention, which stunned her, Mrs R came in touch, not only with the well of anger that was contained inside of her, but with her fear of expressing her rage and destroying needed relationships. That was all to the good, and I began to regard the kind of self-revelation that I had employed as quite a useful tool.

Then I learned something else. About a year later, when, once again, the matter of Mrs R's covert anger and my response to it arose, the patient described the impact that the earlier session had had on her. 'I was shocked and frightened by your response,' she said. 'Not that it wasn't helpful; it was. I realized how much anger I was communicating and that was useful. But since then I realize that I have been holding back. I never thought that I could really get to you and your reaction frightened me. I became afraid that I could anger you to such an extent that you couldn't take it. You would retaliate or, worse, blow up and simply quit the treatment. I didn't want that, so without thinking about it, I realize that I have been very careful about what I say and how I say it.'

Of course I should have picked up on this aspect of Mrs R's response and interpreted her reaction of fear and withdrawal. I did not, in part because the change was a subtle one, but also because I took the reduction in her anger and the shift in her behavior as positive changes that had developed as a result of the insights that she had obtained.

I cite this example to reiterate a truth that is well known to clinicians and that is often forgotten. Patients will hear and respond to our interventions in ways that are quite different from what we intend. And their responses are often expressed in indirect, covert, and subterranean ways that are not readily apparent. If the analyst chooses to employ self-disclosure, therefore, it is necessary to not only be alert to these concealed responses, but to investigate with thoroughness, the unique way that the patient has processed this uniquely powerful type of intervention. A method that can, at times, help open doors that seemed permanently closed, self-disclosure is also one that, if its consequences are insufficiently explored, has the potential to cause much trouble.

CONCLUSION

In this chapter, I have attempted to share some thoughts about aspects of analysis with which I have been concerned in recent years. These are also issues, I believe, to which comparatively little attention has been paid.

Perhaps the most important of these is the flow of non-verbal communication that is an integral part of every analytic hour. Closely connected to the enactments that bring to life the inner conflict of the patient, non-verbal communications are closely linked to key affects that fuel unconscious conflicts and fantasies. Not limited to our patients, non-verbal behavior and enactments constitute an ever-present part of the analyst's communications. Seeking always to use one's own subjective experiences in the service of understanding the inner world of the patient, the analyst must decide when that understanding can be enhanced by sharing with the patient aspects of those experiences. A powerful tool that, at times, proves invaluable, self-disclosure is one that must be used selectively and with great care, for given the enormous impact of the analyst's words, it can have a profound and disruptive effect on the patient's sense of self.

REFERENCES

Chused, J. (1987) 'Panel: Psychoanalysis of the Young Adult, Theory and Technique', *Journal of the American Psychoanalytic Association*, 35: 175–188.

Freud, S. (1910) 'The Future Prospects of Psychoanalytic Theory', in *Standard Edition*, 11: 141–151, London: Hogarth Press, 1957.

Gill, M. M. (1982) *Analysis of Transference: Psychological Issues, Monograph 53*, New York: International Universities Press.

Heimann, P. (1950) 'On Countertransference', *International Journal of Psycho-Analysis*, 31: 81–84.

Jacobs, T. (1973) 'Posture, Gesture and Movement in the Analyst: Cues to Interpretation and Countertransference', *Journal of the American Psychoanalytic Association*, 21: 77–92.

Jacobs, T. (1980) 'Secrets, Alliances and Family Fictions: Some Psychoanalytic Observations', *Journal of the American Psychoanalytic Association*, 27(1): 21–42.

Jacobs, T. (1986) 'On Countertransference Enactments', *Journal of the American Psychoanalytic Association*, 34(2): 289–307.

Jacobs, T. (1991) *The Use of the Self: Countertransference and Communication in the Analytic Situation*, Madison, CT: International Universities Press.

Kohut, H. (1971) *The Analysis of the Self*, New York: International Universities Press.

Kohut, H. (1977) *The Restoration of the Self*, New York: International Universities Press.

McLaughlin, J. (1987) 'The Play of Transference Enactment in the Analytic Situation', *Journal of the American Psychoanalytic Association*, 35: 357–582.

McLaughlin, J. (1988) 'The Analyst's Insights', *Psychoanalytic Quarterly*, 57: 370–389.

McLaughlin, J. (1992) 'Nonverbal Behavior in the Analytic Situation: The Search for Meaning in Nonverbal Cues', in S. Kramer and S. Akhtar (eds.), *When the Body Speaks: Psychological Meanings in Kinetic Clues*, Northvale, NJ: Jason Aronson.

Ogden, T. (1994) 'The Analytic Third – Working with Intersubjective Clinical Facts', *International Journal of Psycho-Analysis*, 75: 3–20.

Pally, R. (2001) 'A Primary Role for Nonverbal Communication in Psychoanalysis', *Psychoanalytic Inquiry*, 21: 71–93.

Poland, W. (1986) 'The Analyst's Words', *Psychoanalytic Quarterly*, 55: 244–271.

Reich, A. (1951) 'On Countertransference', *International Journal of Psycho-Analysis*, 72: 25–31.

Reich, A. (1960) 'Further Remarks on Countertransference', *International Journal of Psycho-Analysis*, 41: 389–395.

Reich, A. (1966) 'Empathy and Countertransference', in *Annie Reich: Psychoanalytic Contributions* (1973), New York: International Universities Press, pp. 344–360.

Searles, H. (1959) 'Oedipal Love in the Countertransference', in *Collected Papers on Schizophrenia and Related Subjects* (1965), New York: International Universities Press, pp. 284–303.

Stern, D. (1985) *The Interpersonal World of the Infant*, New York: International Universities Press.

Epilogue

Michael Stadter and David E. Scharff

Working on this collection of essays has stimulated us to ask an array of questions, and to think in fresh and unexpected ways about our therapeutic work.

We leave this project more curious than ever about the impact of time and space on psychoanalysis and psychotherapy. We are struck with how many contemporary questions about time and space in physics, mathematics and philosophy are relevant to the psychodynamic and subjective domain. Each of these disciplines attempts to grasp 'reality', and this emphasizes for us the under-appreciated connection between psychoanalysis and other disciplines. Certainly, psychoanalytic thought is at the forefront of apprehending subjective and intersubjective 'reality'.

Chaos theory, from mathematics and physics, can help psychoanalytic therapists to understand the oscillations between psychic order and disorder as basic characteristics of complex systems. Such shifts occur in ways that produce unforeseen discontinuities that are both inevitable and necessary for change and development. This finding across disciplines offers support for a framework that allows both patients and therapists to tolerate extended states of disorder and of not knowing. The chapters by Johnson, Hopper, Scharff and Scharff, and Ashbach speak to this key capacity.

It was striking to us – but not surprising – how many of the 19 chapters touched on trauma and narcissism, with many chapters focusing on these subjects. The disintegrating forces of trauma dramatically affect the basic dimensions of life and the sense of self that is fundamentally defined and regulated by time, space and number. Clinicians would do well when studying trauma and self-experience to be sensitively attuned to these dimensions.

A few points about time were especially salient for us. Ravenscroft wrote about internal family life-cycle 'clocks'. We find his perspective intriguing and suggest that it could be extended to examine what occurs when there are different unconscious clock speeds among the various developmental lines within an individual. The presence of different senses of time within a single personality, and within families and societies, is a factor that produces both disorder and new attractors in complex dynamic systems. It would be productive to study couples and families for whom developmental clocks are running at different speeds for each member. We thought, too, about the complementarities and conflicts for couples in which one partner operates predominantly in a time-far state while the other lives in a pre-dominantly time-near mode. The writing in this volume also reinforced our belief that most psychoanalytic work does not pay adequate attention to the concept of the future as a psychic organizer that is on the same representational footing as the past and present.

The role of number in psychological experience has also been under-estimated – perhaps it has been hiding in plain view. However, the different senses of self as a one, a two or a three, Ogden's analytic third, the self in a family in which the numbers are too large to hold in mind, being alone in the presence of another, Bollas's different orders of magnitude of 4 (family), 5 (group), 6 (society) and various numerical shifts and oscillations are important psychological phenomena. Among other characteristics, this 'psychic numeracy' (to use Bollas's term) helps us to appreciate the quali-tative differences produced by quantitative variation and to considered levels of complexity that psychoanalysis has so far ignored.

Finally, we've been reminded yet again that much of the profound impact of psychotherapy and psychoanalysis comes from thorough, receptive attention to the simple, the elemental, and the momentary. The dimensional questions of When? Where? and How many? can vividly illuminate a moment, an interaction, and a therapy. We ask of our patients and of ourselves that we deeply connect – consciously and unconsciously, with thought and feeling, in both the intersubjective and the intrapsychic. To do this takes a great deal of time, time to deeply consider and to encounter together – the basic dimensions of being fully human.

One final question for us now is, 'Where have these considerations left you, the reader?' We hope we'll have the opportunity over time to learn from many of you what has been evoked through your study of these essays.

Index

Printed and bound by CPI Group (UK) Ltd, Croydon, CR0 4YY

23/10/2024

01777671-0013